IAP Q & A on
Vaccines and Vaccinology

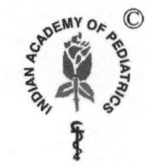

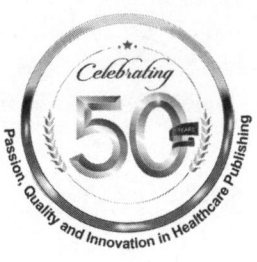

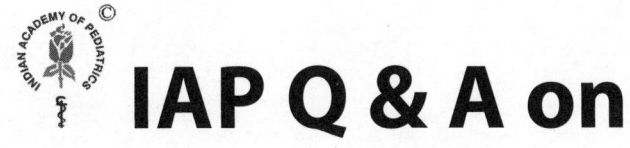

IAP Q & A on
Vaccines and Vaccinology

Editor-in-Chief
Srinivas G Kasi MD DCH
Consultant Pediatrician
Kasi Clinic
Bengaluru, Karnataka, India

Executive Editor
Bakul Jayant Parekh MD DCH FIAP
Senior Pediatrician
Director, BPCH Tertiary Care Center
Mumbai, Maharashtra, India

Editors

Arun Wadhwa MD
Consultant Pediatrician
New Delhi, India

Abhay K Shah MD Dped (UNI FIRST) FIAP
Senior Pediatrician and Infectious Diseases
Consultant Director
Dr Abhay K Shah Children Hospital and
Pediatric Infectious Diseases Centre, Maninagar
Ahmedabad, Gujarat, India

Academic Editors

Nitin Shah MD DCH
Section Head and Consultant
Department of Pediatrics
PD Hinduja Hospital
Mumbai, Maharashtra, India

Bhaskar Shenoy MD
Head
Department of Pediatrics
Chief, Division of Pediatric Infectious
Disease Manipal Hospitals
Bengaluru, Karnataka, India

Sanjay Marathe MD DNB
Director
Colors Intensive Care Hospital and
Marathe Children Hospital
Nagpur, Maharashtra, India

Sanjay Srirampur MD DCH FRCPCH
Head
Department of Pediatrics
Aditya Superspecialty Hospital
Hyderabad, Telangana, India

Alok Gupta MD (Ped) FIAP
Pediatrician and Counselor
Pediatric Specialties Clinic
Jaipur, Rajasthan, India

Foreword
Vinod K Paul

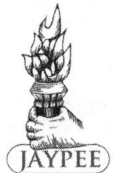

JAYPEE BROTHERS MEDICAL PUBLISHERS
The Health Sciences Publisher
New Delhi | London

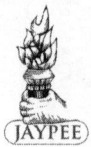 **Jaypee Brothers Medical Publishers (P) Ltd.**

Headquarters

Jaypee Brothers Medical Publishers (P) Ltd
EMCA House, 23/23-B
Ansari Road, Daryaganj
New Delhi 110 002, India
Landline: +91-11-23272143, +91-11-23272703
+91-11-23282021, +91-11-23245672
Email: jaypee@jaypeebrothers.com

Corporate Office

Jaypee Brothers Medical Publishers (P) Ltd
4838/24, Ansari Road, Daryaganj
New Delhi 110 002, India
Phone: +91-11-43574357
Fax: +91-11-43574314
Email: jaypee@jaypeebrothers.com

Overseas Office

JP Medical Ltd
83 Victoria Street, London
SW1H 0HW (UK)
Phone: +44 20 3170 8910
Fax: +44 (0)20 3008 6180
Email: info@jpmedpub.com

Website: www.jaypeebrothers.com
Website: www.jaypeedigital.com

© 2021, Indian Academy of Pediatrics

The views and opinions expressed in this book are solely those of the original contributor(s)/author(s) and do not necessarily represent those of editor(s) of the book.

All rights reserved. No part of this publication may be reproduced, stored or transmitted in any form or by any means, electronic, mechanical, photocopying, recording or otherwise, without the prior permission in writing of the publishers.

All brand names and product names used in this book are trade names, service marks, trademarks or registered trademarks of their respective owners. The publisher is not associated with any product or vendor mentioned in this book.

Medical knowledge and practice change constantly. This book is designed to provide accurate, authoritative information about the subject matter in question. However, readers are advised to check the most current information available on procedures included and check information from the manufacturer of each product to be administered, to verify the recommended dose, formula, method and duration of administration, adverse effects and contraindications. It is the responsibility of the practitioner to take all appropriate safety precautions. Neither the publisher nor the author(s)/editor(s) assume any liability for any injury and/or damage to persons or property arising from or related to use of material in this book.

This book is sold on the understanding that the publisher is not engaged in providing professional medical services. If such advice or services are required, the services of a competent medical professional should be sought.

Every effort has been made where necessary to contact holders of copyright to obtain permission to reproduce copyright material. If any have been inadvertently overlooked, the publisher will be pleased to make the necessary arrangements at the first opportunity. The **CD/DVD-ROM** (if any) provided in the sealed envelope with this book is complimentary and free of cost. **Not meant for sale.**

Inquiries for bulk sales may be solicited at: jaypee@jaypeebrothers.com

IAP Q & A on Vaccines and Vaccinology

First Edition: **2021**

ISBN: 978-93-90595-08-2

Printed at Nutech Print Services - India

Contributors

Aashay Abhay Shah
MBBS MD(UNI FIRST) FISPGHAN
Pediatric Gastroenterologist and Hepatogist at Dr Abhay K Shah Children Hospital and Pediatric Infectious Diseases Centre
Ahmedabad, Gujarat, India

Abhay K Shah MD Dped (UNI FIRST) FIAP
Senior Pediatrician and Infectious Diseases
Consultant Director
Dr Abhay K Shah Children Hospital and Pediatric Infectious Diseases Centre,
Ahmedabad, Gujarat, India

Alok Gupta MD (Ped) FIAP
Pediatrician and Counselor
Pediatric Specialties Clinic
Jaipur, Rajasthan, India

Arun Kumar Manglik
MD (Ped) DNB (Ped)
Consultant Pediatrician
ILS Hospitals
Kolkata, West Bengal, India

Arun Wadhwa MD
Consultant Pediatrician
New Delhi, India

Baldev S Prajapati
MD DPed FIAP MNAMS
HOD and Professor
GCS Medical College
Hospital and Research Centre, Ahmedabad
Aakanksha Children Hospital and Postgraduate Institution
Ahmedabad, Gujarat, India

Bhaskar Shenoy MD
Head
Department of Pediatrics
Chief, Division of Pediatric Infectious Disease Manipal Hospitals
Bengaluru, Karnataka, India

Chetan Trivedi MD DPed
Consultant Pediatrician and Neonatologist
Director
Neha Children Hospital and Neonatal Center, Kankaria
Ahmedabad, Gujarat, India

Dhanya Dharmapalan
MD PG Dip in PID (Oxford)
Consultant in Pediatric Infectious Diseases
Apollo Hospitals Navi Mumbai and Dr Yewale's Multispecialty Hospital for Children
Navi Mumbai, Maharashtra, India

Harish K Pemde MD FIAP
Director Professor
Department of Pediatrics Kalawati Saran Children's Hospital and Lady Hardinge Medical College
New Delhi, India

Jagdish Chinnappa MD
Consultant Pediatrician
Manipal Hospital
Bengaluru, Karnataka, India

Jaydeep Choudhury
DNB(Pediatrics) MNAMS FIAP
Professor
Department of Pediatrics
Institute of Child Health
Kolkata, West Bengal, India

Contributors

Kamlesh Harish MD (Ped)
Senior Consultant
Head, Department of Pediatrics
ESIC Hospital Rohini, New Delhi, India

M Surendranath MD DCH FACI
HOD
Department of Pediatrics
Vijay Marie Hospital
Hyderabad, Telangana, India

Mohit Vohra DNB(Paed)
Director
Sashakt Child Care Centre, Jaipur
Consultant CKS Hospital
Jaipur, Rajasthan, India

Nitin Shah MD DCH
Section Head and Consultant
Department of Pediatrics
PD Hinduja Hospital
Mumbai, Maharashtra, India

NP Singh MBBS MD
HOD and Senior Consultant at
Ayushman Hospital and
Health Services
Dwarka, New Delhi, India

P Sivaraman MD(Pediatrics)
Consultant Pediatrician
Thangam Hospital
Erode, Tamil Nadu, India

Pratima Shah MD DPed
Consulting Pediatrician
Ankur Institute of Child Health
Ahmedabad, Gujarat, India

Pravin Mehta MD DCH
Consulting Pediatrician
Hindu Sabha Hospital
Jack N Jill Nursing Home
Mumbai, Maharashtra, India

Raju C Shah
MD, DPed FIAP FECPCH(UK)
Medical Director
Ankur Institute of Child Health
Ahmedabad, Gujarat, India

Rohit Agrawal MD DCH FIAP
Senior Consultant Pediatrician
Chandra Jyoti Children Hospital and
Rainbow Multispecialty Pediatric Clinic
Mumbai, India
Consultant Pediatrician:
Kohinoor Hospital
Mumbai, Maharashtra, India

Rupesh Masand MD
Senior Professor
Department of Pediatrics
National Institute of
Medical Science and Research
Jaipur, Rajasthan, India

S Balasubramanium
MD DCH FIAP FRCPCH
Medical Director and Head
Department of Pediatrics and IAP
IDCPID Fellowship Coordinator
Kanchi Kamakoti
CHILDS Trust Hospital
Chennai, Tamil Nadu, India

S Shivananda MD
Former, Director
Professor and Head
Department of Pediatrics
Indira Gandhi Institute of Child Health
Former Professor and HOD, Bangalore
Medical College and
Medical Superintendent
Vanivilas Hospital for Women and
Children, Bengaluru
Presently, Academic Head
Department of Pediatrics
Fortis Hospital
Bengaluru, Karnataka, India

Sanjay Marathe MD DNB
Director
Colors Intensive Care Hospital and
Marathe Children Hospital
Nagpur, Maharashtra, India

Sanjay Srirampur MD DCH FRCPCH
Head
Department of Pediatrics
Aditya Superspecialty Hospital
Hyderabad, Telangana, India

Silky Mittal MD
Ex fellow
IAP Pediatric Infectious Diseases
Kanchi Kamakoti Childs Trust Hospital
Chennai, Tamil Nadu, India
Assistant Professor
Sri Aurobindo Institute of Medical Sciences
Indore, Madhya Pradesh, India

Srinivas G Kasi MD DCH
Consultant Pediatrician
Kasi Clinic
Bengaluru, Karnataka, India

Suhas V Prabhu MD DCH MNAMS
Consultant Pediatrician
PD Hinduja Hospital
Mumbai, Maharashtra, India

Sumitha Nayak MD DNB FIAP Adv Cert in Vaccinology (IVI) PGDMLS PGDGC
Consultant Pediatrician
The Children's Clinic
Bengaluru, Karnataka, India

Tanu Singhal MD MSc
Consultant Pediatrics and Infectious Diseases
Department of Pediatrics Kokilaben Dhirubhai Ambani Hospital and Medical Research Institute
Mumbai, Maharashtra, India

Vijay Kumar Guduru
MD (Peds) ACME
Professor of Pediatrics
MGM Hospital/ Kakatiya Medical College
Warangal, Telangana, India

Vijay Yewale MD DCH
Head
Institute of Child Health
Apollo Hospitals, Navi Mumbai
Director
Dr Yewale Multispecialty Hospital for Children
Navi Mumbai, Maharashtra, India

डॉ. विनोद कुमार पॉल
सदस्य
Dr. Vinod K. Paul
MEMBER

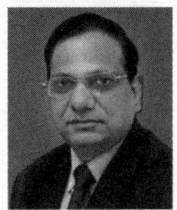

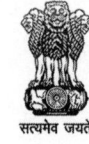
सत्यमेव जयते

भारत सरकार
नीति आयोग, संसद मार्ग
नई दिल्ली-*110 001*
Government of India
NATIONAL INSTITUTION FOR TRANSFORMING INDIA
NITI Aayog, Parliament Street
New Delhi-110 001
Tele. : 23096809 Telefax : 23096810
E-mail : vinodk.paul@gov.in

Foreword

I am happy to note that the Indian Academy of Pediatrics is publishing a book on common queries on immunizations encountered by healthcare professionals involved in childcare.

In India, children below five years account for 10% of the total population, a group which contributes a significant burden to the morbidity and under five mortality rate associated with infectious diseases. The Universal immunization program (UIP) of GOI has contributed significantly to the reduction of Vaccine preventable diseases (VPDs). The Intensified Mission Indradhanush launched on 25 December 2014 has further contributes to the increased coverage of the UIP vaccines. In recent years, many new vaccines have been introduced in the UIP.

Vaccinology is constantly evolving field and it is essential for healthcare professionals to remain updates. I am happy to note that this book discusses the commonly used vaccines and the basics of vaccinology. In addition, newer vaccine technologies, future vaccines and therapeutic vaccines are also discussed. Ethical issues of vaccinations and vaccine hesitancy, which have assumed significance, are also covered.

I am sure that this book will go a long way in a educating those involved in childcare, in the essentials of vaccinology and contribute to the enhancement of quality childcare in India.

Vinod K Paul

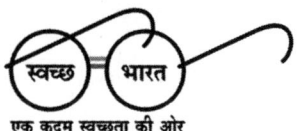
स्वच्छ भारत
एक कदम स्वच्छता की ओर

Preface

Vaccination is widely considered as one of the greatest medical achievements of the 20th century. Childhood diseases that were frequently seen less than a generation ago, are now infrequently seen, largely due to vaccines and vaccination programs. In 1979, Smallpox was declared to have been eradicated. The scourge of polio, which devastated the world, leaving many crippled, is largely controlled. In most of the developed world, the incidence of tetanus, diphtheria, Hib and pneumococcal infections have been drastically reduced. In the words of Dr Stanley Plotkin "next to clean water, no single intervention has had so profound an effect on reducing mortality from childhood diseases as has the widespread introduction of vaccines".

It should be noted that the benefits of newer vaccines were experienced by the developed countries before it could percolate to the lesser developed countries (LDC), where the need was more acute. Till the recent past, it took at least a decade before the newer vaccines were introduced in the LDC. The advent of international health financing agencies like the GAVI and the Bill and Melinda Gates foundation, has hastened the introduction of newer vaccines in the LDC. The rotavirus vaccines and the Pneumococcal Conjugate vaccines (PCV) have been introduced in the LDC almost in parallel with their introduction in the developed countries.

In India, the Expanded Program of Immunizations (EPI) was introduced in 1978 with BCG, OPV, DPT and the whole cell Typhoid vaccines. In 1985, the Universal Immunization program was launched with BCG, OPV, DPT and measles vaccine. TAB vaccine was dropped. For almost two decades no new vaccines were introduced. This was followed by Hepatitis B vaccines, Hib as part of the pentavalent vaccine, IPV and the MR vaccines. Rotavirus vaccines and the PCVs have been introduced sub-nationally.

In the private sector, the introduction of new vaccines has been more rapid and the uptake is also rapid. To date, almost every childhood vaccine in use in the developed countries, are available in the private sector in India.

Every vaccine has its own characteristics, indications, contraindications, interactions with other vaccines, storage conditions and special use recommendations.

Moreover, knowledge about general aspects of vaccinology are also important in day-to-day practice.

Vaccine hesitancy is rearing its ugly head and needs to be tackled in a gentle but effective manner.

Textbooks of vaccines are too lengthy and unsuitable for quick references. For the practitioner, having all this information in a concise and easily readable form is a necessity.

With this objective, the Indian Academy of Pediatrics (IAP), has published this comprehensive book in a question and answer format, brief enough to be easily readable and with adequate information to answer all the questions.

Each chapter has been authored by experts in the field of vaccinology drawn from all over the country. These experts have delved into the literature about vaccines and formulated these all-inclusive chapters.

It is our fervent hope that this book satisfies the needs of postgraduate students, practitioners and everyone involved in the care of children.

Jai IAP, Jai Hind
Editorial Board

Message

Dear Fellow IAPians,

Greetings from Indian Academy of Pediatrics.

It gives me a great honor to write a message from the desk of National President of IAP. I remember discussing the possibility to come up with the first ever IAP's book on various FAQs regarding vaccines with the national convenor of ACVIP committee - Dr Srinivas G Kasi in the beginning of this year. I am very happy to know that Dr Srinivas G Kasi and his team has left no stone unturned in making this dream of mine come true.

We all have heard about the maxim - "Prevention is better than cure". The best example of this maxim that I can think of is for vaccines and immunization. In fact, I believe that immunization is the most cost effective invention of the millennium. We know that immunization and vaccine development is a highly dynamic science. Louis Pasteur invented vaccine to prevent Smallpox and since then many more vaccines are being added every year.

Initially there were just a few vaccines. Now, there are a number of vaccines available, some are included in the UIP by the Government, while some vaccines, not included in the UIP, are strongly recommended by IAP. These differences in recommendations often lead to queries in the minds of parents and the Healthcare workers (HCWs). This book to aims to empower those HCWs, responsible for childcare, to gain the knowledge to answer all queries regarding vaccines and vaccinations.

Vaccine hesitancy is rearing it's ugly head all over the world and India is no exception. I am happy to note a full chapter, discussing this issue.

Keeping the above points in mind, the dynamic team of ACVIP led by Dr S G Kasi et al., have come up with answers to many questions in the minds of practising pediatricians and many other healthcare workers. I am certain that this ready reckoner will find its place in many of our libraries - physical as well as digital. I am certain that this ready reckoner will continue to evolve and help many of us for many generations to come. I believe that this is a must have book in every Pediatrician's clinic.

I congratulate the team of editors and contributors who have burnt the midnight oil to bring this masterpiece to our table and helping me in achieving one more milestone and dream this year. I, as a national president and the Chairman of ACVIP committee, compliment the team for the excellent work in spite of the difficult time due to Covid-19 Pandemic. Kudos and three cheers!

Bakul Jayant Parekh
President, 2020
Indian Academy of Pediatrics

Message

I am delighted to know that the IAP is coming out with a book answering the common and uncommon questions in Vaccinology, with Dr Srinivas G Kasi as the Chief Editor. I am sure that with the expertise of all the contributors, this multiauthor, multifaceted book will prove to be a treasure house of knowledge for both practicing pediatricians and postgraduate students. I wish all the success for this venture.

Piyush Gupta
President, 2021
Indian Academy of Pediatrics

Message

Dear Academician Friends,

It is quite heartening to note our Academy is launching a book on FAQs in Vaccinology. As the title implies, this is certainly a comprehensive reference source for all the vaccines which are in vogue.

Our fraternity being the stake holders of wellness of children of our country, are always passionate to provide the most optimal immunization care to our wards. Keeping updated and leaning back to the basics is mandatory to choose and deliver the vaccines and counsel the care takers appropriately.

I am sure Dr Srinivas G Kasi and Team have delivered the goods on immunization front in a consolidated FAQ pace through this book. The vaccinology experts have gone an extra mile to ensure all anticipated queries on immunization domain have been addressed in this unique scientific venture.

I wish this resourceful book on FAQs on Immunization will be a rich addition to the desktop of our fellow academicians in the pediatric segment. Alongside, I congratulate the Editorial and Central IAP Team for this novel initiative.

Remesh Kumar R
President Elect, 2022
Indian Academy of Pediatrics

Acknowledgments

The Editorial Board acknowledges the efforts of Shri Jitendar P Vij (Group Chairman), Mr Ankit Vij (Managing Director), Ms Chetna Malhotra Vohra (Associate Director–Content and Strategy), Ms Pooja Bhandari (Production Head), and Dr Rajul Jain (Development Editor) of M/s Jaypee Brothers Medical Publishers (P) Ltd., New Delhi, India, for their commendable efforts in ensuring the publication of this book in time, in spite of the difficulties caused by the Covid-19 pandemic, the national lockdown and suspension of all activities for a period of time.

The Editorial Board is ever thankful to Dr Bakul Jayant Parekh, President IAP 2020, for initiation of this project and his continued guidance at all times.

The Editorial Board acknowledges the support and encouragement of Dr Piyush Gupta President, IAP 2021 and Dr G V Basavaraja HSG 2020-22.

The Editorial Board acknowledges the consent of the IAP Advisory Committee on Vaccines and Immunization Practices (ACVIP), for utilizing some excerpts from the "IAP Guidebook on Immunization, 2018-19."

Contents

SECTION 1 BASIC VACCINOLOGY AND GENERAL CONSIDERATIONS

1. **Basic Immunology** 3
   Abhay K Shah

2. **Basic Epidemiology in Vaccinations** 24
   Bhaskar Shenoy

3. **Vaccination Schedules** 37
   Suhas V Prabhu

4. **General Immunization Practices** 43
   Sanjay Srirampur

5. **Documentation of Vaccination** 50
   Chetan Trivedi

6. **Cold Chain Management** 54
   Sanjay Marathe, Srinivas G Kasi

7. **Adverse Event following Immunization** 72
   Arun Wadhwa

8. **Vaccination in Special Situations** 81
   Srinivas G Kasi

9. **Vaccine Safety** 92
   Srinivas G Kasi

10. **Setting Up a Vaccination Clinic** 98
    Vijay Kumar Guduru, Srinivas G Kasi

11. **Combination Vaccines** 102
    P Sivaraman

12. **Immunoglobulins for Passive Protection against Vaccine-Preventable Diseases** 107
    Raju C Shah, Pratima Shah

SECTION 2 INDIVIDUAL VACCINES

13. **BCG Vaccine** 119
    Baldev S Prajapati

14. **Polio Vaccines** 126
    Srinivas G Kasi

15. **Diphtheria, Pertussis, and Tetanus Vaccines** 135
    S Balasubramanium, Silky Mittal

16. **Haemophilus Influenzae Type b Vaccines** 144
    Sumitha Nayak

17. **Hepatitis B Vaccines** 150
    S Shivananda, Arun Wadhwa

18. **Rotavirus Vaccines** 162
    Abhay K Shah, Aashay Abhay Shah

19. **Pneumococcal Conjugate Vaccines** 174
    Sanjay Srirampur

20. **Influenza Vaccines** 189
    Nitin Shah

21. **Measles, Mumps and Rubella Vaccines MR/MMR/MMRV Vaccines** 204
    Rohit Agrawal

22. **Typhoid Vaccines** 215
    Vijay Yewale

23. **Hepatitis A Vaccines** 222
    Jaydeep Choudhury

24. **Varicella Vaccines** 228
    Tanu Singhal

25. **Human Papillomavirus (HPV) Vaccines** 239
    Sanjay Marathe

26. **Rabies Vaccines** 254
    Arun Wadhwa

27. **Meningococcal Vaccines** 263
    M Surendranath

28. **Japanese Encephalitis Vaccines** 270
    Pravin Mehta

29. **Cholera Vaccines** 279
    Arun Kumar Manglik

30. **Yellow Fever Vaccines** 282
    Rupesh Masand

31. **Zoster Vaccines** 290
    Srinivas G Kasi

SECTION 3: Vaccination in Special Groups

32. Adolescent Vaccination 301
Mohit Vohra

33. Adult Vaccination 306
Srinivas G Kasi

34. Vaccinations for Travelers 314
Alok Gupta

SECTION 4: Newer Technologies and Newer Vaccines

35. Newer Vaccine Technologies 323
NP Singh

36. Newer Vaccines in Pipeline 333
NP Singh

37. Vaccines against Novel Viruses 345
NP Singh

38. Covid-19 Vaccines 355
NP Singh, Srinivas G Kasi

39. Therapeutic Vaccines 368
Dhanya Dharmapalan, NP Singh

SECTION 5: Miscellaneous Topics

40. Ethical Issues and Vaccine Refusal 377
Jagdish Chinnappa

41. National Immunization Program 384
Harish K Pemde, Kamlesh Harish

Annexure: Vaccines marketed in India *393*

Index *397*

SECTION 1
Basic Vaccinology and General Considerations

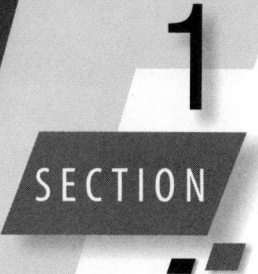

- **Basic Immunology**
  Abhay K Shah

- **Basic Epidemiology in Vaccinations**
  Bhaskar Shenoy

- **Vaccination Schedules**
  Suhas V Prabhu

- **General Immunization Practices**
  Sanjay Srirampur

- **Documentation of Vaccination**
  Chetan Trivedi

- **Cold Chain Management**
  Sanjay Marathe, Srinivas G Kasi

- **Adverse Event following Immunization**
  Arun Wadhwa

- **Vaccination in Special Situations**
  Srinivas G Kasi

- **Vaccine Safety**
  Srinivas G Kasi

- **Setting Up a Vaccination Clinic**
  Vijay Kumar Guduru, Srinivas G Kasi

- **Combination Vaccines**
  P Sivaraman

- **Immunoglobulins for Passive Protection against Vaccine-Preventable Diseases**
  Raju C Shah, Pratima Shah

CHAPTER 1

Basic Immunology

Abhay K Shah

Q1. What is the function of immune system?

Ans. The immune system is an extremely important defense mechanism that can identify an invading organism, from outside the body (e.g., viruses, bacteria, parasites, allergens, etc.) or within the body, e.g., malignant cells, and destroy it.

Q2. What is immunity?

Ans. **Immunity** can be defined as a complex biological system endowed with the capacity to recognize and tolerate whatever belongs to the self, and to recognize and reject what is foreign (non-self).

Q3. What are antigens and antibodies?

Ans. A protein, toxin, or other substances of high molecular weight, to which the body reacts by producing antibodies and stimulates an immune response. Different organisms contain several different antigens.

Antibodies [Ab, immunoglobulins (Ig)] are protein molecules that bind specifically to a particular part of an antigen, called antigenic site or epitope. They are found in low levels in the blood and tissue fluids, including mucus secretions, saliva and breast milk. However, when an immune response is activated greater quantities are produced to specifically target the foreign material.

Q4. What is epitope and paratope?

Ans. An "epitope", also known as antigenic determinant, is the part of an antigen that is recognized by the immune system, specifically by antibodies, B cells, or T cells. The part of an antibody that recognizes the epitope is called a "paratope" **(Fig. 1)**.

Q5. What is the difference between immunization and vaccination?

Ans. Immunization is the immune response to any administered antigen whereas vaccination is the immune response elicited in the body with the help of the vaccine.

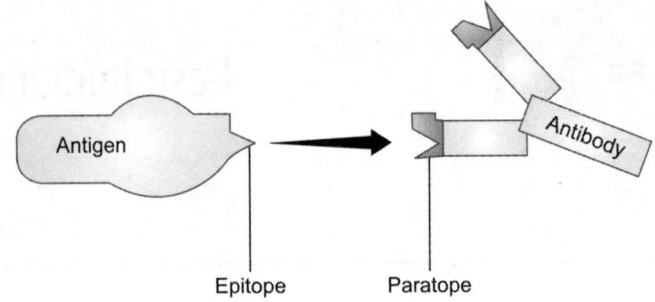

Fig. 1: Epitope and paratope.

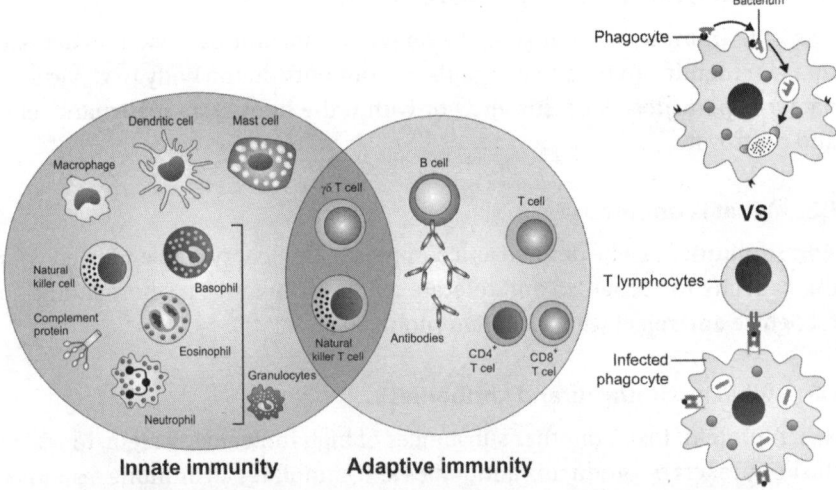

Fig. 2: Differentiation between innate and adaptive immunity.

Q6. What are innate and adaptive of immune response elicited in body in response to an antigen?

Ans. Immunity may be broadly classified as innate and adaptive immunity (**Fig. 2**).

Innate immunity comes into play within hours of the entry of an infective agent. The components of the innate immune system comprise of epithelial and mucosal barriers (mechanical), the antibacterial chemicals in these barriers, phagocytes (neutrophils, macrophages and NK cells) as well as complement. It is not very specific as it is triggered by structures shared by different microbes instead of specific microbial antigens. There is no immune memory. It plays a very important role as it is the first line of defense. It is also the effector pathway of adaptive immunity.

The innate immune system triggers the development of adaptive immunity by presenting antigens to the B lymphocytes and T lymphocytes. Adaptive immunity takes time to develop. The two arms of adaptive immunity are humoral immunity (B lymphocyte mediated) and cell mediated immunity (T lymphocyte mediated). It has intense diversity and is capable of responding to millions of antigens and possesses immune memory. Adaptive immunity takes time to evolve and is pathogen specific.

Q7. What is trained immunity?

Ans. The ability of the innate immune system to develop adaptive features and provide long-term protection against unrelated pathogens is term trained immunity. Epigenetic modification of various transcriptional pathways, as well as metabolic reprogramming of innate immune cells by both endogenous and exogenous stimuli, is the main driving force for trained immunity. Recent studies have revealed that innate immune cells, especially monocytes and macrophages, can develop adaptive features after adequate priming. Akin to adaptive immune response, trained innate immunity is associated with a heightened immune response to reinfections. In general, trained immunity is known to provide relatively short-term protection ranging from about 3 months to 1 year. Monocytes are very short-lived cells; however, the heightened secondary response can be spotted even several months after the primary stimulation. This shows that the immune memory is created at the level of progenitor cells, in the bone marrow.

A wide range of stimuli, such as beta-glucan (fungal ligand) and BCG (Bacillus Calmette-Guérin), are known to induce trained immunity. In humans, BCG vaccination-mediated non-specific protection against secondary infections is believed to be caused by trained immunity. Induction of trained immunity is considered to be a potential therapeutic strategy to manage various health conditions associated with immune system malfunctioning, such as cancer. Moreover, triggering trained immunity via live vaccines, such as BCG, measles, and oral polio vaccines, can be an effective approach in treating patients with severe infectious diseases, such as coronavirus disease 2019 (COVID-19). Long-term boosting of innate immune responses, also termed "trained immunity," by certain live vaccines (BCG, oral polio vaccine, measles) induces heterologous protection against infections through epigenetic, transcriptional, and functional reprogramming of innate immune cells.

Q8. What are B lymphocytes and T lymphocytes? What is their function?

Ans. B cells, also known as B lymphocytes, form the most important component of adaptive immunity (*see* **Fig. 2**). They provide humoral immunity by secreting antibodies. B-lymphocytes are produced in fetal liver and mature in the bone marrow in humans. In other species they mature in "Bursa of Fabricius" and hence named as B cells. B cells activated by the antigen present in the microbes and vaccines. These activated B cells are differentiated into antibody secreting plasma cells. For effective antibody B cells need help from T Helper cells.

T cells or T lymphocytes are mediators of cell mediated immunity. They have a key importance in the immune system and are at the core of adaptive immunity. They originate in thymus and mature in periphery and get activated in spleen/nodes. T cells can be distinguished from other lymphocytes by the presence of a T-cell receptor on the cell surface. T cell does not interact directly with the vaccine antigen unless presented by antigen presenting cells.

Q9. Which are different types of T cells?

Ans. They are as under:

- *CD4+ helper cells*: CD4+ helper cells help in the maturation of B cells into plasma cells and memory B cells. They also help activate cytotoxic T cells and macrophages. They become activated when they are presented with peptide antigens by major histocompatibility complex (MHC) class II molecules, which are expressed on the surface of antigen presenting cells (APCs). Once activated, they divide rapidly and secrete small proteins called cytokines that regulate or assist in the active immune response.
- *CD8+ cytotoxic cells:* CD8+ cytotoxic cells cause lysis of virus-infected and tumor cells. They are also involved in transplant rejection. These cells recognize their targets by binding to antigen associated with MHC class I molecules which are present on the surface of all nucleated cells. Cytotoxic cells secrete hole forming proteins called perforins for its cytolytic action.
- *Natural killer T cells:* They bridge the adaptive immune system with the innate immune system. While most T cells function based on recognition of MHC class molecules, natural killer T cells are able to recognize other antigen classes. Once activated, they are also able to perform the same functions as CD4+ and CD8+ cells.

Q10. Describe clinical implications of Th1, Th2, Th17 and Treg immune responses.

Ans. T cells play a central role in the adaptive immune response. T-helper (Th) cells can be classified into Th1, Th2, Th17 and Tregs cells. Th1 cells produce interleukin (IL)-2 and interferon (IFN) γ and are involved in cellular immunity, which help to eradicate infections by intracellular microbes which include certain viruses, protozoans, and intracellular bacteria, such as the mycobacteria.

Th2 cells, which produce IL-4, IL-5 and IL-13, are involved in humoral immunity, mainly against extracellular microorganisms.

Th17 cells play a role in host defense against extracellular pathogens, particularly at the mucosal and epithelial barriers, e.g., B pertussis, but aberrant activation has been linked to the pathogenesis of various auto-immune diseases. TH17 cells arise when the cytokines IL-6 and transforming growth factor (TGF)-β predominate during naive CD4 T-cell activation.

Regulatory T (TReg) cells are essential for maintaining peripheral tolerance, preventing autoimmunity and limiting chronic inflammatory diseases. However, they also limit beneficial responses by suppressing sterilizing immunity and limiting anti-tumour immunity. Suppression by inhibitory cytokines: interleukin-10 (IL-10), transforming growth factor-β (TGFβ) and the newly identified IL-35 are key mediators of TReg-cell function. Treg cells, which are CD4+/CD25+, regulate the functions of Th1, Th2 and Th17 cells.

Clinical implications: In TB, T helper (Th)1 cytokines provide protection whereas Th2 and T regulatory (Treg) cytokines contribute to the pathogenesis and Th17 cytokines play a role in both protection and pathogenesis.

In respect to the type of cellular immunity, wP-containing vaccine induce a Th1 and Th17 skewed response whereas aP-containing vaccines mostly induce a Th2 skewed response.

Th1 responses have been traditionally elicited by live-attenuated, vector-based or Toll-like receptor ligand-adjuvanted formulations for optimal stimulation of the innate immune system and immunomodulation, while most of the present licensed alum-adjuvanted subunit vaccines fail to elicit Th1/Th17 immune responses.

Q11. What is humoral immunity?

Ans. Humoral immunity is mediated through B lymphocytes by secreting antibodies (immunoglobulins) that act by neutralization, complement activation or by promoting opsonophagocytosis, which results in early reduction of pathogen load and clearance of extracellular pathogens and their toxins. Some humoral antibodies prevent colonization, which is the first step in pathogenesis by encapsulated organisms such as Haemophilus influenzae type B (HIB), pneumococcal, meningococcal and non-capsulated organisms causing diphtheria and pertussis.

Q12. What are immunoglobulins? Which are different types of immunoglobulins? What is their role?

Ans. B cells have immunoglobulin surface receptors which bind with appropriate antigen that stimulates B cell to mature into antibody secreting plasma cells and generate immunoglobulins. Immunoglobulins are of different types (IgG, IgM, IgA, IgD and IgE) and they differ in their structure, half-life, site of action and mechanism of action. Scientists have identified nine chemically distinct classes of human immunoglobulins, four kinds of IgG and two kinds of IgA, plus IgM, IgE, and IgD. Immunoglobulins G, D, and E are similar in appearance.

The role of each type of immunoglobulin is as under **(Fig. 3)**:
1. IgG, the major immunoglobulin in the blood, is also able to enter tissue spaces, able to cross placenta, it works efficiently to coat microorganisms, speeding their destruction by other cells in the immune system.

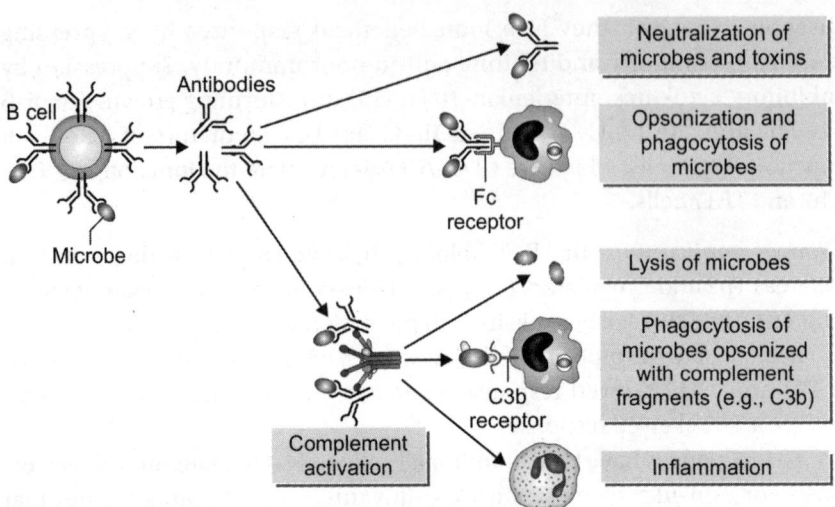

From Abbas, Lichtman, and Pober: Cellular and Molecular Immunology. WB Saunders, 1999.

Fig. 3: Functions of antibodies.

2. IgD is almost exclusively found inserted into the membrane of B cells, where it somehow regulates the cell's activation.
3. IgE is normally present in only trace amounts, but it is responsible for the symptoms of allergy.
4. IgA guards the entrance to the body. It concentrates in body fluids such as tears, saliva, and secretions of the respiratory and gastrointestinal tracts.
5. IgM usually combines in star-shaped clusters. It tends to remain in the bloodstream, where it is very effective in killing bacteria in early phase.

Q13. What is the main function of cell mediated or cellular immunity?

Ans. T cells are the effectors of cell mediated immunity (CMI). It is the principal defense mechanism against intracellular microbes. The T cell responses are more robust, long lasting and more cross protective than humoral responses hence modern vaccinology is being directed in this direction. The inherent T cell mediated immune regulatory mechanisms prevent any vaccines causing autoimmune diseases.

BCG is the only currently used human vaccine for which there is conclusive evidence that T cells are the main effectors.

Q14. What are antigen presenting cells (APC)?

Ans. Antigen-presenting cells (APCs) are a heterogeneous group of immune cells that mediate the cellular immune response by processing and presenting antigens for recognition by certain lymphocytes such as T cells. Classical APCs include dendritic cells, macrophages, Langerhans cells and B cells.

Q15. What are the dendritic cells?

Ans. Dendritic cells (DCs) are antigen-presenting cells (also known as accessory cells) of the mammalian immune system. They act as messengers between the innate and the adaptive immune systems. Dendritic cells are present in those tissues that are in contact with the external environment, such as the skin (where there is a specialized dendritic cell type called the Langerhans cell) and the inner lining of the nose, lungs, stomach and intestines. They can also be found in an immature state in the blood. At certain development stages they grow branched projections, the dendrites that give the cell its name as dendritic cell. Once activated, they migrate to the lymph nodes where they interact with T cells and B cells to initiate and shape the adaptive immune response.

Q16. What role do dendritic cells play in immunity?

Ans. Dendritic cells are the only cells, capable of activating naïve T cells and play a crucial role in the induction of T cell response. They capture antigen, process then into small peptides, display them through MHC molecules and provide costimulation signals to activate antigen-specific T cells.

Vaccine antigens are taken up by immature dendritic cells (DCs) activated by the local inflammation, which provides the signals required for their migration to draining lymph nodes. During this migration, DCs mature and their surface expression of molecules changes. DCs sense "danger signals" through their toll-like receptors and respond by a modulation of their surface or secreted molecules. Simultaneously, antigens are processed into small fragments and displayed at the cell surface in the grooves of MHC (HLA in humans) molecules. As a rule, MHC class I molecules present peptides from antigens that are produced within infected cells, whereas phagocytosed antigens are displayed on MHC class II molecules. Thus, mature DCs reaching the T cell zone of lymph nodes display MHC-peptide complexes and high levels of costimulation molecules at their surface. CD4+ T cells recognize antigenic peptides displayed by class II MHC molecules, whereas CD8+ T cells bind to class I MHC peptide complexes **(Fig. 4)**.

Q17. What are toll-like receptors?

Ans. Toll-like receptors (TLRs) are a class of proteins that play a key role in the innate immune system. They are single-pass membrane-spanning receptors usually expressed on sentinel cells such as macrophages and dendritic cells, that recognize structurally conserved molecules derived from microbes. Innate immunity is induced by exposure to evolutionarily conserved molecular structures termed pathogen-associated molecular patterns (PAMPs) that are expressed by a wide variety of infectious microorganisms. The recognition of PAMPs is mediated by pattern

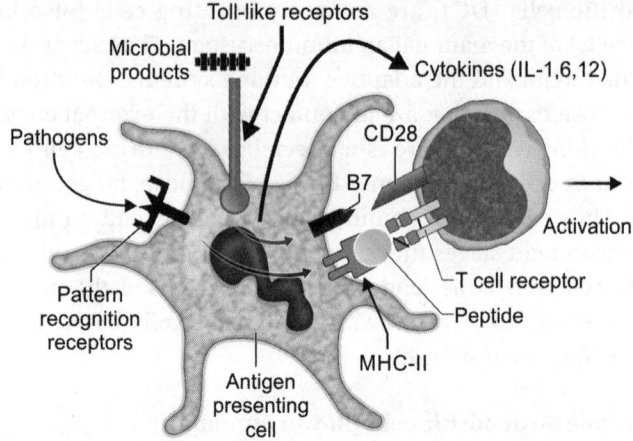

Fig. 4: Role of dendritic cells in immunity.

recognition receptors including TLRs, nod-like receptors and RIG-I-like receptors. Among them TLRs constitute one of the largest and most extensively studied classes of pattern recognition receptors. The innate immune response elicited by TLR activation is primarily characterized by the production of proinflammatory cytokines, chemokines, type I interferons (IFNs) and antimicrobial peptides. The ability of the immune system to recognize molecules that are broadly shared by pathogens is, in part, due to the presence of immune receptors called toll-like receptors that are expressed on the membranes of leukocytes including dendritic cells, macrophages, natural killer cells, cells of the adaptive immunity T cells, and B cells, and nonimmune cells. There are 13 TLRs, TLR 1 to TLR13, though the last three are not found in humans.

Q18. How do vaccines mediate protection?

Ans. Vaccines play a crucial role in prevention, elimination and eradication of vaccine preventable diseases. This is best achieved by immunization programs capable of inducing long-term protection. This can be achieved by the maintenance of antigen-specific immune effectors and/or by the induction of immune memory cells.

Most of the currently available vaccines provide protection through induction of B cells and production of antigen-specific antibodies. Antibodies either neutralize the antigen or promote opsonophagocytosis which results in early reduction of pathogen load and clearance of extracellular pathogens.

The role of cell mediated immunity in currently used vaccines (that have T cell dependent antigens) is mainly by supporting antibody protection. Other less common mechanisms by which cell mediated immunity works is by cytotoxic CD8+ T lymphocytes (CTL) that may limit the spread of infectious agents by recognizing and killing infected cells or secreting specific antiviral cytokines. Cellular immunity is essential for clearance of intracellular pathogens. The generation and maintenance of both B and CD8+ T cell responses is supported by growth factors and signals provided by CD4+ T helper (Th) lymphocytes, which are commonly subdivided into T helper 1 (Th1) and T helper 2 (Th2) subtypes.

BCG is the only currently used human vaccine for which there is conclusive evidence that T cells are the main effectors. Another instance is measles vaccination at 6 months during outbreak. These infants fail to raise antibody responses because of immune immaturity and/or the residual presence of inhibitory maternal antibodies, but generate significant IFN-γ producing CD4+ T cells. As a result these children may remain susceptible to measles infection, but are protected against severe disease because of the viral clearance capacity of their vaccine-induced T cell effectors. Thus, prevention of infection may only be achieved by vaccine-induced antibodies, whereas disease attenuation and protection against complications may be supported by T cells even in the absence of specific antibodies.

Q19. Define active and passive immunity.

Ans. Active immunity is acquired through natural infection/immunization and is long lasting. Passive immunity is conferred by maternal antibodies or immunoglobulin/antitoxin sera preparations and is short lasting.

Q20. Which are main types of vaccines?

Ans. Vaccines may be broadly classified as follows:
1. *Live attenuated vaccines:* BCG, oral polio, measles, MMR, chicken pox, Rota virus yellow fever, live influenza vaccine, live hepatitis A.
2. *Inactivated (Killed vaccines)* may be:
    A. *Whole cell inactivated*: Whole Cell Pertussis vaccines, Rabies, IPV, Hepatitis A.
    B. *Subunit vaccines*: They differ from inactivated whole-cell vaccines, by containing only the antigenic parts which are necessary to elicit a protective immune response. They are as under—
        I. Protein vaccines:
            a. Inactivated toxins/toxoids (diphtheria/tetanus toxoids)
            b. Subunit vaccines: Acellular pertussis, HBV, some influenza.
        II. Polysaccharide vaccines:
            a. Pure polysaccharide: Comprising only of the polysaccharide—typhoid, PPPV, meningococcal
            b. Conjugated Hib, Typhoid, PCV Meningococcal—conjugation of the polysaccharide with a protein carrier (glycoconjugates) significantly improves the immune response.

III. Virus-like particle (VPL): HPV, Influenza
IV. DNA vaccines
V. RNA vaccines.

Q21. What are live vaccines? How immunogenic are they?

Ans. Live attenuated vaccines (LAV) are derived from disease-causing pathogens (virus or bacteria) that have been attenuated under laboratory conditions. LAVs stimulate an excellent immune response as they mimic a natural infection. The vaccine virus/bacteria multiply and disseminate in multiple tissues and results in lymph node stimulation of dendritic cells at multiple sites. It also provides continual antigenic stimulation giving sufficient time for memory cell production. The activated DCs migrate towards the corresponding draining lymph nodes and launch multiple foci of T and B cell activation.

Q22. What are killed vaccines? How immunogenic are they?

Ans. Inactivated vaccines are made from microorganisms (viruses, bacteria, other organisms) that have been killed through physical or chemical processes. They can be whole or fractional subunit vaccines. Inactivated whole-cell vaccines are far less immunogenic as compared to live vaccines and the response may not be long lasting. Several doses of inactivated whole-cell vaccines may be required to evoke a sufficient immune response. In case of killed vaccines, there is only local and unilateral lymph node activation without associated dissemination and replication.

The immunogenicity of killed vaccine can be improved by various methods. Killed vaccines require adjuvants which improve the immune response by producing robust local inflammation and recruiting higher number of dendritic cells/monocytes to the injection site. Inactivated vaccines are more heat stable than live attenuated vaccines.

Q23. What are adjuvants?

Ans. Adjuvant is a substance that potentiates and/or modulates the immune responses to an antigen to improve their immunogenicity. They act by enhancing antigen presentation and/or by providing costimulation signals (immunomodulators). Aluminum salts are the most commonly used adjuvants in human vaccines. A toll-like receptors analog, named CpG ODNs, a new generation adjuvant, improves the function of professional antigen-presenting cells and boost the generation of humoral and cellular vaccine-specific immune responses:
- Adjuvants help in the translocation of antigens to the lymph nodes where they can be recognized by T cells.
- They provide physical protection to antigens which grants the antigen a prolonged delivery, providing additional time for upregulating the production of B and T cells needed for greater immunological memory in the adaptive immune response.

- They increase the capacity to cause local reactions at the injection site (during vaccination), inducing greater release of danger signals.
- They induce the release of inflammatory cytokines which helps to not only recruit B and T cells at sites of infection but also increase transcriptional events leading to a net increase of immune cells as a whole.
- They are believed to increase the innate immune response to antigen by interacting with pattern recognition receptors (PRRs) on or within accessory cells.

Q24. Does the route of administration of vaccines matter with the type of vaccine? How?

Ans. The site and route of administration of killed vaccines is of great importance. For killed vaccines intramuscular route is preferred over the subcutaneous route. As the muscles are well-vascularized and has a large number of patrolling dendritic cells. Hence, the vaccines which are supposed to be given intramuscularly should not be given subcutaneously and even if administered inadvertently that dose should be discounted, e.g., Rabies vaccine, Hepatitis B vaccine.

Intradermal route recruits the abundant dendritic cells in the skin and offers the advantage of antigen sparing, early and effective protection but the GMTs are lower than that achieved with IM and may wane faster. Dendritic cells are in highest number in the skin and hence marked reduction (e.g., 10-fold) of the antigen dose in intradermal immunization, e.g., ARV, IPV.

Finally due to focal lymph node activation, multiple killed vaccines may be administered at different sites with little immunologic interference.

The site of administration is usually of little significance for live vaccines. Immunologic interference may occur with multiple live vaccines unless they are given on the same day or at least 4 weeks apart or by different routes.

Q25. What are the characteristics of T cell independent immune response? Which vaccines do exhibit such response?

Ans. T cell independent immune response is elicited by B cells only and has following characteristics:
1. Only B cell response, T cell independent
2. Poorly immunogenic below 2 years due to immaturity of the marginal zones
3. Do not trigger GC activity
4. Weaker and shorter immune response
5. No induction of immune memory, hence no booster responses
6. There is no local immunity as IgA are not produced
7. Repeated doses lead to hypo responsiveness.

Bacterial (*S. pneumoniae, N. meningitidis, H. influenzae, S. typhi*) polysaccharide (PS) antigens exhibit T cell independent antigens.

Q26. Describe the first steps after immunization.

Ans. Following vaccine injection, the vaccine antigens attract local and systemic dendritic cells, monocytes and neutrophils. Innate immune responses activate these cells by changing their surface receptors and migrate along lymphatic vessels, to the draining lymph nodes where the activation of T and B lymphocytes takes place. The type of response elicited will depend upon type of vaccine, its antigenic type and content and immune status of an individual. Vaccines that stimulate innate immunity effectively are better immunogens. This can be achieved by live vaccines, adjuvants, toll-like receptors (TLR) agonists, live vectors and DNA vaccines. Live vaccines are capable of activating innate immunity in a better way which is helpful for subsequent induction of adaptive immune effectors.

In the lymph nodes, the response to polysaccharide vaccines and protein/protein-conjugate vaccines are different.

Q27. What are the immune responses to polysaccharide vaccines?

Ans. On being released from the injection site they reach the marginal zone of the spleen/nodes and bind to the specific Ig surface receptors of B cells. In the absence of antigen-specific T cell help, B cells activate, proliferate and differentiate in plasma cells without undergoing affinity maturation in germinal centers. The antibody response sets in 2–4 weeks following immunization, is predominantly IgM with low titers of low affinity IgG. The half-life of the plasma cells is short and antibody titers decline rapidly. Additionally the PS antigens are unable to evoke an immune response in those aged less than 2 years. As PS antigens do not induce germinal centers, bona fide memory B cells are not elicited **(Fig. 5)**. Consequently, subsequent re-exposure to the same PS results in a repeat primary response that follows the same kinetics in previously vaccinated as in naïve individuals.

Q28. What is hyporesponsiveness?

Ans. Revaccination with certain bacterial PS, of which Group C Meningococcus is a prototype, may even induce lower antibody responses

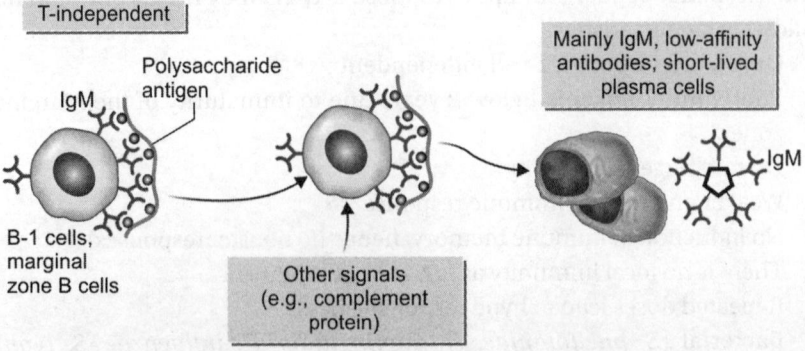

Fig. 5: Immune response to polysaccharide vaccines.

than the first immunization, a phenomenon referred to as hyporesponsiveness. Due to this phenomenon, only a single booster of either Pneumococcal or Meningococcal polysaccharide vaccine is recommended even in patients who require lifelong protection.

Q29. Which are characteristics of T cell dependent vaccines? Which vaccines do exhibit such response?

Ans.
1. Consistently immunogenic in infants beyond 6 months
2. Induces both T cell and B cell response
3. Immune response is robust long lasting and with higher titers of IgG response
4. High quality antibody
5. Booster response with repeated doses
6. No hyporesponsiveness.

Protein antigens which include pure proteins (Hepatitis B, Hepatitis A, HPV, Toxoids) or conjugation of PS antigens with a protein carrier (Hib, Pneumococcal, Meningococcal) are T cell dependent antigens.

Q30. What are the immune responses to protein and conjugated vaccines?

Ans. The immune enhancing effect of protein and of conjugate vaccines is assumed to result from an increase of carrier driven T-helper frequency and T-cell mediated costimulatory signals. Activation of germinal center (GC) is the key to such robust and long lasting immune response **(Fig. 6)**.

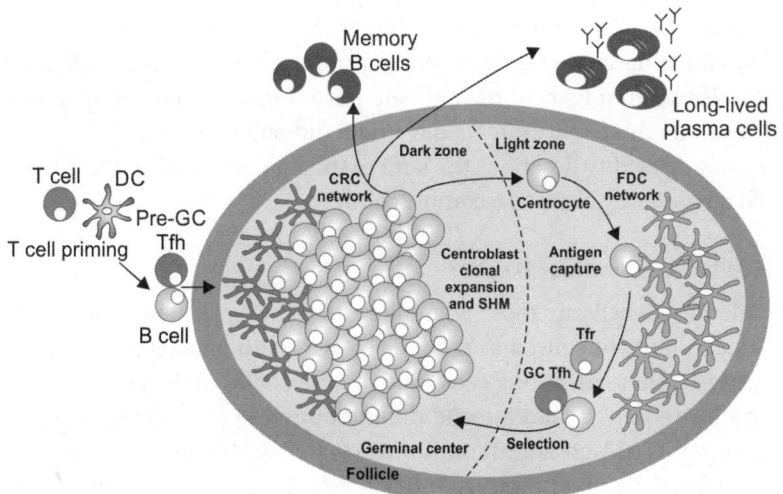

Fig. 6: The germinal center (GC) response.
Source: Stebegg M, Kumar SD, Silva-Cayetano A, Fonseca VR, Linterman MA, Graca L. Regulation of the germinal center response. Front Immunol. 2018;9:2469.

In response to a protein antigen reaching lymph nodes or spleen, B cells capable of binding to this antigen with their surface immunoglobulins undergo a brisk activation. In an extrafollicular reaction, B cells rapidly differentiate in plasma cells that produce low-affinity antibodies (of the IgM ± IgG/IgA isotypes) that appear at low levels in the serum within a few days after immunization (similar to PS antigens). Additionally, antigen-specific helper T cells that have been activated by antigen-bearing dendritic cells trigger some antigen-specific B cells to migrate toward follicular dendritic cells (FDCs) initiating the GC reaction. FDCs play an essential role in B cell responses: they attract antigen-specific B and T cells and capture/retain antigen for extended periods. B cells that are attracted by Ag-bearing FDCs become the founders of GCs. In GCs, B cells receive additional signals from follicular T cells and undergo massive clonal proliferation. This intense proliferation is associated to two major events: Ig class-switch from IgM toward IgG, IgA or IgE, and affinity maturation of the of B cells for their specific antigen which differentiate into plasma cells secreting large amounts of antigen-specific antibodies. At the end of the GC reaction, a few plasma cells exit nodes/spleen and migrate to survival niches mostly located in the bone marrow, where they survive through signals provided by supporting stromal cells.

The development of this GC reaction requires a couple of weeks, such that hypermutated IgG antibodies to protein vaccine antigens first appear in the blood 10–14 days after priming. It is the magnitude of GC responses, i.e., the quality of DC, B cell, Tfh cell and FDC interactions, which controls the intensity of B cell differentiation into plasma cells, and thus the peak of IgG vaccine antibody reached within 4–6 weeks after primary immunization.

Q31. What is antibody affinity and avidity?

Ans. Antibody affinity refers to the strength with which the epitope binds to an individual paratope (antigen-binding site) on the antibody. High affinity antibodies bind quickly to the antigen, permit greater sensitivity in assays and maintain this bond more readily under difficult conditions.

Antibody avidity describes the sum of the epitope specific affinities with which an antibody binds to a complex antigen.

Q32. What are memory B cells?

Ans. Memory B cells are those B lymphocytes that are generated in response to T-dependent antigens, during the GC reaction, in parallel to plasma cells. They persist there as resting cells until re-exposed to their specific antigens when they readily proliferate and differentiate into plasma cells, secreting large amounts of high-affinity antibodies that may be detected in the serum within a few days after boosting. Antigen-specific memory cells generated by primary immunization are much more numerous than naïve B cells initially capable of antigen recognition.

Memory B cells do not produce antibodies, i.e., do not protect, unless re-exposure to antigen drives their differentiation into antibody producing plasma cells. This reactivation is a rapid process, such that booster responses are characterized by the rapid increase to higher titers of antibodies that have a higher affinity for antigen than antibodies generated during primary responses. The reactivation, proliferation and differentiation of memory B cells occur without requiring the induction and development of GC responses. This process is thus much more rapidly completed than that of primary responses.

Q33. Why do we need more than one dose, even for live vaccines?

Ans. The older concept that single dose of live vaccine induces life-long immunity is not true. The live vaccines induce an immune response similar to that seen with protein vaccines. However, live vaccines have limitations in the form of primary and secondary failures. Sometimes the take up of live vaccines is not 100% with the first dose (primary failure). Hence, more than 1 dose is recommended with these live vaccines. Once the vaccine has been taken up, immunity is robust and lifelong or at least for several decades. This is because of continuous replication of the organism that is a constant source of the antigen. The second dose of such live vaccine will take care for primary vaccine failures (no uptake of vaccine). Secondary vaccine failures are associated with decline in antibody titers with passage of time and here also second dose of live vaccine becomes necessary. The examples are varicella and mumps vaccines.

Q34. What is primary and secondary (booster) immune response?

Ans. When an antigen is introduced for the first time, the immune response starts after a lag of 10 days or so. This is called primary response. Such response is short-lived, has a lag period, mainly IgM type with low titers of antibodies. In primary immune response, the antigen exposure elicits an extrafollicular response that results in the rapid appearance of low IgG antibody titers. As B cells proliferate in GCs and differentiate into plasma cells, IgG antibody titers increase up to a peak value usually reached 4 weeks after immunization. The short-life span of these plasma cells results in a rapid decline of antibody titers, which eventually return to baseline levels 3.

Secondary immune responses start on subsequent exposure (booster) to the same antigen. There is no lag phase, response starts in less than 7 days, persists for a long time, mainly IgG type with high antibody titers. Booster exposure to antigen reactivates immune memory B cells and results in a rapid (<7 days) increase of IgG antibody titer by a rapid proliferation of memory B cells and their evolution into abundant antibody secreting plasma cells. Short-lived plasma cells maintain peak Ab levels during a few weeks, after which serum antibody titers decline initially with the same rapid kinetics as

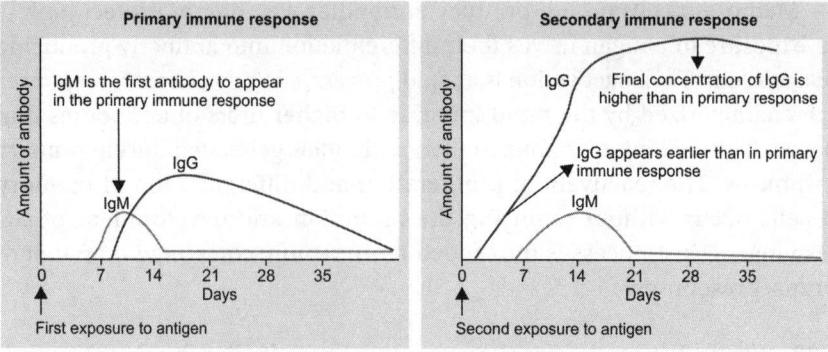

Fig. 7: A schematic diagram showing a primary and secondary response.

following primary immunization. Long-lived plasma cells that have reached survival niches in the bone marrow continue to produce antigen-specific antibodies, which then decline with slower kinetics. This generic pattern may not apply to live vaccines triggering long-term IgG antibodies for extended periods of time **(Fig. 7)**.

Q35. Which are the determinants of intensity and duration of immune responses?

Ans. Both, primary and secondary immune responses after vaccination depend on various factors such as vaccine type, nature of antigen, vaccination schedule, genetic and environmental factors and age at immunization.

Vaccine Type
Broadly speaking live vaccines are superior (exception BCG, OPV) to protein antigens which in turn are superior to polysaccharide vaccines.
- *Live vs. inactivated:* Higher intensity of innate responses, higher antigen content following replication and more prolonged antigen persistence generally result into higher antibodies (Ab) responses to live than inactivated vaccines.
- *Protein vs. polysaccharide:* Recruitment of T cell help and induction of germinal centers (GCs) results into higher antibody responses to protein or glycoconjugate than to pure polysaccharide vaccines.
- *Adjuvants:* Adjuvants improve immune responses to inactivated vaccines by either modulation of antigen delivery and persistence (depot or slow-release formulations) or enhancement of Th responses (immunomodulator) which may support or limit antibody responses.

Antigen Content
- *Polysaccharide antigens:* Failure to induce GCs limit immunogenicity.
- *Protein antigens:* Inclusion of epitopes readily recognized by B cells (B cell repertoire), inclusion of epitopes readily recognized by follicular

CHAPTER 1: Basic Immunology

helper T cells, elicitation of efficient follicular T cell help and the capacity of antigen to associate/persist in association to follicular dendritic cells (FDCs) result into higher antibody responses.
- *Antigen dose:* As a rule, higher antigen doses (e.g., Hepatitis B vaccine) increase the availability of antigen for B/T cell binding and activation, as well as for association with FDCs however there is a limiting dose for each.

Vaccination Schedule

The immune response improves with increasing number of doses and increased spaces between doses.

Other Factors
- *Age at immunization:* Early life immune immaturity or age-associated immune senescence impairs immune responses to an administered vaccine.
- *Genetic factors:* The capacity of antigen epitopes to associate to a large panel of MHC molecules increases the likelihood of responses in the population. MHC restriction may limit T cell responses. Gene polymorphisms in molecules critical for B and T cell activation/differentiation are likely to affect Ab responses. T cell responses differ markedly between individuals and populations because of genetic variability of MHC molecules (HLA A2).
- *Environmental factors:* Mostly yet to be identified.

Q36. What is priming and boosting mechanism for killed vaccines?

Ans. The immune response improves with proper spacing of vaccine doses. Traditionally, "0-1-6" month schedule (prime and boost) is considered as a most immunogenic schedule than 6-10-14 week or 2,3,5 month or 2,4,6 month schedules for non-live T-cell dependent vaccines such as Hepatitis-B, vaccine. Here there is adequate time interval between first few doses for priming and inducing the immune responses and last dose that works as boosters. Since, affinity maturation of B-cells in GCs and formation of memory-B cells take at least 4–6 months, this schedule quite well fulfills these requirements.

More than one dose is needed for better induction and recruitment of more number of GCs in young age considering young age limitations of immune system. A 4 week minimal interval between primary doses avoids competition between successive waves of primary responses.

Q37. What should be the spacing between two or more vaccines?

Ans. The spacing between two or more live and/or killed vaccines is vaccines is given in **Table 1**.

Table 1: Timing and minimal period of spacing between two doses of vaccines.

Antigen combination	Minimal interval between doses
2 or more inactivated antigens	None, can be administered simultaneously or at any interval between 2 doses
Inactivated and live antigens	None, can be administered simultaneously or at any interval between 2 doses
2 or more live	28 days minimum interval if not administered at the same visit

Q38. What is the importance of immune memory in immunization programs?

Ans. Immune memory allows one to complete an interrupted vaccine schedule without restarting the schedule. Immune memory is seen with live vaccines/protein antigens due to generation of memory B cells which are activated on repeat vaccination/natural exposure. Activation of immune memory and generation of protective antibodies usually takes 4–7 days. Diseases which have incubation periods shorter than this period such as Hib, tetanus, diphtheria and pertussis require regular boosters to maintain protective antibody levels. However, diseases such as Hepatitis A, Hepatitis B do not need regular boosters as the long incubation period of the disease allows for activation of immune memory cells.

Q39. What are limitations of immune responses during early life?

Ans. Transplacentally acquired maternal antibodies, and immaturity of immune system limit the immune responses during young age. IgG antibodies are actively transferred through the placenta, via the FcRn receptor, from the maternal to the fetal circulation. Upon immunization, maternal antibodies bind to their specific epitopes at the antigen surface, competing with infant B cells and thus limiting B cell activation, proliferation and differentiation. The inhibitory influence of maternal antibodies on infant B cell responses affects all vaccine types, although its influence is more marked for live attenuated viral vaccines that may be neutralized by even minute amounts of passive antibodies. Hence, antibody responses elicited in early life are short lasting. The extent and duration of the inhibitory influence of maternal antibodies increase with gestational age, e.g., with the amount of transferred immunoglobulins (Ig), and declines with postnatal age as maternal antibodies wane.

Early life immune responses are characterized by age-dependent limitations of the magnitude of responses to all vaccines. Antibody responses to most PS antigens are not elicited during the first 2 years of life, which is likely to reflect numerous factors including: the slow maturation of the spleen marginal zone; limited expression of CD21 on B cells; and limited availability of the complement factors. Although this may be circumvented in part by the use of glycoconjugate vaccines, even the most potent glycoconjugate vaccines elicit markedly lower primary IgG responses in young infants.

Although maternal antibodies interfere with the induction of infant antibody responses, they may allow a certain degree of priming, i.e., of induction of memory B cells. This likely reflects the fact that limited amounts of unmasked vaccine antigens may be sufficient for priming of memory B cells but not for full-blown GC activation, although direct evidence is lacking.

Maternal antibodies inhibit only B cell induced antibodies responses but not T-cell response, which remain largely unaffected or even enhanced, e.g.,:
1. BCG may be given as the maternal antibodies actually enhance T cell responses.
2. OPV may be given as there are no maternal IgA in the gut to neutralize the virus.
3. Measles vaccine if given at the age of 6 months (in an outbreak situation) may work by inducing T cell immunity.

Q40. How are these limitations of young age immunization overcome?

Ans. This issue can be addressed favorably to a certain extent by increasing the number of a vaccine doses for better induction, use of adjuvants to improve immunogenicity of vaccines, and by use of boosters at later age when immune system has shown more maturity than at the time of induction. Increasing the dose of vaccine antigen may also be sufficient to circumvent the inhibitory influence of maternal antibodies, as illustrated for hepatitis A or measles vaccines.

Q41. Why do we offer birth doses of BCG, OPV, HBV in spite of presence of maternal antibodies?

Ans.
1. BCG can be given as maternal antibodies actually enhance T cell responses. (BCG is T cell response and not affected by circulating maternal antibodies)
2. OPV may be given as there is no maternal IgA in the gut to neutralize the virus as maternal Ab are only IgG type. (Priming, so better seroconversion to subsequent doses)
3. Birth dose of HBV acts as priming dose so that subsequent doses are capable of eliciting immune response even in presence of maternal antibodies. This is because maternal antibodies do not interfere with induction of memory B cells allowing certain degree of much needed priming. (Important for prevention of both vertical and horizontal transmission)

Q42. Why do we practice early accelerated schedule of 6-10-14 weeks despite young age limitations on immunization schedules?

Ans. Immunization schedules, practiced in developed world, commencing at 2 months and having 2 months spacing between the doses are considered technically appropriate. However, we do not follow it in our country. Disease epidemiology of vaccine-preventable diseases (VPDs) in a country often determines a particular vaccination schedule. Since, majority of childhood infectious diseases cause morbidity and mortality at an early age in developing countries, there is need to protect the children at the earliest opportunity through immunizations. This is the reason why early, accelerated schedules are practiced in developing countries despite the known limitations of young age immunization. So for both, operational reasons and for early completion of immunization, the 6, 10, 14 week's schedule is chosen in developing countries. Such a schedule has shown to give adequate protection in recipients.

Q43. Why do we have different number of doses for different age groups for inactivated vaccines?

Ans. For killed vaccines such as DPT, Hib, Pneumococcal and Hep B which are administered as early as birth/6 weeks, the first dose acts only as a priming dose while subsequent doses provide an immune response even in presence of maternal antibodies. However a booster at 15–18 months is required for durable immunity. As the age of commencement of vaccination advances the number of doses reduces (2 doses at 6–12 months followed by a booster dose and 1–2 doses between 12 and 23 months for Hib and Pneumococcal vaccines).

Q44. Do we need a vaccine after getting recovered from a particular disease?

Ans. In general natural infection with viral illness provides very long lasting or life-long immunity. Hence, viral vaccines such as MMR, Varicella, etc., are not advised after such diseases. On the other hand bacterial illnesses do not impart such protection, justifying the need for vaccination, e.g., diphtheria, tetanus, typhoid.

■ SUGGESTED READING

1. Balasubramanian S. IAP Guidebook on Immunization 2018–2019, 3rd edition. Advisory Committee on Vaccines and Immunization Practices, Indian Academy of Pediatrics. New Delhi: Jaypee Brothers Medical Publishers (P) Ltd.; 2020.
2. Hong Kong Measles Vaccine Committee. Comparative trial of live attenuated measles vaccine in Hong Kong by intramuscular and intradermal injection. Bull World Health Organ. 1967;36:375-84.

3. Indian Academy of Pediatrics. Advanced Science of Vaccinology (IAP Module 2009). Mumbai: IAP; 2009.
4. Indian Academy of Pediatrics. IAP Practical Vaccinology (module 2018). Mumbai: IAP; 2018.
5. Kamat D, Madhur A. Vaccine Immunology. In: Vashishtha VM (Ed). IAP Textbook of Vaccines. New Delhi: Jaypee Brothers Medical Publishers (P) Ltd.; 2013.
6. Kobrynski LJ, Sousa AO, Nahmias AJ, Lee FK. Cutting edge: antibody production to pneumococcal polysaccharides requires CD1 molecules and CD8+ T cells. J Immunol. 2005;174:1787-90.
7. Lee CJ, Lee LH, Lu Cs, Wu A. Bacterial polysaccharides as vaccine-immunity and chemical characterization. Adv Exp Med Biol. 2001;491:453-71.
8. MacLennan IC, Toellner KM, Cunningham AF, Serre K, Sze DM, Zúñiga E, et al. Extrafollicular antibody responses. Immunol Rev. 2003;194:8-18.
9. Netea MG. 2020. Trained Immunity: a Tool for Reducing Susceptibility to and the Severity of SARS-CoV-2 Infection. Cell. https://www.sciencedirect.com/science/article/pii/S0092867420305079.
10. Plotkin SA. Vaccination against the major infectious diseases. CR Acad Sci III. 1999;322:943-51.
11. Rowe J, Poolman JT, Macaubas C, Sly PD, Loh R, Holt PG, et al. Enhancement of vaccine-specifi C cellular immunity in infants by passively acquired maternal antibody. Vaccine. 2004;22:3986-92.
12. Siegrist CA. Mechanisms by which maternal antibodies influence infant vaccine responses: review of hypotheses and definition of main determinants. Vaccine. 2003;21:3406-12.
13. Saito S, Nakashima A, Shima T, Ito M. Th1/Th2/Th17 and regulatory T-cell paradigm in pregnancy. Am J Reprod Immunol 2010.
14. Siegrist CA. Neonatal and early life vaccinology. Vaccine. 2001;19:3331-46.
15. Siegrist CA. Vaccine Immunology. In: Plotkin SA, Orenstein W, Offit P (Eds). Vaccines, 5th edition. Philadelphia: Saunders Elsevier; 2008.
16. Stebegg M, Kumar SD, Silva-Cayetano A, Fonseca VR, Linterman MA, Graca L. Regulation of the germinal center response. Front Immunol. 2018;9:2469.
17. Timens W, Boes A, Rozeboom-Uiterwijk T, Poppema S. Immaturity of the human splenic marginal zone in infancy. Possible contribution to the deficient infant immune response. J Immunol. 1989;143:3200-6.

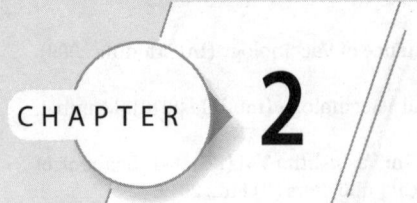

Basic Epidemiology in Vaccinations

Bhaskar Shenoy

Q1. What is epidemiology?

Ans. The term epidemiology, literally meaning "the study of what is upon the people", is derived from Greek language: *epi* meaning "upon, among", *demos* meaning "people, district" purpose of surveillance is to monitor aspect of disease occurrence and spread that are pertinent to effective control.

Epidemiology is defined as "study of the distribution and determinants of health-related states or events in specified populations and the application of this study to the control of health problems," The term "disease" encompasses all unfavorable health changes, including injuries and mental health.

Epidemiological methods help us in identifying target pathogens, their sources and transmission pathways. This information is utilized to design disease-specific control, elimination and/or eradication strategies. This guides the policy makers, planning bodies and healthcare providers, not only in formulating policies and planning specific health interventions, but also in prioritizing resource allocation.

Q2. What is the importance of epidemiology in vaccinology?

Ans. The learning and study of vaccine epidemiology is significant in the following ways:
- To assess the disease burden
- To identify target pathogens for vaccine research
- To identify sources and transmission pathways of disease-causing agents
- To determine vaccination strategies
- To make a choice of choose vaccines for inclusion in a public health program
- To design disease-specific control, elimination, and eradication strategies
- To monitor performance indicators
- To take steps to improve surveillance
- To measure the progress and impact of vaccination strategies.

Q3. What are measures of disease frequency?

Ans. Incidence and prevalence are measures of disease frequency. Incidence rate is defined as the number of new cases occurring in a defined population during a specified period of time. It is calculated by the following formula:

Table 1: The difference between incidence and prevalence.

	Incidence	Prevalence
Numerator	Number of new cases of disease during a specified period of time	Number of existing cases of disease at a given point of time
Denominator	Population at risk	Population at risk
Focus	Whether the event is a new case	Presence or absence of a disease
Uses	Expresses the risk of becoming ill	Estimates the probability of the population being ill at the period of time being studied

$$\text{Incidence} = \frac{\text{Number of new cases} \times 10^n}{\text{Population at risk}}$$

Prevalence is defined as all current cases (old as well as new) exiting at a given point of time (point prevalence) or over a period of time (period prevalence) in a specified population. Prevalence is actually a ratio which is estimated as follows:

$$\text{Prevalence} = \frac{\text{Total number of cases: Old and new} \times 100}{\text{Total population at risk}}$$

The difference between incidence and prevalence is described in **Table 1**.

Prevalence is dependent on both incidence and disease duration. Provided that the prevalence (P) is low and does not vary significantly with time, it can be calculated approximately as:

P = incidence × average duration of disease

Q4. What is burden of disease and how it is measured?

Ans. The term "disease burden" or burden of disease (BoD) occupies a key place in epidemiology. Several parameters are utilized to quantify the BoD. These include incidence or prevalence of a disease (prevaccine and postvaccine); severity/mortality (measured as case fatality ratio, hospitalization, and disease sequelae); disability [measured by disability-adjusted life years (DALYs) and quality-adjusted life years (QALYs)]; economics (measured by cost-effectiveness, cost benefit, and cost utility); and social aspects (measured by societal disruption, economic disruption, and household impact).

Q5. What is "descriptive epidemiology"?

Ans. Descriptive epidemiology is the subdivision of epidemiology which describes the occurrence and distribution of disease by time, place and person.

Q6. Define endemic disease?

Ans. A disease, or an infectious agent that is constantly present in a defined geographical area or a population, is defined as an endemic disease, e.g., cholera, tuberculosis, etc.

Q7. What is a holoendemic disease?

Ans. It is disease which has a high prevalence of infection in early life so that it affects majority of the pediatric population, leading to a state of population immunity with advancing age. This results in a much lower incidence of the disease in the adults as compared to children. Malaria is holoendemic in some regions of Sub-Saharan Africa, as is trachoma in few areas of Saudi Arabia.

Q8. What is a hyperendemic disease?

Ans. Hyperendemic disease is a disease that is constantly present at a high incidence and/or prevalence and affects all age groups equally. Dengue is hyperendemic in India.

Q9. What is an epidemic?

Ans. Epidemic refers to an increase, often sudden, in the number of cases of a disease above what is normally expected in that population in that geographical area. Examples of infectious agents that can give rise to epidemics are measles, influenza, meningococcal disease. The number of cases indicating the presence of an epidemic of a particular disease is variable. It depends on the characteristics of the agent, the characteristics of the population exposed such as previous exposure to the disease and time and place of occurrence.

Q10. Differentiate between outbreak and epidemic.

Ans. Outbreak carries the same definition of epidemic, but is often used for a more limited geographic area, e.g., outbreak of *Salmonella* in a neonatal unit.

Q11. Define epizootic disease?

Ans. It is epidemic of a disease occurring in an animal population; often with the potential of spreading in the human populations. Influenza A viruses are known to infect a large number of warm-blooded animals such as birds, pigs, horses, along with humans.

Q12. Define pandemic disease with examples?

Ans. It is an epidemic occurring over a very large area which generally extends beyond international boundaries, and affects a large number of people worldwide. In other words, it is a global epidemic, e.g., acquired immunodeficiency syndrome (AIDS), H1N1 influenza, severe acute respiratory syndrome coronavirus 2 (SARS–CoV 2).

Q13. Define index case and primary case?

Ans.

Index case: It is the first case in a defined group or population to come to the attention of the investigator.

Primary case: It is the individual who introduces the disease into the group or the population. The primary case is not necessarily the first diagnosed case in the group; hence, it must be distinguished from the term "index case". The cases infected by the primary case are known as "secondary cases" which in turn infect other susceptible individuals to produce the "tertiary cases".

Q14. Define secondary attack rate?

Ans. It is the number of cases of an infection occurring among the susceptible contacts of a primary case within the incubation period of the pathogen; the denominator includes only those contacts that are susceptible. It is a measure of contagiousness of the disease. It can be utilized as a tool in evaluating the disease control measures.

Q15. What is the meaning of basic reproductive number and how is it calculated?

Ans. Basic reproductive number or R_0, measures "the average number of secondary cases generated by one primary case in a susceptible population." A number of factors determine its magnitude, including the course of infection in the patient and the factors that determine transmission between people. The magnitude of R_0 varies according to location and population. It is strongly influenced by birth rate, population density, and behavioral factors. The magnitude of R_0 can be ascertained by cross-sectional and longitudinal serological surveys.

For organisms to survive:
- $R_0 = 1$ (A primary case must attempt to generate at least one new case)
- $R_0 > 1$ (Expansion of infected individuals)
- $R_0 < 1$ (Shrinking pool of infected individuals).

To calculate the magnitude of R_0, a few key epidemiological, demographic, and vaccination program-related parameters should be known. Parameters such as average age at infection prior to mass vaccination, life expectancy of the study population, and the average duration of protection by maternal antibodies should be considered. A number of studies have been conducted in different parts of the world to assess the average age of infections and to derive the basic reproductive number.

Q16. What is the effective reproductive rate (R)?

Ans. It is the number of secondary cases generated by the index case in a mixed population of susceptible and immune individuals.

$R = R_0 \times X$, where X is the proportion of susceptible in a population.

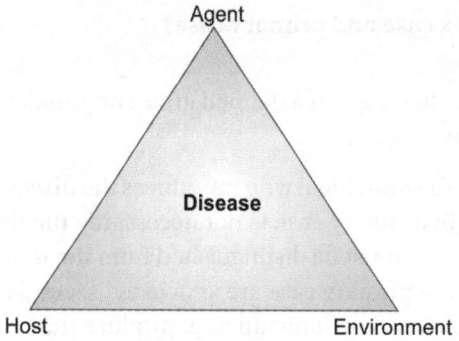

Fig. 1: Epidemiological triad.

Q17. What is epidemic threshold?

Ans. It is the number or the density of susceptible hosts required in a population for an epidemic to occur.

Q18. What is epidemiological triad?

Ans. The concept of "epidemiological triad" refers to a complex interaction between the agent, the host and the environment that determines the natural history of the disease **(Fig. 1)**.

Q19. Define seroconversion?

Ans. It is defined as more than or equal to four-fold increase in the antibody titer from prevaccination to postvaccination level or a detectable post vaccination titer in a vaccine who had no detectable antibody before vaccination. It is calculated to find the efficacy of a vaccine or a vaccination schedule. It is also described as antibody concentration changing from prevaccination seronegative to postvaccination seropositive. Seroconversion does not necessarily mean seroprotection.

Q20. Define seroprotection?

Ans. It is the state of protection (from disease), due to the presence of humoral immunity, or antibody detectable in plasma or serum. This term is usually used in the context of the level of such antibody necessary for protection.

Q21. What is seropositivity?

Ans. It is the presence of detectable antibodies against an antigen. The sensitivity of antibody detection depends on the serological technique used.

Q22. Define vaccine immunogenicity?

Ans. It is the ability of a vaccine to induce specific immunity against a particular pathogen. The level of antibodies signifying the protective threshold for majority of the vaccines is defined for many diseases. This is known as the "correlate of protection".

CHAPTER 2: Basic Epidemiology in Vaccinations

Q23. Define vaccine effectiveness (VE)?

Ans. Vaccine effectiveness is the sum of the reduction in the clinical events that might be expected to be associated with the disease in conditions of population usage.

It is a combination of vaccine efficacy, coverage, conditions under which vaccine administered (including maintenance of cold chain), presence of immunocompromising conditions in the population, e.g., HIV and herd effect.

The most commonly used study design to assess a vaccine's effectiveness is a retrospective case-control analysis, and the odds ratio thus obtained can be used to calculate vaccine effectiveness, as follows:

$$\text{Effectiveness} = (1 - OR) \times 100$$

Vaccine effectiveness could be assessed by observational studies: Cohort studies, household contact study, case-control study and screening.

Q24. Define vaccine efficacy?

Ans. It is the percentage reduction of cases among the vaccinated individuals. It denotes the direct protective effect of a vaccine in the vaccinated population.

Vaccine efficacy is calculated by means of the following equation:

$$VE\,(\%) = \frac{(RU - RV)}{RU} \times 100 \quad \text{or} \quad VE = \frac{1 - RV}{RU} \times 100$$

Where, RU = the incidence risk or attack rate in unvaccinated people, and RV = the incidence or attack rate in vaccinated people.

The vaccine efficacy is usually measured by double blind, randomized placebo controlled clinical trials. The vaccine efficacy for a number of vaccines is known, such as measles 90–95%; mumps: 72–88%; and rubella 95–98%. In vaccine trials, the vaccine's efficacy (among other things, including safety) is assessed. This is an important criterion for licensing of the vaccines and for making decisions on programmatic use. Vaccine efficacy is dependent on internal or individual factors, e.g., the efficacy of the measles vaccine depends on the presence of inhibitory maternal antibodies, the immunologic maturity of the vaccine recipient, and the dose and strain of the vaccine virus.

Q25. What are the types of population level effects of vaccination?

Ans.

Direct effect: The reduction of disease in the vaccinated cohort.

Indirect effect: The population level effect of widespread vaccination on people not receiving vaccine.

Total effect: Combination of population level effect and effect of vaccination on individuals receiving vaccine.

Overall public health effect: The effect of vaccination program based upon weighted average of indirect effect on the individual not receiving vaccine and total effect on individual receiving vaccination. It takes into consideration all the population level effects of the vaccination program.

Q26. What is vaccine impact?

Ans. The impact of immunization is measured by evaluating effects directly on the vaccinated individual, indirectly on the unvaccinated community (herd protection), the epidemiology of the pathogen (such as changing circulating serotypes or prevention of epidemic cycles), and the additional benefits arising from improved health.

Q27. How vaccination perturbs epidemiology?

Ans. Vaccination results in disturbances in the natural transmission pathways of the pathogen, resulting in alteration in the epidemiology of that infectious disease.

This perturbation results in herd immunity, herd effect and epidemiologic shifts.

Q28. Define herd immunity?

Ans. It is defined as the resistance of a group or a community in total, against the invasion and spread of an infectious agent as a result of a large proportion of individuals in the group being immunized.

The proportion of immune subjects in a population, beyond which the incidence of the infection decreases, is known as "herd immunity threshold". The herd immunity threshold for various infectious diseases has been calculated and shown in **Table 2**.

Q29. Define Herd effect?

Ans. Herd effect" or "herd protection" is "the reduction of infection or disease in the unimmunized segment as a result of immunizing a proportion of the population" or is "the change induced in epidemiology (incidence reduction)

Table 2: Herd immunity threshold for various diseases.

Disease	R0	Threshold (%)
Mumps	4–7	75–86
Polio	5–7	80–86
Smallpox	5–7	80–85
Diphtheria	6–7	85
Rubella	6–7	83–85
Pertussis	12–17	92–94
Measles	12–18	83–94

(R_0: basic reproduction number)

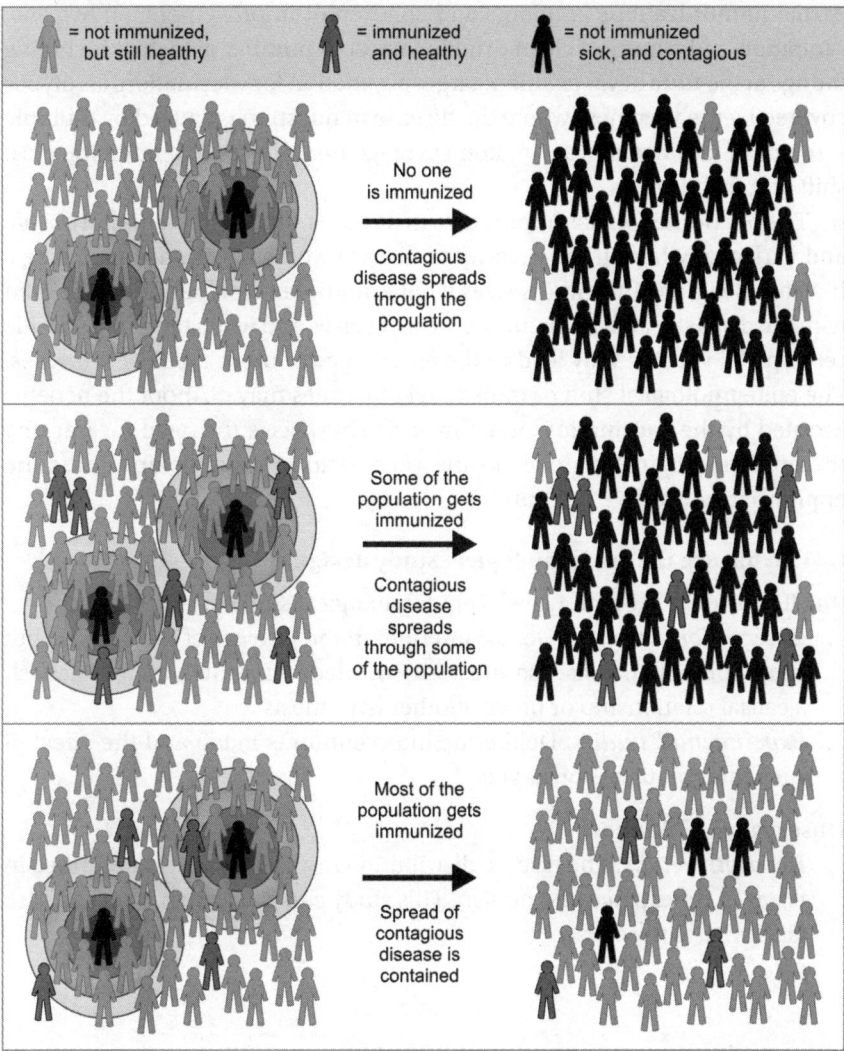

Fig. 2: Disease outbreak pattern in a community showing unimmunized and healthy people, immunized and healthy people, and sick and contagious people.

among unvaccinated members when a good proportion is vaccinated (**Fig. 2**)." Herd effect is seen only for infections where humans are the source, and it extends beyond the age the vaccine is given, i.e., *Haemophilus influenzae* type B (Hib) vaccine is given to infants and protected other under-5 children, flu vaccine to children and beneficial effect among other family members.

Q30. What do you mean by epidemiological shift?

Ans. Epidemiological shift is defined as an upward shift in the age of acquisition of a particular infection. This may occur due to a state of partial immunizations of infants and children or improvements in hygiene, sanitation and supply of clean drinking water. A number of factors including the age at the time of vaccination, target population for vaccination, serotypes covered by the vaccines (where the disease in question is caused by multiple serotypes), and overall vaccination coverage may affect the epidemiological shift or transition.

The phenomenon has importance in diseases such as hepatitis A, rubella, and varicella, wherein the severity of disease worsens with advancing age. It also has significance in diseases where multiple serotypes are associated with the diseases such as pneumococcal diseases and when targeting specific serotype by vaccine may lead to the emergence of other types of serotypes. The epidemiological shift or transition sometimes may offshoot the benefits accrued by the vaccination program. This showcases the need for tracking the epidemiological changes in the vaccination programs and initiating appropriate corrective measures.

Q31. What are the epidemiological study designs?

Ans. There are two broad types of epidemiological studies (**Fig. 3**):
1. *Observational studies:* Do not interfere in the process of the disease, but simply observe the disease and the associated factors. It does not establish a causal relationship or prove another hypothesis.
2. *Experimental studies:* Deliberate intervention is made and the effect of such intervention is observed.

Observational Studies
1. *Descriptive study*: The disease distribution in a community is described in terms of time, place and person. This study can give clues about the "risk factors" and the cause.

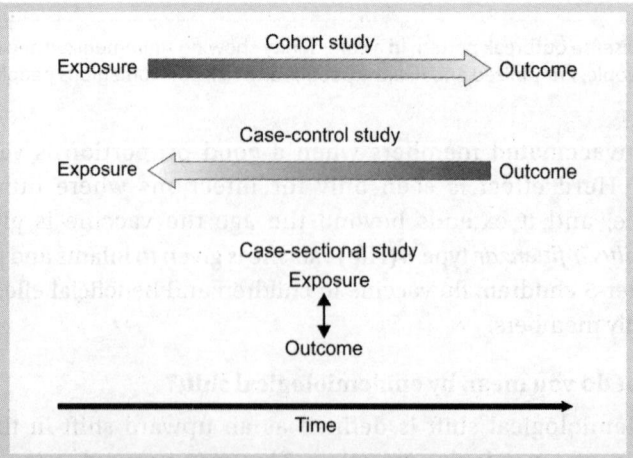

Fig. 3: Schematic diagram showing temporal directions of the 3 study designs.

2. *Analytical study*: Case control and cohort studies are the two types of analytical observational studies.

2a. *Case control study*: Observational study that starts with the researcher/investigator identifying groups (cases and controls) by an outcome/disease of interest (e.g., Rotavirus diarrhea): do participants have (case) or do not have (control) a disease/outcome. Then looking backward to establish the level of exposure (e.g., Rotavirus vaccination). For case-control studies, researchers determine the proportion of cases with the exposure, cases without the exposure, controls with the exposure, and controls without the exposure. Case control studies are generally retrospective.

2b. *Cohort study*: Study that follows subjects over time. Observational study that starts by the researcher/investigator selecting groups by their exposure status, e.g., Rotavirus vaccination (exposed individuals and nonexposed individuals) and then following the groups over time to see if an outcome develops (e.g., disease, rotavirus gastroenteritis). Cohort studies are generally prospective.

2c. *Cross-sectional study*: Study that provides a "snap-shot" of a population. Observational study that measures the outcome/disease and exposure at the same time.

Experimental Studies

There are three main types of experimental studies:

1. *Randomized controlled trials (RCT)*: These use patients as units of study, mostly for assessing a new therapy. Double-blind, randomized, placebo-control trials—The ideal vaccine efficacy study is a clinical trial starting with persons susceptible to disease.
2. *Field trials*: These use healthy individuals as units of study, mostly for assessing preventive agents such as vaccines.
3. *Community trials*: These use communities as units of study for assessing community-based interventions such as health status in villages with a training program versus in those without.

Stepped wedge design studies: These are used when previous studies have indicated that the intervention is likely to be beneficial and the public health needs to introduce the intervention precludes withholding it from a population. The intervention is introduced in phases, group by group, until the entire target population is covered. The groups form the unit of randomization.

Q32. Describe vaccine-preventable disease surveillance.

Ans. Disease surveillance is another public health and epidemiology tool. A functioning disease surveillance system helps in understanding disease epidemiology before vaccines are introduced. Thereafter, it guides how well the vaccination program is doing in reducing the burden of disease (BoD). It helps in decision-making on the introduction of vaccines and also in assessing the impact of interventions. Unfortunately, the disease surveillance

system in the majority of the low- and middle-income countries (LMICs) requires a major boost:
- Disease modeling.
- The models are often referred to as "tools for thinking and simplification of systems," suitable for analysis.
- Epidemiology aims to measure the disease burden; however, where measurement is not practical, estimates must be developed. The modern epidemiological methods and disease modeling have reached the level where accurate projection can be made based on existing knowledge and information. The estimates derived from various sources are often used in vaccination programs. The estimates are used for decision-making at local levels (i.e., state and national levels), for deriving estimates for neighboring countries (with similar settings) and for global (or international) levels. The estimates, if done with similar methods can provide useful information for interstate, intercountry, and inter-disease comparisons, to observe the disease trend over a period of time, and for comparison of choices between intervention versus none versus others.
- In vaccination programs, a number of models are used:
  - A static or decision analysis model is used on the assumption of a constant force of infection (or fixed risk). These models are more commonly used for noninfectious diseases. The static models are usually applied to a single cohort
  - Markov models
  - Dynamic model used for infectious diseases. Suspected, infected, and recovered (SIR) approach is an example of a dynamic model. These models are applied to multiple cohorts.

Q33. What are the modes of disease transmission?

Ans. Modes of transmission of disease may be of two major types:
1. *Direct transmission*: Direct contact, droplet infection, through soil, inoculation into skin or mucosa and transplacental transmission.
2. *Indirect transmission*: Vehicle borne, airborne, vector borne, fomite borne.

Q34. Define control of diseases?

Ans. The reduction of disease incidence, prevalence, morbidity or mortality to a locally acceptable level. Continued intervention measures, e.g., diarrheal diseases are necessary to maintain control.

Q35. Define elimination of disease and elimination of infection?

Ans.
Elimination of disease: Reduction to zero of the incidence of a specified disease in a defined geographical area. Continued intervention measures are to be continued. e.g., neonatal tetanus.

Elimination of infections: Zero incidence of infection as a result of deliberate efforts. Continued measures to prevent re-establishment of transmission are required. *Example:* measles, poliomyelitis.

Q36. Define eradication and extinction of disease/infectious agent?

Ans. Eradication: Permanent reduction to zero of the worldwide incidences of infection caused by a specific agent as a result of deliberate efforts. Intervention measures are no longer needed. *Example:* smallpox.

Extinction: The specific infectious agent no longer exists in nature or in the laboratory.

Q37. Define epidemiological shift?

Ans. Natural epidemiologic shift (in age):
- Improving economic, environmental conditions
- *Example:* Hepatitis A virus (HAV) infection—large outbreaks in China, Mauritius.

Vaccination associated shift:
- An upward shift in age of infection/disease in communities with partial immunization coverage
- *Significance:* Important for diseases such as rubella, varicella and hepatitis A wherein severity of disease worsens with advancing age.

Q38. Define clinical trial?

Ans. An experimental study carried out on humans to assess the safety and efficacy of a regimen is termed as "clinical trial". Whenever a new vaccine or a drug is introduced, it undergoes a series of trials before it is established for the purpose it is meant for.

Q39. What are the phases of clinical trials?

Ans.
- *Phase I trial:* It is the first testing of a new vaccine or a drug in a small group of healthy human volunteers (generally <100) to determine its safety and pharmacological profile.
- *Phase II trial:* It is the trial to evaluate the efficacy, immunogenicity and safety in 200–500 volunteers.
- *Phase III trial:* In this phase, extensive analysis is done to evaluate the safety and efficacy using a large number of subjects with the disease or the condition of interest (in thousands) with random allocation to study and control groups, e.g., a randomized control trial (RCT). It is the final testing done before a vaccine/drug is approved for marketing.
- *Phase IV trial:* It is the post-approval study which is done after the regulatory authority has approved registration and the marketing has

been started. Its purpose is to estimate the incidence of any rare adverse effects. It is a part of post marketing surveillance.

Q40. Describe vaccine failure.

Ans. When a person who has been fully vaccinated develops the disease against which she/he has been vaccinated, it is referred to as vaccine failure. This could be of two types:
1. *Primary vaccine failure*: It occurs when the recipient does not produce enough antibodies when first vaccinated. Infection can therefore occur at any time post vaccination. For example, this occurs in about 10% of those who receive the measles, mumps, and rubella (MMR) vaccine.
2. *Secondary vaccine failure*: It occurs when adequate protective levels of antibodies are produced immediately after the vaccination, but the levels fall over time. The incidence of secondary vaccine failure therefore increases with time after the initial vaccination and hence booster doses are required. This is a characteristic of a number of the inactivated vaccines.

Q41. How is economic evaluation of vaccines done?

Ans. Economic evaluation in health care addresses the question whether an intervention or procedure is worth doing when compared with other possible uses of the same resources for other intervention measures. This is based on the premise that resources are finite and there are opportunity costs. In such analysis, both costs (resources used) and outcomes (benefits) are considered. There are number of analyses including cost-effective analysis, cost-benefit analysis, cost analysis, and cost utility analysis.

■ SUGGESTED READING

1. Black RE, Cousens S, Johnson HL, Lawn JE, Rudan I, Bassani DG, et al. Child Health Epidemiology Reference Group of WHO and UNICEF. Global, regional, and national causes of child mortality in 2008: a systematic analysis. Lancet. 2010;375:1969-87.
2. Lahariya C. A brief history of vaccines and vaccination in India. Indian J Med Res. 2014;139:491-511.
3. Weinberg GA, Szilagyi PG. Vaccine epidemiology: efficacy, effectiveness, and the Translational Research Roadmap. J Infect Dis. 2010;201(11):1607-10.

CHAPTER 3

Vaccination Schedules

Suhas V Prabhu

Q1. What is meant by vaccination schedule?

Ans. This is a timetable of vaccinations against various pathogens as recommended by various recommendation agencies, that every normal child should receive to prevent infectious diseases. The list will generally include the following: the name of the vaccine/disease for which the vaccine is given, the dose and route of administration, the recommended age (or age group). If multiple doses are required, the number and interval between doses and the age (or age ranges) for booster doses are specified. Some comments about the type and usage of the vaccine may also be added. If there are various different types of vaccines available for a particular infectious disease, the preferred choice of vaccine (e.g., OPV vs. IPV or conjugated vaccine vs. nonconjugated vaccine) is stated. If more than one brand of vaccines is available, the schedule may also indicate the preferred brand based on formulation, availability of local seroconversion or efficacy data, reactogenicity, or other considerations.

Q2. What are the determinants of an optimum immunization schedule?

Ans. The determinants include:
- *Immunological*: The earliest age at which an acceptable immune response is elicited by a vaccine.
- *Epidemiological*: The earliest age at which the disease and its complications exert a significant health burden.
- *Programmatic*: The schedule should be able to be piggy-backed on to the existing schedule without creating need for additional contacts.
- *Safety*: The vaccine should be safe in the age at which it is administered.
  Thus, any schedule is a fine balance between epidemiological needs and immunological determinants.

Q3. Why does the schedule recommend only a single dose for some vaccines while others need to be given in multiple doses?

Ans. The number of doses required depends on the type of vaccine used. Many live vaccines such as BCG or hepatitis A confer lifelong immunity even after a single dose. However not all live vaccines give lifelong immunity after a single dose, e.g., OPV or Varicella vaccine. These require more than one dose. Most killed vaccines and toxoids require multiple doses for effective long-term protection. Sometimes, the vaccine needs to be repeated at intervals to adjust for and afford protection against organisms with antigenic drift (e.g., influenza). The number of doses required for protection may also vary with the age at which the administration is started. In case of PCV, the primary series is 3 doses if started before 6 months of age, 2 doses if started between 6 and 12 months of age and only one dose if started after 1st birthday.

Q4. When we look at the schedules, for some vaccines, it lists primary series and boosters. What is the difference between the two?

Ans. Primary series of vaccination is the one at the end of which a large majority (usually over 90%) of the recipients have developed protective immunity to that particular disease. This may occur after a single dose or after 2 or even 3 doses. The number of doses required to achieve this constitutes the primary series. However, this immunity which has developed as a result of the primary series may wane over a period of time. Then, in such cases, (usually 1 year or more after the primary series is completed) the vaccine has to be readministered to boost the protective antibody titers or immunological memory. These are referred to as boosters. Some vaccines may require more than one booster at designated intervals.

Q5. Who decides the schedule?

Ans. The schedule is generally decided by the health ministry of the government of the country and is applicable to the immunization program undertaken by the public health department for all children in the country. In India, this is referred to as the National Immunization Program (NIP). Vaccines listed in this schedule are given free of cost to all children.

A schedule may also be announced by the academic body of pediatricians of a country (or by a committee constituted specifically for this purpose). This acts as a directive to pediatricians and other clinicians in the private medical sector to administer vaccines to children receiving vaccines in the private sector in a particular sequence. This list would normally include all the vaccines that are advised in the public health schedule and additional vaccinations that the body feels are of benefit to protect individual children, beyond those recommended by the public health department. It is important that these two schedules should not be in direct conflict. In India, the Indian Academy of Pediatrics (IAP) committee, Advisory Committee on Vaccines and Immunization Practices (ACVIP) recommends a schedule that is revised every 2 years or so. This is referred to as the IAP schedule.

Q6. How often are the schedules revised?

Ans. The IAP's committee, the ACVIP usually issues a revision of the schedule every 2 years. The revision is based on several factors such as availability of newer vaccines, new data about existing vaccines, outbreaks or increased prevalence of infections, etc.

The NIP is revised at irregular intervals as decided by the health ministry. Like the IAP, they will decide revisions based on availability and disease prevalence but also financial considerations and advisories from international health organizations such as World Health Organization (WHO).

Very occasionally a vaccine may be totally dropped from an earlier schedule because a particular disease is no longer a threat or has been eradicated. Examples of this are the Smallpox vaccine and the Type 2 oral polio vaccine.

It is important to follow only the latest schedule issued.

Q7. Which schedule should the pediatrician follow, the NIP or the IAP schedule?

Ans. As stated earlier, the NIP and IAP schedules are not in conflict with each other. The IAP schedule only contains additional vaccines for individual protection of children who can afford it. For example, the NIP does not include the chickenpox vaccine as the Indian Health Ministry does not think that the cost-benefit ratio for this disease warrants the high expenditure for administering this vaccine, as the morbidity and mortality from chickenpox is low. However, there are undesirable social consequences and occasional serious morbidity due to complications from chickenpox that make chickenpox vaccinations desirable for those who can afford it. In the past, the term "optional vaccines" was used for these vaccines. But this is not a desirable term. All vaccines provide protection against diseases and are generally very safe with minimal undesirable adverse reactions and therefore should be offered to all who can afford them.

Q8. Are the schedules applicable to a country as a whole and are they the same in each country?

Ans. The schedules will vary from country to country. In some cases, in large countries, the schedule may change from region to region, e.g., in India, Japanese encephalitis (JE) vaccines are recommended only in certain states and not for the whole country depending on regional endemicity of JE. In some countries, the schedule may also vary by the ethnicity of the population, e.g., in New Zealand, at one time, the schedule was different for the native Maori population from that for the white population. Sometimes, the schedule will vary from one part of a country to another because a vaccine is being introduced in a phased manner. This is true for the Rotavirus and Conjugated Pneumococcal vaccines in the NIP for India.

Q9. Why are the schedules different in different countries? Why is this so?

Ans. The reasons for this are many. The major determinant of a schedule is the prevalence of the disease in that particular region. So if a disease (such as tuberculosis) is uncommon in the US, the vaccination for that (BCG) will not form a part of the recommended schedule. Similarly Yellow fever vaccine is routinely administered in many countries in Africa but not elsewhere. Variation in age prevalence of a disease will also lead to a different timing of the vaccination in the schedules in different countries. Primary DPT immunization is started (and completed) earlier in tropical countries such as India and later in the developed Western nations precisely because of such epidemiological considerations.

Another reason for trimming a schedule is nonavailability of a vaccine for a particular infection in adequate quantity. IPV is desirable in India but a full course of three or four doses is not listed in the schedule by the Indian government because of shortage of the vaccine. Instead two fractional doses of the vaccine are administered intradermally.

One more consideration is cost, which is an important factor in resource limited countries. While the Indian Health Ministry agrees that administration of PCV and Rotavirus vaccines to all children is desirable, it has been introduced only in some parts of the country with a plan to include the rest of the country in a phased manner in view of limited financial resources.

When a country's health authority decides to introduce a vaccine in the national immunization schedule, the primary aim is to benefit a large majority of the children of the country by preventing infections that result in morbidity and mortality. But it also has to weigh this benefit against the total cost of administration of the vaccine (not just the actual purchase cost of the vaccine but also the delivery program costs). The medical and social costs of possible adverse effects of a vaccine to the recipient (such as convulsions or death after DTwP vaccination) or to the community (VAPP from oral polio) also need to be factored in. This exercise of cost-benefit analysis is the essential foundation of the decision to add a new vaccine in the schedule. The underlying principle is "the greatest good of the greatest number".

Q10. Can vaccine schedules change with changes in disease epidemiology?

Ans. Yes. Alteration in schedules may be necessary with changes in disease epidemiology or new data regarding immunogenicity/efficacy.

In countries with low measles transmission rates, where the exposure to measles in infancy is low, the measles containing vaccine may be administered at 12 months, instead of 9 months, to obtain better seroconversion rates.

Other examples are the changes in the polio immunization schedule with eradication of polio, hepatitis A vaccine at 1 year instead of 18 months due to lower seroprevalence rates in pregnant women, 2 dose schedule of HPV vaccine in those <15 years of age.

Q11. If a foreigner comes to India, which schedule should his child follow?

Ans. Each countries schedule is based on local epidemiology. The purpose of immunization is to protect children from locally prevailing diseases. Hence, in such a situation, it is better to use the Indian schedule. In some cases, it is prudent to administer the vaccine to the child even before entering India (e.g., Typhoid and Hepatitis A vaccine) if these are not part of the home country's schedule. However, if the child is planning to return to the homeland, certain mandatory vaccines of the home country may have to be additionally given. This is so that the child does not face any problem such as quarantine or school admission on return to the home country.

Q12. Is the schedule sacrosanct or can it be modified in individual cases? If so, under what circumstances?

Ans. The recommended schedule is applicable to all children with certain exceptions which are usually indicated in the schedule. This would include conditions such as prematurity, low birth weight and immunocompromised states such as HIV, immunosuppressive therapy, etc. In such cases, the vaccines may have to be deferred or avoided altogether in view of the recipient's immune status. The schedule recommended for each such situation may different.

Another situation is a case where a child has missed taking the doses at the appropriate age specified in the schedule. In such cases a "catch-up" schedule is advised which may include some or all of the vaccines that he child has missed and the number of doses recommended will also be different (usually reduced).

Q13. What is the latest schedule recommended by the IAP ACVIP?

Ans. The latest schedule recommended by the IAP ACVIP is given in **Table 1**.

Table 1: IAP recommended vaccine schedule for routine use (2020–21).

Age	Vaccine	Comments
Birth	BCG OPV Hepatitis B-1 (BD)	• *BCG*: Before discharge • *OPV*: As soon as possible after birth • Hep B should be administered within 24 hours of birth
6 weeks	DTwP/DTaP-1 IPV-1 Hib-1 Hep B-2 Rotavirus-1 PCV-1	• DTwP or DTaP may be administered in primary immunization • *IPV*: 6–10–14 weeks is the recommended schedule; if IPV, as part of a hexavalent combination vaccine, is unaffordable, the infant should be sent to a government facility for primary immunization as per UIP schedule.
10 weeks	DTwP/DTaP-2 IPV-2 Hib-2 Hep B-3 Rotavirus-2 PCV-2	*RV1*: 2-dose schedule; all other rotavirus brands: 3-dose schedule

SECTION 1: Basic Vaccinology and General Considerations

Age	Vaccine	Comments
14 weeks	DTwP/DTaP-3 IPV-3 Hib-3 Hep B-4 Rotavirus-3 PCV-3	An additional 4th dose of Hep B vaccine is safe and is permitted as a component of a combination vaccine
6 months	Influenza (IIV)-1	Uniform dose of 0.5 mL for DCGI approved brands
7 months	Influenza (IIV)-2	To be repeated every year, in pre-monsoon period, till 5 years of age
6–9 months	Typhoid conjugate vaccine	As of available data, there is no recommendation for a booster dose
9 months	MMR -1	
12 months	Hepatitis A	Single dose for live attenuated vaccine
15 months	MMR-2 Varicella -1 PCV booster	
16–18 months	DTwP/DTaP- B1 Hib-B1 IPV-B1	
18–19 months	Hep A-2 Varicella-2	Only for inactivated Hep A vaccine
4–6 years	DTwP/DTaP-B2 IPV-B2 MMR-3	
10–12 years	Tdap HPV	• Tdap is to be administered even if it has been administered earlier (as DTP-B2) • *HPV*: 2 doses at 6 months interval between 9–14 years • *3 doses*: From 15 years or immunocompromised of any age (0–1–6 months for HPV2, 0–2–6 months for HPV4)

(BCG: Bacillus Calmette–Guérin; OPV: oral poliovirus vaccine; Hep B: hepatitis B; DTwP: diphtheria, tetanus and whole-cell pertussis; DTaP: diphtheria, tetanus and acellular pertussis; DTP: diphtheria, tetanus toxoids and pertussis; IPV: inactivated polio vaccine; PCV: pneumococcal conjugate vaccine; RV: rotavirus vaccine; IIV: inactivated influenza vaccine; MMR: measles, mumps, and rubella; Tdap: diphtheria toxoid and acellular pertussis; Td: tetanus and diphtheria; HPV: human papillomavirus)

■ SUGGESTED READING

1. History of Vaccine Development. Plotkin SA (Ed). Springer 2011.
2. IAP Guidebook on Immunization 2018-19. Indian Academy of Pediatrics. Jaypee Brothers Medical Publishers.
3. Immunization Handbook for Medical Officers. Department of Health and Family Welfare, Government of India 2008
4. Red Book. Center for Diseases Control 31st Ed. 2018-21.

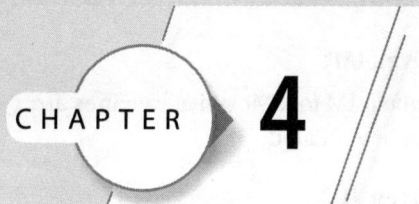

General Immunization Practices

Sanjay Srirampur

■ COMMUNICATION WITH PARENTS/CARE GIVERS

Q1. What are the issues you discuss with parents before vaccination?

Ans. Uniform issues to be discussed are:
- The disease which the vaccine prevents
- Efficacy of the vaccine
- Safety/expected reactions after vaccination
- Schedule of the vaccine
- Cost of the vaccine
- Address any concerns.

■ VACCINATION: THE PROCEDURE

Q2. Is a written consent necessary before vaccination?

Ans. Consent is implied in vaccination. In private practice when a patient is brought by the parent for vaccination written consent is not necessary. The legal issues come up only if the practitioner goes against standard of care or is negligent.

Q3. How do you observe asepsis during vaccination?

Ans.
- Wash hands with soap and water using the 6-step procedure, before starting the session and/or if hands are visible dirty
- Alcohol based hand rubs can be used between patients
- Gloves only if there is a risk of contact of infectious fluids between vaccinee or vaccinator or vaccinator has any infected lesions on the hands.

■ VACCINE ADMINISTRATION

Q4. What are the various routes of administration?

Ans.
- Intramuscular (IM)
- Subcutaneous (SC)
- Intradermal (ID)
- Oral
- Intranasal.

Q5. What happens if SC vaccines are given IM?

Ans. Generally, vaccines given SC can be given IM too. Most live vaccines are given SC. The doses are valid and need not be repeated.

Q6. What happens if IM vaccines are given SC?

Ans. Vaccines containing adjuvants can be reactogenic if given SC, hence, adjuvanted vaccines are given IM. For inactivated vaccines the site of administration is crucial. Moreover, the immunogenicity may be suboptimal for some inactivated vaccines. Inadvertent administration by SC route of inactivated Hepatitis A vaccine, meningococcal conjugate vaccine, IPV and PPSV23 is acceptable and the dose need not be repeated.

Q7. What is the recommended site for vaccination?

Ans. Gluteal should not be used for two reasons: Sciatic nerve injury and reduced efficacy because of administration in thick intermuscular fat planes:
- *Children less than 3 years*: Anterolateral part of the thigh
- *Children more than 3 years*: Anterolateral thigh or deltoid for IM. IM injections are to be given at 90° to the skin. Subcutaneous injections should be given 45° to the skin.

Q8. How long is it mandatory to observe children after vaccination?

Ans. Children should be observed for 15 minutes after vaccinations for occurrence of serious adverse reactions.

Q9. Is it required to withdraw the piston after injection to check whether any blood vessel is injured?

Ans. If given at the proper site there is no need to withdraw the piston. If blood appears, withdraw needle and use fresh vaccine for administration.

Q10. Is it necessary to rub the injection site after vaccination?

Ans. The site of vaccination should not be rubbed. Firm pressure should be given at the site of vaccination till the bleeding stops.

Q11. What should be the standard length and gauge of the needle for IM injections?

Ans. The gauge should be 22/25, the length should be 5/8 inch. For intradermal injections the length should be 0.5 inch. Some experts believe that the length of the needle for IM injections should be 5/8 inch if the skin is stretched but if the skin and the subcutaneous tissue are bunched up then the length of the needle should be 1 inch.

Q12. How to administer multiple vaccines?

Ans. When multiple vaccines are administered, the thigh is the ideal place in view of the large surface area and greater muscle mass. When different vaccines are administered, use different limbs. If the same limb is used to administer different vaccines 1-inch distance or more is to be maintained between two injections.

Q13. What should be done if a part of the vaccine dose spills out?

Ans. If the vaccine is given below the standard dose the dose should be repeated. Can be given same day if inactivated vaccine or after 4 weeks if live vaccine.

Q14. Can all vaccines be administered simultaneously? What are the exceptions?

Ans. Yes. All vaccines can be administered at the same visit as all other vaccines. This will increase the compliance. The only exceptions are:
- Menactra™ and PCV13. Simultaneously administering of both vaccines for those children with asplenia or hyposplenia reduces the immunogenicity of PCV13. The serotypes with reduced immunity are (4,6B and 18C). PCV13 is to be given first followed by 4 weeks later with Menactra™. This does not apply to Menveo™
- PCV13 and PPSV23 should not be administered simultaneously. PCV13 is to be administered first followed by PPSV23 after an interval of 8 weeks in the immunocompromised and 6–12 months in the immunocompetent.

Q15. What should be the minimum interval between 2 doses of live parenteral vaccines?

Ans. Live vaccines are administered simultaneously or if they are separated then the minimum duration between two live vaccines should be 4 weeks. If 2 live, parenteral vaccines are administered at an interval of less than 4 weeks, the vaccine given second should be considered as an invalid dose and should be repeated 4 weeks after the invalid dose. This rule does not apply to orally-administered live attenuated vaccines. It applies to intranasally-administered live attenuated vaccines.

Q16. What should be the minimum interval between 2 doses of different inactivated vaccines?

Ans. Two doses of different inactivated vaccines can be given at any interval (see Q14 for exception).

Q17. What should be the minimum interval between 2 doses of the same inactivated vaccine?

Ans. The minimum interval between two doses of the same inactivated vaccine is 4 weeks. Vaccines administered up to 4 days before 4 weeks are valid, but if 5 or more days earlier, should be considered invalid and repeated. This 4-day margin is called the "grace period". The repeated dose should be after the minimum interval of 4 weeks.

Q18. What should be the minimum interval between an inactivated vaccine and a live vaccine?

Ans. An inactivated and a live parenteral vaccine can be administered on the same day or at any interval between them.

Q19. Some combination vaccines result in an extra dose of an antigen. Is this justified?

Ans. It is justified when: (1) when the extra antigen is not contraindicated; (2) products that contain only the antigen are not available; (3) benefits outweigh the risks. An extra dose of many live virus vaccines, hepatitis B and Hib vaccines has not been found to be harmful.

Q20. Are diluents interchangeable?

Ans. No. Diluents vary widely in composition, and therefore only the diluent assigned by the manufacturer for the specific vaccine and presentation should be used. Unless otherwise specified by the manufacturer, the correct temperature for long-term storage of diluents is +2°C to +8°C.

Q21. If a child is brought for the 2nd dose of hepatitis A vaccine after 1 year, should the series be restarted?

Ans. No. The vaccine series should be continued. Increasing the interval between doses of a multidose vaccine does not diminish the effectiveness of the vaccine.

Q22. Are vaccine brands interchangeable?

Ans. Certain vaccines that provide protection from the same diseases are available from different manufacturers, and these vaccines usually are not identical in antigen content or method of formulation. Manufacturers use different production processes, and their products might contain different concentrations of antigen per dose or a different stabilizer or preservative.

All brands of Hib conjugate, hepatitis B, inactivated hepatitis A, are interchangeable within their respective series.

As far as possible, HPV, Rotavirus, DTaP, PCV brands should not be interchanged.

For vaccines in general, vaccination should not be deferred because the brand used for previous doses is not available or is unknown.

Q23. Is it necessary to wait for the vaccine to reach room temperature before administering it to a patient?

Ans. There is no recommendation to wait until a vaccine reaches room temperature before administration. The vaccine should be administered as soon as it is prepared.

Q24. What is the meaning of "simultaneous administration" of vaccines?

Ans. Simultaneous means the same day—the same clinic day. If someone receives a vaccine in the morning and then another that same afternoon, it would be considered simultaneous administration.

Q25. When a manufacturer states "to be used immediately after reconstitution", what is "immediately" here?

Ans. The definition of "immediately" varies from manufacturer to manufacturer. CDC considers "immediately" to be the reasonable time it takes to prepare and transport the vaccine to the patient to be administered. Consensus states the "immediately" can be up to 30 minutes.

Q26. Some prefilled vaccines come with an air pocket in the syringe chamber. Do we need to expel the air pocket before vaccinating?

Ans. No. there is no need to expel the air pocket. The small amount of air (0.2-0.3 cc) would not cause a problem. The air will be absorbed. When the syringe is inverted during an injection, the air bubble moves to the top and ensures clearance of the entire content of the medication from the needle.

Q27. Is it recommended to change needles after a vaccine dose has been drawn into a syringe from a vial?

Ans. No. It is not necessary to change the needle when a lyophilized vaccine is reconstituted the needle has passed through two stoppers. Changing needles is a waste of resources and increases the risk of needle stick injury.

Q28. Which vaccines are contraindicated in egg allergic individuals?

Ans. Only yellow fever vaccine is contraindicated in egg-allergic children.

Q29. What rules are to be followed when vaccine and its antibody are administered?

Ans. If a vaccine is given first then the antibody preparation should be administered after an interval of 2 weeks.

If antibody is administered first then the interval for administration of vaccine is 3 months or longer for administering a live attenuated vaccine. See table below:

Indication	Dose	Interval (months)
Blood transfusion		
Washed RBCs	10 mL/kg	0
Packed RBCs	10 mL/kg	6
Whole blood	10 mL/kg	6
Plasma or platelet products	10 mL/kg	7
Hepatitis A prophylaxis (as IGIM)	0.1 mL/kg	3

Indication	Dose	Interval (months)
Hepatitis B prophylaxis (as HBIG)	0.06 mL/kg	3
Measles prophylaxis (as IGIM)	0.5 mL/kg	6
Rabies prophylaxis (as RIG)	20 IU/kg	4
Rabies prophylaxis (as Mabs)		0
RSV prophylaxis (palivizumab monoclonal antibody		0
Tetanus prophylaxis (as TIG)	250 IU	3
IVIG	400 mg/kg	8
IVIG	800–1000 mg/kg	10
IVIG	1600–2000 mg/kg	11
Replacement (or therapy) of immune deficiencies (as IVIG)	300–400 mg/kg	8

Situations when both vaccine and antibody are administered together are: Rabies vaccine and antibody, hepatitis B vaccine and antibody and tetanus vaccine and antibody.

■ PAIN RELIEF

Q30. Why is pain relief important for vaccination?

Ans. This is necessary to reduce anxiety and improve compliance. If not addressed, this pain can lead to preprocedural anxiety in the future, needle fears and health care avoidance behaviors, including nonadherence with vaccination schedules.

It is estimated that up to 25% of adults have a fear of needles, with most fears developing in childhood.

About 10% of the population avoids vaccination and other needle procedures because of needle fears.

Q31. How should we relieve pain with immunizations?

Ans. 24% sugar solution, distraction, pretreatment with 5% topical lidocaine plus prilocaine, fast injection technique, administering the less painful vaccine first, cooling at the injection site are some of the techniques used to reduce the pain of vaccination.

Q32. Should antipyretics be routinely administered with vaccinations?

Ans. Evidence does not support the use of routine antipyretics following vaccination. They may interfere with the immunogenicity of some vaccines. Even in children with febrile seizures routine prophylactic use of antipyretics does not prevent the occurrence of febrile seizures. They may be used if there is discomfort or fever following vaccination.

CONTRAINDICATION/PRECAUTION

Q33. What are contraindications to vaccination?

Ans. A condition in a recipient which greatly increases chances of serious adverse effects after vaccination is defined as a contraindication. There are only a few contraindications.

Permanent
- Serious allergic reactions after the administration of a vaccine
- Encephalopathy after the administration of pertussis vaccine
- Severe combined immunodeficiency (SCID) for a child who receives Rota vaccine and other live vaccines.

Temporary
- Pregnancy
- Immunosuppression.

Q34. What is a precaution?

Ans. Precaution is a condition in the recipient which might increase the chances of a serious adverse reaction or it might compromise the ability of a vaccine to produce immunity.

Some precautions may be permanent:
- High fever more than 105°F
- Persistent crying for more than 3 hours after vaccination
- Seizures within 3 days of vaccination
- Hypotonic-hyporesponsive episodes (HHE) after administration of DPT.

Some precautions may be temporary:
- Severe acute illness
- Receipt of antibody containing product.

SUGGESTED READING

1. Balasubramanian S. IAP Guidebook on Immunization 2018-2019 (Advisory Committee on Vaccines and Immunization Practice). New Delhi: Jaypee Brothers Medical Publishers (P) Ltd.; 2020. pp. 56-66.
2. CDC. General Best Practice Guidelines for Immunization Best Practice Guidance of the Advisory Committee on Immunization Practices (ACIP). [online] Available from: www.cdc.gov/vaccines/hcp/acip-recs/generalrecs/downloads/general-recs.pdf. [Last Accessed November, 2020].
3. Plotkin S, Orenstein W, Offit P, Edwards KM. General Immunization Practices. In: Plotkin's Vaccines, 7th edition. Gurugram: Elsevier India Limited; 2017. pp. 96-120.
4. WHO (2010). Best Practices for Injections and related procedures toolkit. [online] Available from: https://www.who.int/infection-prevention/publications/best-practices_toolkit/en/. [Last Accessed November, 2020].
5. WHO. Policy Statement: Multidose Vial Policy (MDVP). [online] Available from: https://apps.who.int/iris/handle/10665/135972. [Last Accessed November, 2020].

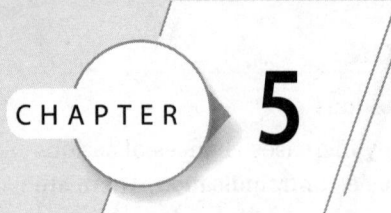

Documentation of Vaccination

Chetan Trivedi

Q1. Why is "documentation of vaccination" an important issue?

Ans. Immunization records are necessary:
- To know whether the child has received the appropriate vaccines in the past
- To know whether the child is receiving the appropriate vaccines at present
- To advise regarding future vaccinations
- To have details regarding vaccine and vaccinee in the event of adverse events following immunization (AEFI)
- Documentation for insurance purposes
- Documentation for purposes of establishing coverage rates in the community, state or country
- Immunization records may be required for children to attend school or child care centers. They may be required for admission into foreign universities. Adults may be required to provide immunization records to be eligible to work in certain professions, such as health care, teaching or occupations requiring international travel.

Q2. What are the parameters to be documented during the vaccination procedure?

Ans. These parameters are in four major categories:
1. Documentation of vaccine recipient.
2. Documentation of vaccine.
3. Documentation of vaccination.
4. Documentation of AEFI.

Documentation of Vaccine Recipient
- *Name*: Full correct name which is must for further data, record and certification
- *Age/DOB*: Correct date of birth is must as the whole vaccination schedule will be planned according to age of the child
- *Weight*: Important for certain vaccination such as hepatitis B
- Birth weight and maturity at birth (newborn)
- Maternal HBsAg status (newborn) for need for immunization dose and schedule of hepatitis B vaccination
- Any existing precaution or contraindication for vaccination.

Documentation of Vaccine
- *Name*: Generic/brand name/components of a combination vaccine
- *Volume*: Important for Influenza
- Lot number, batch number and date of expiry
- Name of manufacturer
- Best option is to stick adhesive labels supplied with vaccines or stuck on vials.

Documentation of Vaccination
- Site of vaccination, e.g. left thigh–LT, right deltoid–RD, immunization site map **(Fig. 1)**
- When more than one vaccination single site such as thigh RUT–right upper thigh and RLT–right lower thigh
- Date and time of vaccination, dose number in a schedule
- Next date of vaccination and plan of vaccination schedule, e.g., 2 +1, 0, 1, 6, etc.
- Name of vaccinator or vaccine provider with signature.

Documentation of AEFI
- This will include the nature of AEFI, past and present, details regarding symptoms/signs, treatment given, hospitalization done and outcome
- Whether reported and outcome of investigations.

Q3. Where should the documentation be done?

Ans. Documentation should be done in two places:

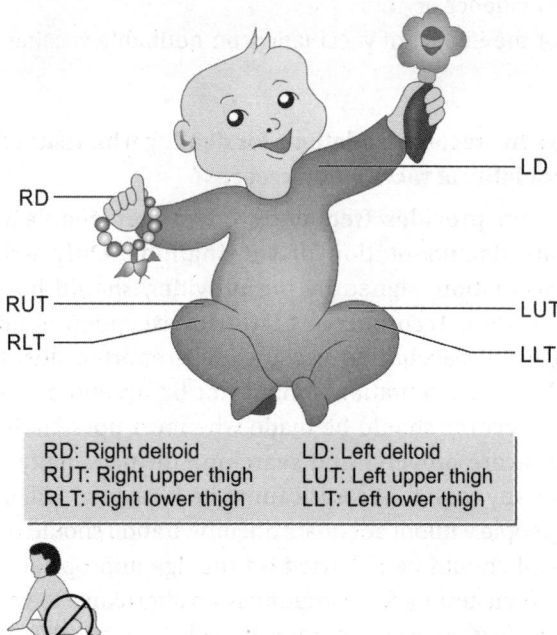

RD: Right deltoid
RUT: Right upper thigh
RLT: Right lower thigh
LD: Left deltoid
LUT: Left upper thigh
LLT: Left lower thigh

Fig. 1: Sites for vaccinations in infants and children.

1. Personal immunization card/chart (in patient file) and prescription which is given to parents.
2. Healthcare provider's records: Which may be on a case/file or an electronic record on the computer (soft copy).

Electronic immunization record keeping that allows online access by vaccine recipients and health care providers should be encouraged.

Documentation should be completed before the patient leaves the clinical setting.

Q4. What are best practice guidelines for documentation of Immunization?

Ans. Document maximum possible details clearly on the vaccination card and keep a record with you too.

Q5. Is documentation of consent or decision not to vaccination needed?

Ans.
- Till date, in India, written consent is not required. A verbal consent is usually adequate
- In the event of a parent's decision not to vaccinate, it should be recorded at all sites where vaccination records are maintained.

Q6. Should you report the vaccine administered in your clinic, to the appropriate health authorities?

Ans. Yes. This is necessary to:
- Reliably estimate vaccination coverage
- Know the incidence of AEFI
- To monitor the impact of vaccination on notifiable vaccine-preventable diseases.

Q7. What are the recommendations for dealing with issues arising from nonavailability of vaccination records?

Ans. Vaccination provides frequently encounter people who do not have adequate documentation of vaccinations. Only written, dated records of vaccination, signed by the provider, should be accepted as proof of vaccination. According to CDC with exception of influenza and pneumococcal polysaccharide vaccine, self-reported doses of vaccine without written documentation should not be accepted. An attempt to locate missing records should be made whenever possible by contacting previous healthcare provider and searching for personally held record. However, if for any reason, records cannot be located or will definitely not be available, people without adequate documentation should be considered susceptible and should be restarted on the age appropriate vaccination schedule. Serologic testing for immunity is an alternative to vaccination for certain antigens (e.g., measles, mumps, Rubella hepatitis B, hepatitis A, and varicella).

In general, receiving extra doses of vaccine poses no medical problem. Receiving excessive doses of tetanus containing vaccines (DTaP, DT, Tdap or Td) can increase the risk of a local adverse reaction.

Q8. Is there any authorized format for recording vaccination details?

Ans. Not in India. But formats exist in other countries, which can be suitably adapted for our situation.

Summary:
- Documentation of vaccination is a must!
- Document all details about vaccinee, vaccine vaccination and AEFI clearly
- Document immunization at office-based card as well as home-based cards
- Documentation helps for smooth, safe and error free vaccination.
  Figure 1 can be utilized for documenting the sites of vaccination.

■ SUGGESTED READING

1. American Academy of Pediatrics. Immunizations. [online] Available from: http://www2.aap.org/immunization/pediatricians/refusaltovaccinate.html. [Last Accessed October, 2020].
2. American Academy of Pediatrics. Immunization Training Guide and Practice Procedure Manual, 3rd edition revised 2017. Illinois: American Academy of Pediatrics; 2017.
3. Centers for Disease Control and Prevention. Appendices. [online] Available from: https://www.cdc.gov/vaccines/pubs/pinkbook/appendix/index.html. [Last Accessed October, 2020].
4. Centers for Disease Control and Prevention. Finding and Updating Vaccine Records. [online] Available from: https://www.cdc.gov/vaccines/parents/records/find-records.html?CDC_AA_refVal=https%3A%2F%2Fwww.cdc.gov%2Fvaccines%2Fparents%2Frecords-requirements.html. [Last Accessed October, 2020].
5. Pemde H. General aspects of vaccination. In: Balasubramanian S (Ed). IAP Guidebook on Immunization 2018-19. Mumbai: IAP: 2020. pp. 48
6. Rajput M, Sharma L. Informed consent in vaccination in India: medicolegal aspects. Hum Vaccin. 2011;7:723-37.

CHAPTER 6: Cold Chain Management

Sanjay Marathe, Srinivas G Kasi

"Cold Chain is the lifeline of any immunization program."

Q1. What is cold chain?

Ans. Cold chain is a system of storing and transporting vaccine at the recommended temperature range from the point of manufacture to point of use **(Fig. 1)**.

Q2. What is the importance of maintaining this cold chain?

Ans. Vaccines are biologicals and are sensitive to heat and light, and some are sensitive to freezing. They need to be stored at an optimum temperature range to maintain potency throughout the shelf life. Therefore, vaccines should be kept at an appropriate temperature range from the time of manufacture to

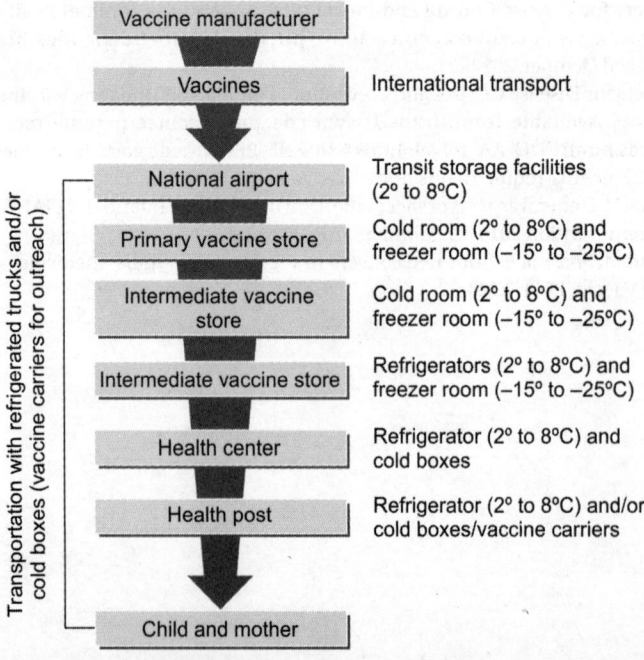

Fig. 1: Representation of cold chain.

the time of use. Improperly stored vaccines may lose potency and result in vaccine failures which may have a negative impact on the immunization program apart from incurring significant financial losses.

It should be remembered that once vaccines lose their potency due to heat or freezing, they can no longer protect individuals from a disease and therefore are useless. Vaccine-potency once lost cannot be restored.

Q3. What are the key elements of the cold chain?

Ans. Personnel: To manage vaccine storage and distribution (vaccine and cold-chain handler at each cold-chain point).

Equipment: To store and transport vaccine and monitor temperature—Walk-in-Coolers (WIC), Walk-in-Freezers (WIF), Deep Freezers (DF), Ice-lined Refrigerators (ILR), Refrigerated trucks, Vaccine vans, Cold boxes, Vaccine carriers and icepacks.

Procedures: To ensure correct utilization of equipment and ensure vaccines are stored and transported safely.

It is not just the fridge or the ILRs, but includes the personnel who manage it and the standard operating procedures followed, which are equally important.

Q4. Which is more harmful for vaccines, heat exposure or freezing?

Ans. Both are equally harmful and common. A single exposure to freezing temperature [0°C (32°F) or colder] can totally inactivate vaccine containing an adjuvant. While heat sensitivity is cumulative, freeze damage is an all or none phenomenon.

Generally, live attenuated, freeze dried vaccines tolerate freezing while inactivated vaccines are rapidly inactivated by freezing.

Q5. Are all vaccines equally heat sensitive of freeze sensitive?

Ans. No. Vaccines have varying degrees of heat stability and sensitivity to freezing. The World Health Organization (WHO) has classified vaccines into groups according to their heat sensitivity in descending order.

Most sensitive:
- *Group A*: OPV, Rotavac
- *Group B*: Influenza, VZV.

Moderately sensitive:
- *Group C*: IPV, JE, M/MR/MMR
- *Group D*: Cholera, DTaP/DTwP combos, Hib, Rotarix, Yellow fever.

Least sensitive:
- *Group E*: HPV, BCG, TT, Td
- *Group F*: Hepatitis B vaccine, HPV, Rabies, Menc-A, PCV, TCV.

Table 1: Sensitivity of vaccines to heat, light and freezing.*

Vaccine	Exposure to heat/light	Exposure to cold
Heat and light sensitive vaccines		
OPV	Sensitive to heat	Not damaged by freezing
Measles/MR	Sensitive to heat and light	Not damaged by freezing
BCG, RVV and JE	Relatively heat stable, but sensitive to light	Not damaged by freezing
Freeze sensitive vaccines		
HepB/Penta/PCV	Relatively heat stable	Freezes at −0.5°C (should not be frozen)
IPV, DPT and TT	Relatively heat stable	Freezes at −3°C (should not be frozen)

At the PHC level, all vaccines are kept in the ILR for a period of 1 month at temperature of +2°C to +8°C

Vaccines sensitive to heat
- BCG (after reconstitution)   ← Most sensitive
- OPV, Ro
- IPV
- MR
- Rotavirus
- JE
- DPT
- BCG (before reconstitution)
- TT
- Penta, HepB, PCV   ← Least sensitive

Vaccines sensitive to freezing
- HepB   ← Most sensitive
- PCV
- Penta
- IPV
- DPT
- TT   ← Least sensitive

*This knowledge has implications in storage of vaccines in the fridge/ILR.

Generally, all vaccines are to be stored between +2°C and +8°C.

Q6. Which are the vaccines which should never be frozen?

Ans.
- DTaP-Hepatitis B-Hib-IPV (hexavalent)
- DTwP or DTwP-Hepatitis B-Hib (pentavalent)
- Hepatitis B (HepB)
- Hib (liquid)
- Human papilloma virus (HPV)
- Inactivated poliovirus (IPV)
- Influenza
- Pneumococcal
- Rotavirus (liquid and freeze-dried)
- Tetanus, DT, Td.

CHAPTER 6: Cold Chain Management

Table 2: Recommended ranges of storage temperature for Vaccines.

Vaccines	National level stores Maximum duration of storage: 6–12 months	State and district level stores Maximum duration of storage: 3 months	Health facility level Maximum duration of storage: 1 month
OPV	−15°C to −25°C OPV is the only vaccine that can be repeatedly frozen and thawed		+2°C to +8°C
BCG, measles, MMR, MR, yellow fever, Hib lyophilized, meningitis, JE	+2°C to +8°C Under exceptional circumstances (shortage of storage space), can be stored at −15°C to −25°C, for short periods		+2°C to +8°C
HepB, DTP-HepB, DTP-HepB-Hib liquid, Cholera, Hib liquid, DTP, DT/TT/Td Pneumococcal, Rotavirus, HPV, Pneumococcal, Rabies, Influenza, IPV	+2°C and +8°C.		

Q7. What are the devices used for storage of vaccines in office practice?

Ans.
- Domestic refrigerator
- Purpose built refrigerator
- Ice-lined refrigerators (ILRs).

While the purpose built refrigerator is the ideal storage devices for vaccines, the most common device used is the domestic refrigerator. ILRs are preferred in areas with unreliable power supply.

Q8. Why is the purpose-built refrigerator the ideal storage devices for vaccines (Fig. 2)?

Ans.
- A stable, controlled temperature between +2°C and +8°C, from the top to the bottom of the cabinet.
- Internal temperature is not much affected by the ambient temperature.
- An evaporator operates at +2°C, preventing the vaccine from freezing.
- Automatic defrost cycle which prevents significant temperature excursions beyond the recommended range.
- Standard alarm and safety features to alert to temperature fluctuations in the cabinet.
- Inbuilt digital temperature monitoring (inbuilt data logger) and/or digital temperature indicators (minimum and maximum temperature displays).

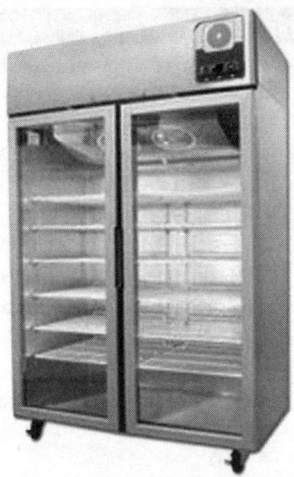

Fig. 2: Purpose-built refrigerator.

- Effective temperature recovery after the refrigerator door has been opened.
- Most of the internal space can be used for vaccine storage.

Q9. What are the types of domestic refrigerators?

Ans.
- Cyclic defrost
- Manual defrost
- Auto defrost.

In both cyclic defrost and manual defrost types, during the defrost process, the temperature excursions may occur beyond the safe zone and hence not recommended for vaccine storage.

They can also be classified as:
- Bar-type fridge
- Single door fridge
- Double door fridge.

In both, bar-type and single door refrigerators, temperature excursions are wider during door opening and closing. Freezing may occur more frequently. Hence, these types are not recommended for vaccine storage.

Direct cool refrigerators are to be avoided as in this type of refrigerator, the air in circulation is cooled inside the fridge compartments by means of the natural convection process. As the process is natural, there is uneven temperature distribution and formation of ice from the water vapor inside the refrigerator.

Hence, the choice should be a frost-free fridge with separate doors for the freezer and main compartments.

Q10. What is the difference between automatic and manual defrost?

Ans. In an automatic defrost refrigerator, heating of the interior refrigerator coils occurs at regular intervals. This prevents frost from building up and allows for effective cooling of the refrigerator or freezer. Temperature excursions are minimal. However, the automatic defrost refrigerator consumes more electricity than the manual defrost refrigerator.

A manual defrost refrigerator does not contain automatic heating elements. As frost builds up on the coils, airflow is restricted and the coils will not cool as efficiently. Defrosting should be done when necessary, but should be done as soon as necessary. Because the defrost process can take a variable time, temperature excursions are far more with a manual defrost than in an automatic defrost refrigerator.

Q11. What are the disadvantages of a domestic fridge for vaccine storage?

Ans.
- Domestic fridge is designed for storage of food and liquids. It does not satisfy the criteria for vaccine storage.
- Significant temperature variations occur every time if the door is opened.
- Since cooling occurs from the freezer at the top, the temperature may be higher in the lower compartments.
- Internal temperature may be significantly affected by ambient temperature.

Q12. What are the prerequisites for a good domestic fridge?

Ans.
- Separate freezer and cabinet compartments: Double door
- Door seals should close snugly
- Free from leakages of water and coolant
- Auto door closure on leaving free
- Auto defrost
- No temperature fluctuations in danger zones
- Quiet operation.

Q13. What are the standards regarding placement of fridge?

Ans.
- It should be placed in a corner away from direct sunlight and away from doors and windows.
- A distance of 10 cm should be maintained all around to permit air circulation.
- It should be placed on a stand at least 5 cm in height.
- Studies find most units work best when placed in an area with standard indoor room temperatures, usually between 20°C and 25°C (68°F and 77°F).

- The electric socket should be switchless or the switch should be taped to avoid accidental switching off.
- Access to the fridge should be restricted to 1–2 persons only.

Q14. What is the order of storage of vaccines in the fridge (Fig. 3)?

Ans.

Top compartment (below chiller tray): The most freeze resistant vaccines should be stored in the top compartment, which is the coldest part of the main compartment. Measles, MR, MMR, BCG, OPV, YF, live-JE, Varicella, Rotavac vaccine, live hepatitis A vaccine, should be stored in this compartment.

Middle compartment: All the pertussis containing combination vaccines, other rotavirus vaccines, inactivated hepatitis A vaccines should be stored here. All the most heat resistant vaccines, which include HepB, HPV, Rabies, PCV, and TCV are to be stored in this compartment. ROTAVAC 5D®, is the liquid formulation which can be stored at 2–8°C.

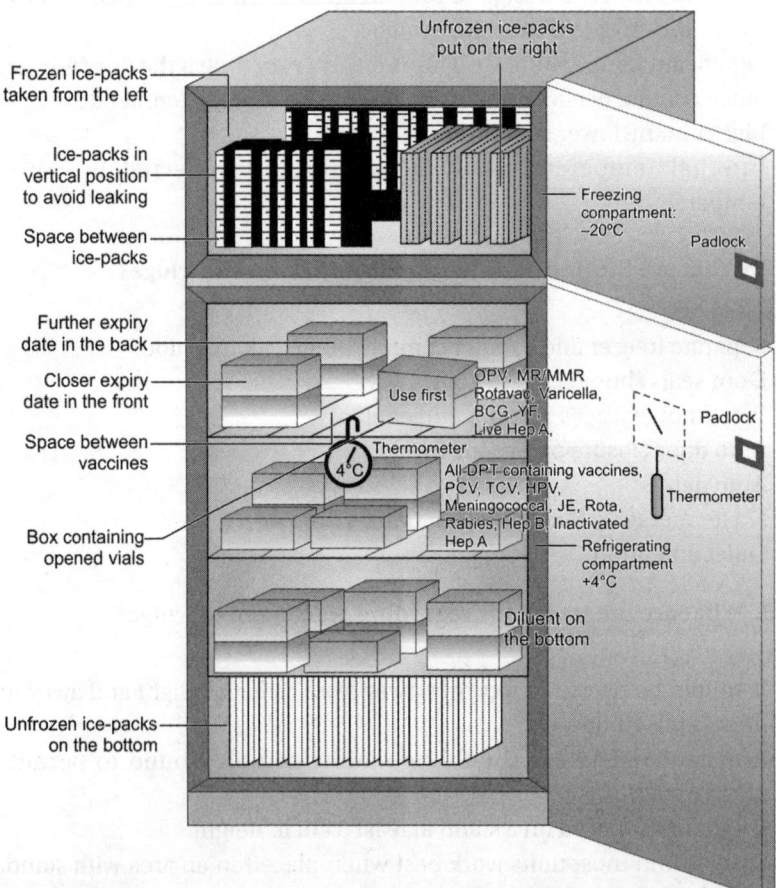

Fig. 3: Front-loading refrigerator with separate freezer compartment.

Lower compartment: Only diluents. Ice packs are to be stored in the freezer compartment. Water bottles can be stored in the lowest tray and door racks to increase the cold mass, which will help to maintain temperature during short periods of power outages. Vaccines should not be stored here.

Q15. What is the standard procedure for storage of diluents?

Ans. Diluents should be stored between +2° and +8°C. However, diluents may be stored outside the cold chain as it may occupy the space of ILR but should be kept in ILR for at least 24 hours before use, to ensure that vaccines and diluents are at +2° to +8°C when being reconstituted. Otherwise, it can lead to thermal shock that is, the death of some or all the essential live organisms in the vaccine.

Q16. What other precautions are to be observed for storage of vaccines in the fridge?

Ans.
- Place individual vaccines in separate trays, label tray mentioning vaccine stored.
- Keep 4 cm distance between trays, trays and front, back and walls of fridge. This is to permit cool air circulation between trays.
- Vaccines with the shortest expiry dates are to be stored in front.
- Fresh stocks should be kept at the back and the older stocks moved to the front. "first in, first out (FIFO)".

Q17. How should you prepare a new fridge or a repaired fridge for vaccine storage?

Ans.
- When the refrigerator is first installed, set the thermostat so that the refrigerator compartment stays between +2°C and +5°C during the coldest part of the day (typically the morning). It is essential to avoid freezing temperatures and the freezing risk is greatest when the ambient room temperature is low.
- Once the daily temperature range remains consistently between +2°C and +8°C, the thermostat is correctly adjusted and the setting should not be changed, even if electrical power is lost.
- The thermostat should not be readjusted if the temperature occasionally rises a degree or so above +8°C after a power cut, or in very hot weather.

The fridge should be used for storing vaccines only and nothing else.

Q18. What measures are to be taken regularly to keep the fridge in top running condition?

Ans.
- Use a vacuum or broom to remove dust buildup from the fridge coils.

- Inspect the door seals to see if there are any areas that are cracked or otherwise damaged. Close the fridge door on a small piece of paper. If you can pull it out easily, the seal is not effective and you should consider replacing it. If the door seal is in good shape, clean it with warm soapy water and then wipe it dry.
- Most fridges rely on a drain hole and drip pan to remove condensation. This area should be kept clean and unobstructed.
- Refrigerators that are not "frost-free" should be defrosted regularly to prevent ice build-up. An ice build-up of more than 0.5 cm is associated with reduced cooling efficiency. During defrosting, the vaccines are to be kept in a prepared cold box.

Q19. What are the advantages of an ILR?

Ans.

- There are coils all around the interior walls of the ILR **(Figs. 4A and B)**, wherein the water freezes and maintains the requisite range of temperature without any electricity supply.
- ILR can maintain a temperature from +2°C to +8°C with as little as 8 hours of power supply in 24 hours.
- An ILR has a top-opening lid which prevents loss of cold air during door opening.
- It has inbuilt thermometers and alarm for temperature excursions beyond the safe range.
- The "holdover time" is at least 24 hours and can extend up to 72 hours.

"Holdover time" is the duration that the ILR can maintain temperature between +2°C and +8°C, in the absence of any power supply.

Hence, this is the ideal storage device especially in areas with unreliable power supply.

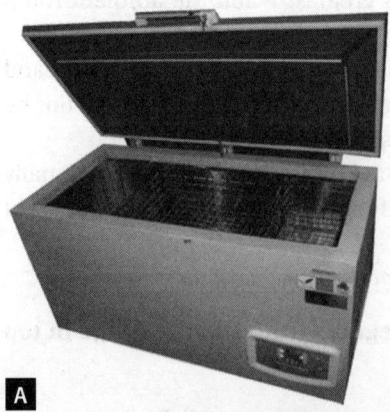
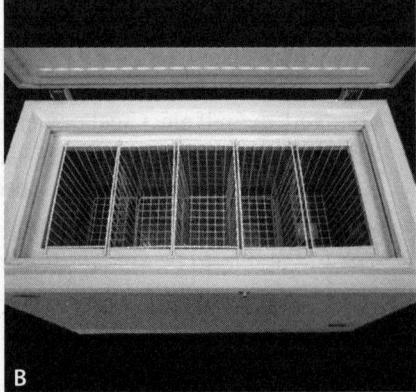

Figs. 4A and B: Ice-lined refrigerators.

Table 3: Specifications of cold chain equipment.

Equipment	Temperature	Storage capacity	Holdover time
Electrical			
Deep freezer (large)	−15°C to −25°C	Ice packs or OPV stock for 3 months (275–300 L)	At 43°C for 2 hours 30 min (minimum)
ILR (large)	+2°C to +8°C	BCG, OPV, IPV, RVV, DPT, TT, Measles/MR, Hep-B, Penta, IPV, Vaccine stock for 3 months (135 to 160 L)	At 43°C for 20 hours (minimum)
Deep freezer (small)	−15°C to −25°C	Ice packs (105 to 125 L)	At 43°C for 2 hours 30 min (minimum)
I LR (small)	+2°C to +8°C	BCG, OPV, IPV, RVV, DPT, TT, Measles/MR, Hep-B vaccine stocks for one month (90-105 L)	At 43°C for 20 hours (minimum)
Nonelectrical			
Cold box (large)	+2°C to +8°C	All vaccines stored for transport or in case of power failure (20–25 L)	At 43°C for 96 hours (minimum)
Cold box (small)	+2°C to +8°C	All vaccines stored for transport or in case of power failure (5–8 L)	At 43°C for 48 hours (minimum)
Vaccine carrier (1.7 liters)	+2°C to +8°C	All vaccines carried for 12 hours (4 conditioned Ice packs and 16–20 vials)	At 43°C for 36 hours (minimum)

Q20. How should vaccine be stored in an ILR?

Ans.
- Vaccines should be stored in baskets to avoid direct contact with the sides and the bottom **(Fig. 4B)**.
- The bottom of the ILR is its coldest part.
- Hence, the most heat sensitive vaccines should be stored at the bottom and the most heat resistant vaccines in the top compartment. This is reverse of the domestic refrigerator.
- *Bottom*: Measles, MR, MMR, BCG, OPV, YF, live-JE, Varicella, 116E-RV.
- *Middle*: All the pertussis containing combination vaccines, other rotavirus vaccines, inactivated hepatitis A vaccines.
- *Top*: HepB, HPV, Rabies, PCV, TCV and the diluents.

It needs to be emphasized that only adequately trained persons should be authorized to handle the cold chain equipment and vaccines.

Q21. What is a vaccine vial monitor (VVM) (*see* **Fig. 5**)?

Ans. This is a time-temperature indicator which contains a heat-sensitive, color changing compound called Diacetylene, which is colorless. On exposure to temperatures, it polymerizes and undergoes serial color changes, depending on the temperature and duration of exposure to that temperature. As the container moves through the supply chain, the VVM records its cumulative heat exposure through a gradual change in color. If the color of the inner square is the same color or darker than the outer circle, the vaccine has been exposed to too much heat and should be discarded.

Q22. Are the VVMs on all vaccines the same?

Ans. No. There are four types of VVMs, to match the heat sensitivity of the vaccine. There are VVM2, VVM7, VVM 14 and VVM30. The VVM number is the time in days that it takes for the inner square to reach the color indicating a discard point, if the vial is exposed to a constant temperature of 37°C. In combination vaccines the VVM corresponds to the most heat sensitive component of the vaccines, e.g., in DPT vaccine the VVM corresponds to the pertussis component of the vaccine.
- VVM2: OPV, Rotavac
- VVM14: All DPT containing vaccines, other rotavirus vaccines, MR/MMR
- VVM30: BCG, HPV, Rabies, monocomponent HB vaccine, PCV.

Q23. How is the VVM interpreted?

Ans.
- *If the inner square is lighter than the outer circle*: Vaccine can be used
- If the inner square is of the same color as the outer circle or darker, the vaccine has reached the discard point and cannot be used (**Fig. 5**).

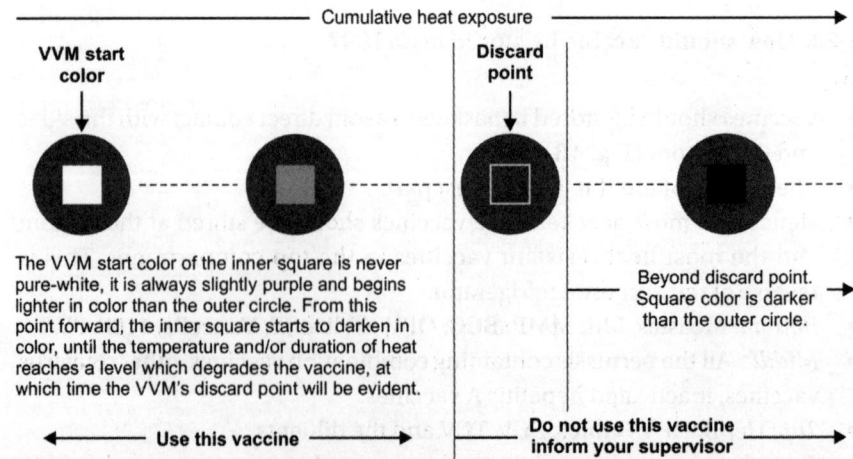

Fig. 5: Interpretation of vaccine vial monitor.

Q24. What is the significance of the position of the VVM on the vaccine vial?

Ans. There are two different locations for VVMs and each is associated with specific guidance for handling opened multidose vials of vaccine:
1. *WHO-prequalified vaccines, where VVM is attached over the label*: The vaccine vial once opened can be used for next 28 days (liquid or freeze-dried).
2. *The VVM is attached anywhere other than label (cap or neck of ampoule)*: The vaccine vial, once opened, must be discarded after immunization session or within 6 hours of opening, whichever comes first.

Q25. What are the other recommended temperature monitoring devices?

Ans.
1. *Integrated digital thermometers (Fig. 6)*: Current prequalified vaccine refrigerators and freezers are equipped with devices such as the one shown in **Figure 6**. An internal temperature sensor monitors the storage compartment and an instantaneous temperature reading is displayed on the unit's control panel. The sensing device of the temperature monitor should be placed in the center of the vaccine storage unit away from the coils, walls, door, floor, and fan. The monitor portion should be easily accessible, preferably mounted on the outside of the vaccine storage unit to minimize the number of times the door of the unit is opened. These are battery operated. They require calibration and change of batteries at 6-month intervals.
2. *Digital maximum-minimum thermometers (Fig. 7)*: The maximum-minimum thermometers provide three readings—the current temperature, the maximum temperature reached since it was last reset and the minimum temperature since it was last reset. Similar to the above, a probe with sensor is placed in the middle of the main compartment, not touching any contents.
3. *Digital data loggers (Fig. 8)*: The data loggers are continuous temperature recording devices, which record the temperature at fixed intervals over a prolonged period of time. These readings can be downloaded onto a

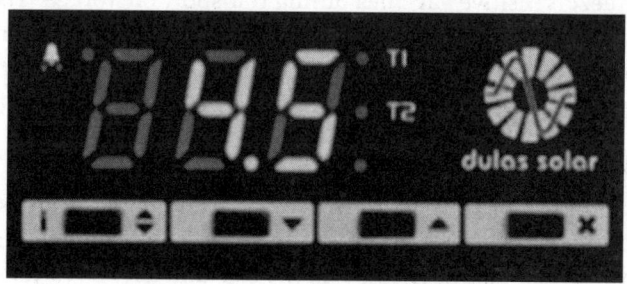

Fig. 6: Integrated digital thermometers.

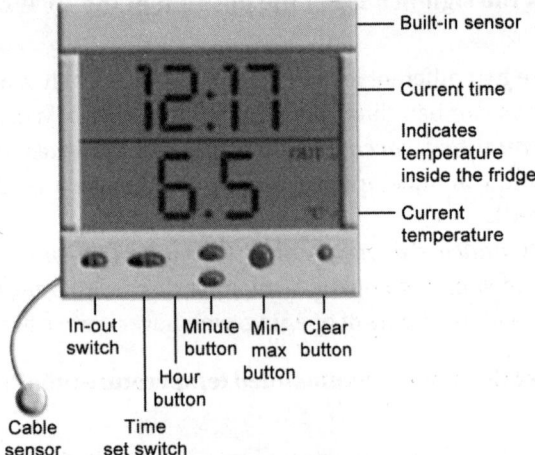

Fig. 7: Digital maximum-minimum thermometers.

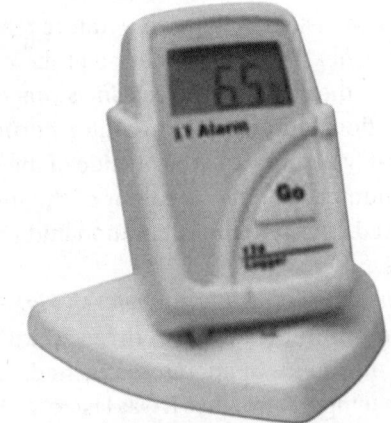

Fig. 8: Digital data loggers.

computer. The data loggers should record temperature increments by 0.1°C. The unit is placed inside the cold storage equipment **(Fig. 8)**.

4. *Electronic freeze indicators*: These are small digital devices that are placed with freeze-sensitive vaccines during transport or storage. The devices have a visual indicator that shows whether the vaccine has been exposed to freezing temperatures. Electronic freeze indicators are not needed in refrigerators where there is a continuous temperature monitor **(Fig. 9)**.

Q26. How often should the temperature be recorded?

Ans. Temperature of ILRs/freezers used for storage of vaccines must be recorded twice daily. A break in the cold chain is indicated if temperature rises above +8° C or falls below +2°C in the ILR; and above −15°C in the deep freezer. These readings should be recorded in a log book.

CHAPTER 6: Cold Chain Management

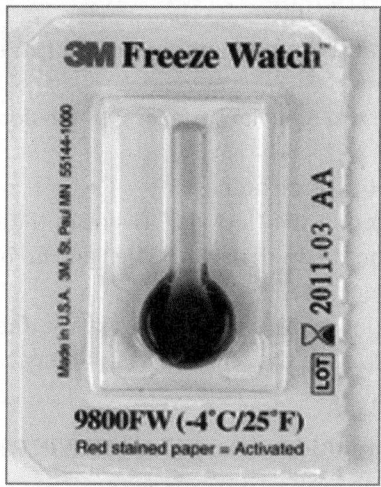

Fig. 9: Electronic freeze indicators.

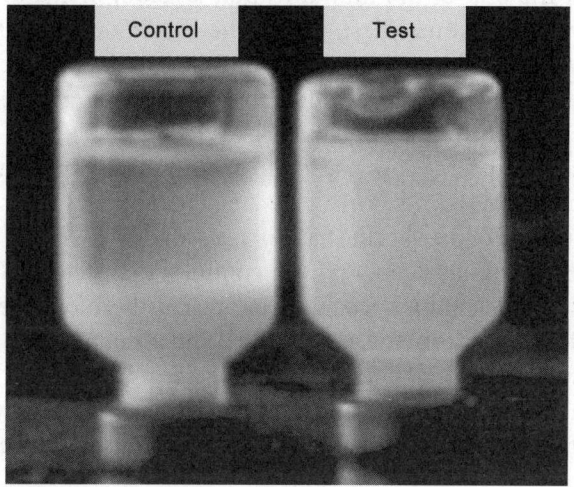

Fig. 10: This is a "negative" shake test.

Q27. What is "Shake test" and how is it performed?

Ans. The "Shake test" is performed to assess whether an adjuvanted vaccine has been frozen. It is a validated test. If a freeze indicator is activated, or temperature recordings show negative temperatures, the "Shake test" should be performed to decide whether the freeze-exposed vials can be used **(Fig. 10)**.

Take a vaccine vial you suspect may have been frozen – this is "test" sample:
- Take a vaccine vial of the same type, same manufacturer, same batch number as the suspect vaccine vial you want to test and freeze it overnight. This is the "control" sample.

- Let it thaw. Do *not* heat it.
- Hold the control and the test sample together in hand and vigorously shake the samples.
- Place both vials to rest on a flat surface, side-by-side observe them for 30 minutes.
- Compare the rate of sedimentation.
- If the sedimentation in the "test vial" is slower than in the "frozen vial": The vaccine has not been damaged. The vaccine batch is not damaged and can be used.
- If the sedimentation is similar in both the vials or if sedimentation is faster in the "test" vial than in the "frozen" vial: The vaccine is damaged and should not be used.

Q28. What is WHO's multidose vial policy (MDVP) 2014?

Ans. WHO multidose vial policy (MDVP) 2014:

All opened WHO-prequalified multidose vial of vaccine should be discarded at the end of the immunization session, or within 6 hours of opening, whichever comes first, unless the vaccine meets all four of the criteria listed here. If the vaccine meets the four criteria, the opened vial can be kept and used for up to 28 days after opening. The criteria are as follow:
1. The vaccine is currently prequalified by WHO.
2. The vaccine is approved for use for up to 28 days after opening the vial, as determined by WHO.
3. The expiry date of the vaccine has not passed.
4. The vaccine vial has been, and will continue to be, stored at WHO – or manufacturer-recommended temperatures; furthermore, the VVM, if one is attached, is visible on the vaccine label and is not past its discard point, and the vaccine has not been damaged by freezing.

If all of the criteria cited above are present, the vaccine vial may be kept and used for up to 28 days after opening, or until all the doses are administered.

Q29. What is electronic Vaccine Intelligence Network (eVIN)?

Ans. Electronic Vaccine Intelligence Network (eVIN) is India's solution for ensuring effective management of the immunization supply chain. It answers three crucial questions for cold-chain handlers:
1. Where are my vaccines?
2. Are they available in adequate quantities?
3. Are they being stored in the appropriate conditions?

With data answering these questions, cold-chain handlers will be able to make effective vaccine storage and stock management decisions. eVIN was conceptualized and piloted by the Immunization Technical Support Unit (ITSU), MoHFW.

Electronic Vaccine Intelligence Network is made up of three components—processes, technology, and human resources, which are all required to ensure vaccine stock, temperature data visibility and improved immunization supply chain performance.

Q30. What are the equipment available for temporary storage of vaccines?

Ans. Cold box/coolers: A cold box is an insulated container that can be lined with water packs to keep vaccines and diluents in the required temperature range during transport or short-term storage. Cold boxes can be used to store vaccines for periods of up to 2 days when there is no electricity available. Cold boxes should be lined with conditioned ice packs on all sides, bottom and top, before storing vaccines.

Q31. What precautions are to be taken while "packing a cold box"?

Ans. Precautions:
- Place conditioned ice packs at the bottom and sides of the cold box **(Figs. 11A and B)**.
- Load the vaccines in cardboard cartons or polythene bags.
- Never place freeze-sensitive vaccines in direct contact with the ice packs. Surround them with OPV/BCG/JE vaccines.

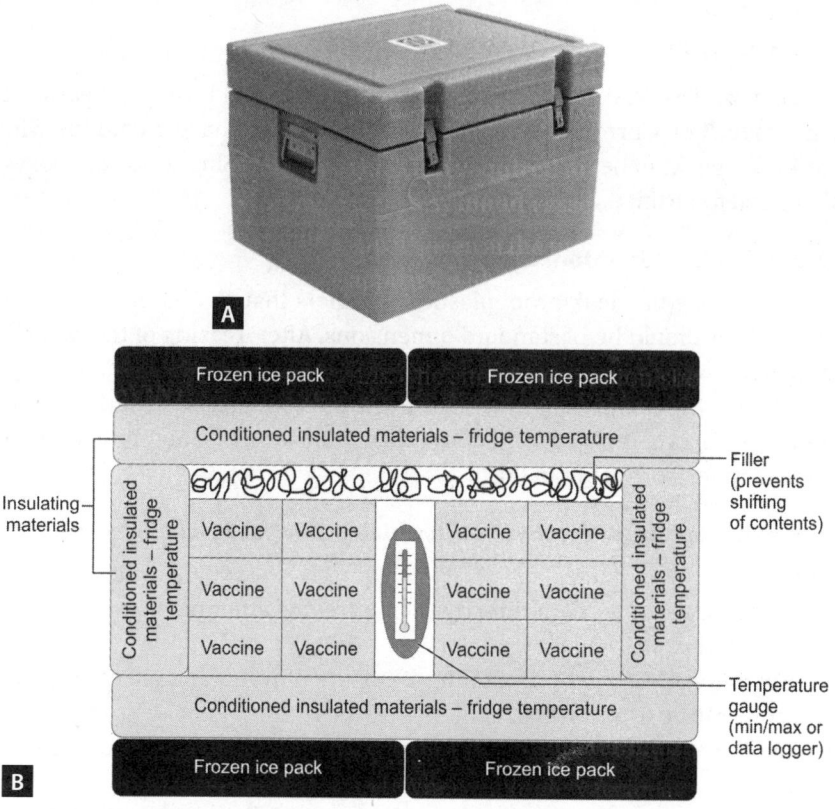

Figs. 11A and B: (A) Cold box; (B) Packing of a cold box for transporting vaccine.

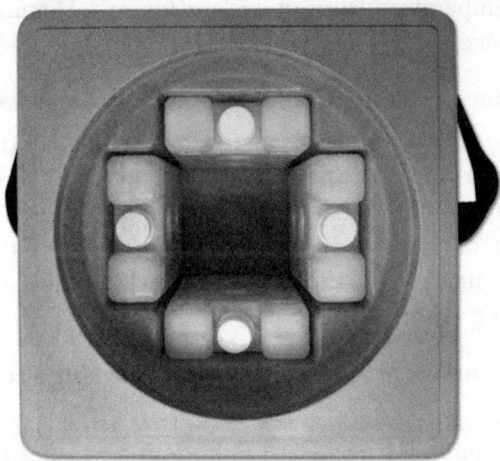

Fig. 12: Vaccine carrier.

- Keep a thermometer in the cold box.
- Place two rows of conditioned ice packs above the vaccine vials.
- Place a plastic sheet to cover the ice packs kept on top to ensure full hold over time.
- Securely close the lid of the cold box.

Vaccine carriers: Vaccine carriers are smaller than cold boxes and easier to carry **(Fig. 12)**. Current prequalified vaccine carriers have a cold life with frozen ice packs of between 18 and 50 hours at +43°C. Similar to cold boxes, they need to be lined with conditioned ice packs.

Q32. What are conditioned ice packs?

Ans. These are flat, leak-proof plastic containers that can be filled with tap water. They should be of standard dimensions. After freezing of the water in deep freezers, the ice packs are to be kept at room temperature till "sweating" occurs, the icepack has begun to melt and some condensation, or droplets of water appears on the surface. They contain a mixture of water and ice at an initial temperature of about 0°C.

Q33. What are the different ways in which water packs can be used?

Ans.
- *Frozen ice packs,* taken directly from a freezer at temperatures between 10°C and –25°C.
- *Conditioned ice packs* containing a mixture of water and ice at an initial temperature of about 0°C.
- *Cool water packs,* containing liquid water at an initial temperature of +5°C or less.
- *Warm water packs,* containing liquid water, initially at room temperature, and between +18°C and +24°C.

Q34. What is the "cold life" of a cold box?

Ans. The "cold life" of a cold box is the maximum length of time that a closed cold box can maintain temperatures below +10°C when it is lined with frozen ice packs. Current prequalified cold box models have a maximum cold life of 2–7 days when tested at a constant +43°C.

The "cool life" "of a cold box is the maximum length of time the closed cold box can maintain temperatures below +20°C if lined with cool water packs that have been stored in a refrigerator. Current prequalified cold box models have a maximum cool life of 12 hours to 2 days when tested at a constant +43°C.

Q35. How do you maintain vaccines properly during power failure?

Ans.
- For power failure <4 hours, keep the fridge shut. Increasing the cold mass, as discussed before, will assist maintenance of required temperature.
- For power loss of >4 hours, without power backup, vaccines must shifted to a prepared cold box or an alternate location where power supply is uninterrupted.

Q36. How is a "cold chain breach" to be managed?

Ans.
- Strictly, the vaccines should be isolated, kept at +2°C to +8°C, and not used.
- In private practice inform the manufacturer/supplier.
- In government set up, inform the health authorities.
- Arrange to get fresh stocks.
- Do not overstock vaccines.

■ SUGGESTED READING

1. Balasubramaniam S. IAP Guidebook on Immunization 2018–2019. Advisory Committee on Vaccines and Immunization Practices, Indian Academy of Pediatrics. New Delhi: Jaypee Brothers Medical Publishers (P) Ltd.; 2020.
2. CDC. Vaccine Storage and Handling. Epidemiology and Prevention of VPDs. Atlanta: CDC; 2011.
3. CDC. Vaccine Storage and Handling Toolkit. Washington DC: US deptt. of Health and Human Services; 2019.
4. Galazka A, Milstien J, Zaffran M. Thermostability of Vaccines. WHO (Global Programme for Vaccines and Immunization). Geneva: WHO; 1998.
5. Handbook for Vaccine and Cold Chain Handlers. New Delhi: MOHFW (GOI)/Unicef/WHO; 2010.
6. Strive for 5, national vaccine storage guidelines. Phillip, Australian Capital Territory: Australian government department of health and ageing; 2019.
7. WHO. The vaccine COLD CHAIN Module 2, WHO 2015. [online] Available from: https://www.who.int/immunization/documents/IIP2015_Module2.pdf?ua=1#:~:text=About%20this%20module%E2%80%A6,workers%20at%20health%20facility%20level. [Last Accessed November, 2020].

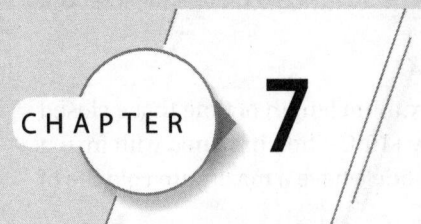

CHAPTER 7: Adverse Event following Immunization

Arun Wadhwa

Q1. What is AEFI?

Ans. Adverse event following immunization (AEFI): By definition, AEFI is any untoward medical occurrence which follows immunization and which does not necessarily have a causal relationship with the usage of the vaccine. The adverse event may be any unfavorable or unintended sign, abnormal laboratory finding, symptom or disease. It might not have been caused by vaccine ingredients or the process of vaccination or immunization but have a temporal relationship with administration of vaccine.

Like any other drug, no vaccine is 100% effective or 100% safe, 100% of time. As with other drugs, adverse events can occur with vaccines too. In addition to the vaccines themselves, the process of administration of vaccines is a potential source of an adverse event following immunization.

Q2. What are the possible different types of AEFI?

Ans. There are five different types of AEFI:
1. *Vaccine product-related reaction:* An AEFI that is caused or precipitated by a vaccine due to one or more of the inherent properties of the vaccine product (or ingredients), e.g., extensive limb swelling following DTP vaccination. In this scenario, vaccine might have been used correctly without any compromise in the manufacturing process, transport, or storage. Thus, correct use of vaccine may also cause this type of AEFI.
2. *Vaccine quality defect-related reaction:* An AEFI that is caused or precipitated by a vaccine that is due to one or more quality defects of the vaccine product including its administration device as provided by the manufacturer, e.g., failure by the manufacturer to completely inactivate a lot of IPV leads to cases of paralytic polio. Syringe, needle defects are included in this category.
3. *Immunization error-related reaction:* An AEFI that is caused by inappropriate vaccine handling, prescribing, or administration and thus by its nature is preventable, e.g., transmission of infection by contaminated multidose vial.
4. *Immunization anxiety-related reaction:* An AEFI arising from anxiety about the immunization, e.g., vasovagal syncope in an adolescent

following vaccination. The anxiety may spread to community too, at times like school immunization camp.
5. *Coincidental event:* An AEFI that is caused by something other than the vaccine product, immunization error, or immunization anxiety, e.g., fever after vaccination (temporal association) and malarial parasite isolated from blood.

Q3. What is the most common AEFI encountered in daily practice?

Ans. Immunization error related reactions are the most common type of AEFI. These are also the ones which can be easily avoided.

Q4. What are the possible causes of immunization errors?

Ans.
- *Nonsterile injection:* Reuse of syringes/needles, contaminated vaccine vial.
- *Reconstitution/administration errors*: Inadequate shaking of vaccine, reconstitution with incorrect diluent, other drug substituted for vaccine or diluent, reuse of reconstituted vaccine at subsequent session.
- *Injection at incorrect site:* BCG given subcutaneously, DTP/DT/TT applied too superficially, injection into buttocks.
- *Improper cold chain maintenance:* Freezing vaccine during transport, failure to keep vaccine in cold chain, exposing to excessive heat or cold.
- *Contraindication ignored:* Live vaccine administered to an immunocompromised child.

Q5. Are there any grades of AEFI?

Ans. Vaccine reactions can be classified into minor reactions or severe, some of which can be serious reactions:
- *Minor AEFI*: Minor AEFIs can be local reactions (pain, swelling, and redness) or systemic reactions (fever >38°C, irritability, malaise, etc.), which can be managed with antipyretics and anti-inflammatory and resolves within 2–3 days.
- *Severe AEFI*: Severe AEFIs are minor AEFIs with increased intensity/severity, e.g., high-grade fever following pentavalent vaccination or post-DPT swelling extending beyond nearest joint. The patient may not be hospitalized and will not have sequelae.
- *Serious AEFI*: An AEFI is considered serious if it: (1) results in death, hospitalization, or persistent or significant disability/incapacity, (2) occurs in clusters, (3) causes parental/community concern, or (4) results in congenital anomaly/birth defect.

Q6. What is the difference between severe and serious AEFI?

Ans. A 14-week-old infant develops more than 20 mm induration after DPT vaccine, it is a severe reaction but not serious as it is unlikely to leave sequalae.

A 5-year-old develops Guillain–Barré syndrome (GBS) after influenza vaccine, it is a serious reaction. All serious reactions are severe but all severe reactions may not be serious.

Q7. Which AEFI do we need to report?

Ans.
1. All serious AEFIs.
2. Events associated with newly introduced vaccine.
3. AEFI that may have been caused by immunization error.
4. Significant events of unexplained cause occurring within 30 days of vaccination.
5. Events causing significant parental or community concern.

AEFIs are to be reported following use of any vaccine including vaccines given in government sector, private sector, travel vaccines, etc.

Q8. Who do we report to?

Ans. In rural areas inform the medical officer in charge of the nearest Public Health Center (PHC).

In urban areas inform the medical officer in charge of the nearest Urban Health Center or the District Immunization Officer (DIO).

If internet available, inform at the website www.IDsurv.org.

Q9. What is the timeline by which we need to do so?

Ans. Most vaccinations in India are given through the government system through outreach sessions by auxiliary nurse midwives (ANMs) and sessions in health facilities. To make reporting simple and to get as many cases reported, health workers and medical personnel are asked to notify serious and severe AEFIs immediately to the nearest PHC medical officer (MO) or the District Immunization Officer (DIO). Private practitioners are also encouraged to notify AEFIs similarly to the DIO. The MO at the PHC then reports the case in the case reporting format (CRF) within 24 hours to the DIO who has another 24 hours to verify the case and send it to the State Immunization/EPI (Expanded Program of Immunization) Officer and the Immunization Division, Ministry of Health and Family Welfare (MOHFW) simultaneously. The CRF gives only the most basic details of the affected person, vaccines and session details, and status of the patient (brief clinical summary) at the time of filling the format.

As soon as the AEFI is reported, case investigation begins. The preliminary case investigation format (PCIF) acts as a checklist and records the details of the investigations done with relation to the case. The investigation involves verifying personal details, vaccine and program details, a clinical examination, interviews with the treating physicians, caregivers, service providers, volunteers, etc., to understand the sequence of events. An epidemiological investigation is also conducted. The cold chain and vaccine transportation

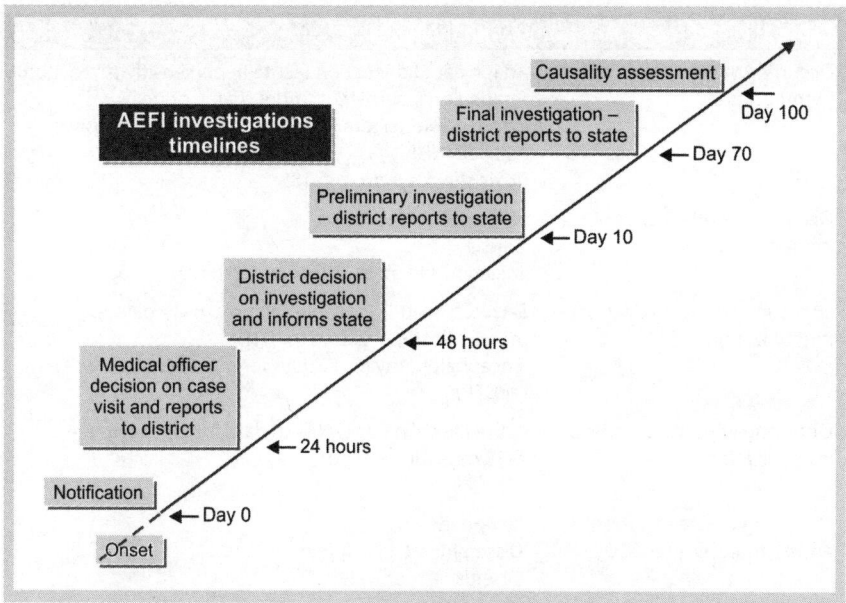

Fig. 1: Investigations timelines of adverse events following immunization (AEFI).

conditions are studied. Hospital records, laboratory test reports, and other relevant documents are collected. In case of death, postmortem is recommended. Verbal autopsies formats have been designed specifically for finding the cause of AEFI deaths. These forms should be used whenever a death is alleged to be associated with vaccine. These, along with the filled PCIF are submitted simultaneously to the state and the national level within 10 days of notification. Whenever required, experts of the District/State AEFI Committees are requested to participate in the investigation.

The causality assessment should be done by 100 days **(Fig. 1 and Table 1)**.

Q10. Is there a specific reporting format?

Ans. The pediatrician should use the case reporting form (CRF) or the "first information report (FIR)" form for reporting serious AEFI cases to the district officials **(Fig. 2)**. The form has three sections for writing details of the patient, vaccine and event related data. Once an AEFI is reported from private sector, the DIO and district AEFI committee members would then investigate the reported AEFI case. The pediatrician should help the investigation team in collection of all the related information. If AEFI occurs save the vial maintaining the cold chain, save needles and syringes if possible and write a log of events.

Q11. Is the causality assessment done by the reporting doctor? What is the pediatrician's role in AEFI?

Ans. Causality assessment is the systematic evaluation of the information obtained about an AEFI to determine the likelihood of the event having been

Table 1: List of reportable events with timelines.

Occurring within 3 hours of immunization	Anaphylactoid reaction (acute hypersensitivity reaction) Anaphylaxis, persistent (more than 3 hours) inconsolable screaming, hypotonic hyporesponsive episode (HHE) Toxic shock syndrome (TSS)
Occurring within 5 days of immunization	Severe local reaction Sepsis Injection site abscess (bacterial/sterile)
Occurring within 15 days of immunization	Seizures, including febrile seizures (6–12 days for measles/MMR; 0–2 days for DTP) Encephalopathy (6–12 days for measles/MMR; 0–2 days for DTP)
Occurring within 3 months of immunization	Acute flaccid paralysis (4–30 days for OPV recipient; 4–75 days for contact)
Occurring between 1 month and 12 months after BCG	Lymphadenitis Disseminated BCG infection Osteitis/Osteomyelitis
No time limit	Any death, hospitalization, or other severe and unusual events that are thought by health workers or the public to be related to immunization

caused by the vaccines received. The causality assessment is conducted at state and national levels by trained experts in the AEFI committees within a month of receipt of all records and reports of the AEFI case. The criteria for causality in the causality assessment process includes proof of temporal relationship, biological plausibility, strength of association, consistency of association, specificity, definitive proof that the vaccine caused the event, consideration of alternate explanations, and prior evidence that the vaccine in question could cause a similar event.

Pediatricians, relying on experience and intuition, are the first to suspect a medical product problem and bring it to the attention of public health and regulatory officials. Other than reporting, pediatricians and other clinicians can be members of the AEFI committees and contribute to investigations and causality assessments. Representatives of professional bodies such as Indian Academy of Pediatrics (IAP) and Indian Medical Association (IMA) as AEFI Committee Members can also help in assisting the immunization program manager to give correct messages to the media in times of crisis. Medical colleges and large hospitals have huge catchment areas and can contribute to AEFI surveillance by reporting AEFI cases to the immunization program manager.

Q12. How do you define a cluster of adverse events?

Ans. Clusters of events is two or more cases of the same adverse event related in time, place or vaccine administered. Clusters are usually associated with

AEFI CASE REPORTING FORM (CRF)			
AEFI reporting ID: IND (AEFI) /__ ST__/DIS__YR__/NUM__(to be allotted by DIO)			
Section A (To be submitted by MO within 24 hours of case notification to DIO)			
State	District		
Block/ward	Village/urban area		
Name of reporting MO (person filling this form):		Today's date:	
Posted at:	Designation:	Time of preparing this form: am/pm	
Contact phone number: e mail:		Date case visited and examined/interviewed: __/__/____	
Notified by [name]: Date notified to MO: __ __/__ __/__ __ __ __	Designation (please circle): health worker/government doctor/private practitioner/community/media/others (specify) ________ ________		
Patient's name			
Date of birth DD/MM/YYYY	Age (in months):________months	Sex	Male Female
Mother's name			
Father's name			
Complete address of the case with landmarks (street name, house number, village, block, tehsil, pin no, telephone no.)			
Pin:	Phone:		
Date of vaccination__ __/__ __/__ __ __ __ Time of vaccination: __ : __ __ am/pm		Address of session site:	
Session: Routine (including SIW)* **Compaign** (SIA)-IPPI/MR/JE/others (specify):________ Other________		**Place of vaccination:** Govt health facility/outreach/ private health facility/others______	

Name of vaccines received (write vaccine and diluent details in separate rows)	Dose no (zero/first/ second/ etc. as applicable)	Name of manufacturer	Batch/lot no.	Expiry date	Date of opening of vial	Time of opening the vial (for reconstituted vaccine)	No. of other beneficiaries who received vaccine from the SMAE vial in this session

Date of first symptom	D D M M Y Y Y Y	Time of first symptom	H H M M am pm
Hospitalization: No/Yes - (Date)	D D M M Y Y Y Y	Time of hospitalization	H H M M am pm
Name and address of hospital [if hospitalized]:			

*Special immunization week

Fig. 2: AEFI—Case reporting form.

a particular provider or health facility or if a vial has been prepared or stored inappropriately or has got contaminated.

Q13. Is vaccine associated paralytic poliomyelitis (VAPP) a form of AEFI?

Ans. Yes, it is a vaccine product related reaction. It is not because of poor quality of OPV nor is an immunization error.

Q14. A new born develops severe diarrhea after birth dose of Hepatitis B. Can it be called AEFI? A child of 6 weeks develops bloody diarrhea after Rotavirus vaccine. Is it a case of AEFI?

Ans. Both are cases of AEFI. By definition any untoward medical occurrence which follows immunization and which does not necessarily have a causal relationship with the usage of the vaccine.

Q15. An infant was well-restrained but the needle breaks during administration of the pentavalent vaccine. What is the possible type of AEFI?

Ans. It is a quality defect related type of AEFI as the needle broke because of its poor quality. As the infant was well-restrained it is not an immunization error.

Q16. A 12-year-old girl complains of giddiness and falls to the ground within a minute of receiving HPV vaccine. Is it AEFI?

Ans. It is an anxiety related AEFI. It is commonly seen in adolescent age group, more in girls than boys.

Q17. What are the possible anxiety related reactions?

Ans. The anxiety related reactions can be:
1. *Fainting*: It is relatively common and affects older children and adults. The patient should be made to lie down with legs elevated and the child recovers in 2–3 minutes. Care should be taken while giving injection next time – best given lying down.
2. *Vomiting*: Younger children can have a breath holding spell or actually vomit at the site of injection as an avoidance reaction.
3. *Hyperventilation*: It is related to the anxiety related to injection and causes light headedness, dizziness and tingling sensation around the mouth.
4. *Convulsions*: Very rarely extreme anxiety related to injection can cause convulsions.

Q18. How common is anaphylaxis following vaccinations?

Ans. Anaphylaxis is very uncommon following vaccinations. Studies have shown an incidence of 0.65–1.0 per 1 million doses. Vaccine antigens very rarely cause anaphylaxis. Other constituents, egg protein, gelatin, neomycin, streptomycin, thiomersal, contribute to a large extent. Gelatin is believed to be the main factor in the majority of vaccine induced anaphylaxis.

Q19. How do we differentiate anxiety related fainting and anaphylaxis?

Ans. The differentiation between anxiety related fainting and anaphylaxis is given in **Table 2**.

Table 2: Distinguishing anaphylaxis from a fainting.

	Fainting	Anaphylaxis
Onset	Usually soon after injection	Usually 5–30 minutes after injection
System		
Skin	Pale sweaty, cold and clammy	Generalized, red raised and itchy rash. Swollen eyes
Respiratory	Normal to deep breaths	Noisy breathing from airways obstruction – wheeze or stridor
Cardiovascular	Bradycardia, transient hypotension	Tachycardia, hypotension
Gastrointestinal tract (GIT)	Nausea, vomiting	Abdominal cramps
Neurological	Transient loss of consciousness, good response once prone	Loss of consciousness, poor response when prone

Q20. How does a clinician treat anaphylaxis if it happens in his clinic?

Ans.
1. Make child lie flat with legs elevated.
2. If needed, immediately begin cardiopulmonary resuscitation (CPR).
3. Give 0.01 mL/kg 1:1,000 adrenaline by deep IM injection into the opposite limb to that in which the vaccine was given. If no improvement in 5 minutes repeat the dose to a maximum of three shots. Usually the response to adrenaline is very quick.
4. Give oxygen if required and available.
5. Any child who has had anaphylaxis should be kept under observation for 24 hours even if there was immediate recovery.

Q21. What are coincidental AEFIs?

Ans. Most vaccines are scheduled early in life when infections, other illnesses and underlying congenital and neurological may also present themselves. Coincidental events are unrelated to immunization but the community may blame the vaccine, especially if the child was previously healthy. An event is more likely to be coincidental if other children of similar age group show same symptoms but have not received the vaccine. It is important for the medical officer to investigate the cause of such an event to prove that AEFI was not because of the vaccine.

Q22. What is AEFI surveillance?

Ans. It is about detecting, monitoring and responding to adverse events following immunization. It helps in implementing appropriate and immediate action to correct any unsafe practices detected through the surveillance system. It thus reduces the negative impact on the individual and the immunization program.

An AEFI surveillance system is usually a passive system to enable spontaneous reporting of all adverse events. It is a part of the National Regulatory Authority for vaccines. The primary purpose of spontaneous AEFI reporting is to monitor the known adverse events associated with vaccine use, and to identify the new adverse events, i.e., safety signals after a product is marketed.

Q23. What minimum equipment should a clinician have in his clinic?

Ans.
1. Injectable epinephrine (adrenaline) 1:1,000; check expiry dates regularly as usually short expiry. Do not use if solution has changed to brownish color.
2. Oral airway, bag mask and endotracheal tubes.
3. Oxygen, and equipment to administer it.
4. Equipment for IV fluid administration.
5. Ringer's lactate.
6. Corticosteroids for IV injection.

Q24. As an individual pediatrician, what does "vaccine safety" mean to me?

Ans.
- Use approved vaccines with multiple peer reviewed, published immunogenicity/efficacy studies
- Use the right vaccines at the right age
- Observe valid precautions and contraindications
- Follow safe injection practices
- Maintain records
- Observe every vaccinated child for 15 min following vaccination
- Be ready for emergencies: Adrenaline, O_2, steroids, IV apparatus
- Have a plan of action ready for any eventuality.

■ SUGGESTED READING

1. Government of India. Adverse Events following Immunization: Surveillance and Response Operational Guidelines. New Delhi: Ministry of Health and Family Welfare, Government of India; 2010.
2. Government of India. Multi Year Strategic Plan (MYP) for UIP of India 2005–10. New Delhi: Ministry of Health and Family Welfare, Government of India; 2010.
3. World Health Organization. Surveillance of Adverse Events following Immunization, Field guide for managers of immunization programs. Geneva: World Health Organization; 1997.

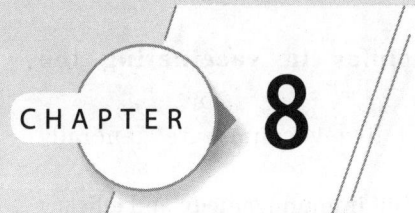

CHAPTER 8

Vaccination in Special Situations

Srinivas G Kasi

Q1. What is a special situation (SS)?

Ans. A special situation is a clinical situation in which, vaccination may result in a suboptimal vaccine response and/or an increased incidence of adverse effects following vaccination.

Q2. What is the importance of vaccinations in SS?

Ans. As mentioned earlier, SS are associated with increased risk and severity of infections. Many of these infections are vaccine preventable. This population is often under vaccinated due to uncertainty or misconceptions about the safety and efficacy of vaccination among patients, parents and health care providers.

Q3. What are the SS encountered in day-to-day practice?

Ans. **Immunocompromised**
- *Congenital:* B cell disorders, T cell disorders, phagocytosis defects, complement disorders.
- *Acquired:* Children on steroids, children on chemotherapy for malignancies, hematopoietic stem cell transplantation (HSCT) recipients, solid organ transplant (SOT) recipients, infant of a HIV +ve mother/HIV+ve child, asplenia/splenectomy.

Immunocompetent
Children with bleeding disorders, children scheduled for cochlear implants, CSF leaks, children with chronic systemic diseases, pregnancy, lactation, preterms, etc.

Q4. What are not SS?

Ans. The following are not special situations:
- Mild illnesses, febrile or afebrile
- Current antimicrobial therapy
- Recent exposure to an infectious disease
- Convalescent phase of illness
- Allergy to products not present in vaccine
- Family history of adverse effects.

Q5. What are the general principles in vaccinating the immunocompromised?

Ans. In severe immunodeficiency, all live vaccines are generally contraindicated:
- All inactivated vaccines may be given, but immunogenicity and efficacy may be low
- Higher doses, a greater number of doses may be required (hepatitis B)
- Antibody titers should be checked postimmunization.
- Regular boosters may be needed.

Q6. What are the recommendations regarding vaccination of contacts of persons with altered immunocompetence?

Ans. Immunocompetent individuals who live in a household with immunocompromised patients should be current with all routinely recommended immunizations to minimize the exposure of the immunocompromised patient to vaccine-preventable infections. All susceptible contacts should receive MMR, varicella, rotavirus and annual influenza vaccines. OPV is to be avoided.

Direct contact should be avoided with susceptible household contact, who has developed a rash after varicella vaccine, until the rash resolves.

Hand hygiene measures should be employed by all members of the household, after contact with feces of a rotavirus-vaccinated infant, for at least 1 week, postvaccination.

Q7. What are the recommendations regarding vaccination of children with congenital immunodeficiency disorders?

Ans.

B-lymphocyte (Humoral) Deficiency Disorders

In severe disorders, e.g., X-linked agammaglobulinemia and common variable immunodeficiency, all live vaccines are contraindicated, inactivated vaccines may not elicit an adequate response, the effectiveness of any vaccine is uncertain if it depends only on the humoral response (e.g., PPSV23 or MPSV4). Administered IVIG may interfere with the immune response to vaccines.

In mild disorders, e.g., selective IgA deficiency and IgG subclass deficiency, OPV, BCG and yellow fever (YF) vaccines are contraindicated. Other live vaccines appear to be safe. All vaccines are likely to be effective, however the immune response might be attenuated.

T-lymphocyte (Cellular) Deficiency Disorders

In severe disorders, e.g, SCID, complete DiGeorge syndrome, all live vaccines are contraindicated while inactivated vaccines are safe and may be effective.

In partial defects (e.g., most patients with DiGeorge syndrome, Wiskott–Aldrich syndrome, ataxia-telangiectasia), all live vaccines are contraindicated while inactivated vaccines may be effective.

In interferon-gamma/interleukin-12 axis deficiencies, all live vaccines are generally contraindicated.

Complement Deficiency

In persistent complement, properdin, or factor B deficiency all vaccine scan be administered as per schedule and are effective.

Phagocytic Function Disorders

In chronic granulomatous disease, leukocyte adhesion deficiency (LAD), and myeloperoxidase deficiency all live bacterial vaccines are contraindicated. Live viral vaccines and all inactivated vaccines are safe and effective.

In phagocytic deficiencies that are undefined or accompanied by defects in T-cell and NK cell dysfunction such as Chediak–Higashi syndrome, all live bacterial and viral vaccines are contraindicated while inactivated vaccines are safe and effective.

Q8. What are the recommendations regarding vaccination of children on steroids?

Ans.
- Children on alternate day steroid therapy, inhaled corticosteroid formulations, intra-articular steroids and topical steroids are not immunosuppressed and can receive all vaccines.
- Children receiving <2 mg/kg (if <10 kg) or <20 mg/day (if >10 kg) of prednisolone or equivalent are not immunosuppressed and can receive all vaccines.
- Children receiving >2 mg/kg (if <10 kg) or >20 mg/day (if >10 kg) of prednisolone or equivalent, for less than 2 weeks should not receive live vaccines during therapy with steroids. All live vaccines can be administered immediately after stopping steroids.
- Children receiving >2 mg/kg (if <10 kg) or >20 mg/day (if >10 kg) of prednisolone or equivalent, for more than 2 weeks are immunosuppressed. No live vaccines should be administered till 1 month after stopping steroids.
- Killed vaccines are safe but may be less efficacious.

Q9. What are the recommendations for vaccination of children on other immunosuppressive drugs/biologicals for nonmalignant conditions?

Ans. Children receiving methotrexate at a dosage of ≤0.4 mg/kg/week, azathioprine at a dosage of ≤3 mg/kg/day, or 6-mercaptopurine at a dosage of ≤1.5 mg/kg/day are not immunosuppressed and can receive all vaccines.

Other immunosuppressive medications include human immune mediators such as interleukins and colony-stimulating factors, immune modulators, and medicines such as tumor necrosis factor-alpha inhibitors and anti-B cell antibodies. In these conditions all live vaccines should be administered at least 3 months after stopping therapy.

Rituximab therapy results in profound B-cell depletion. Once B-cell and immunoglobulin levels have recovered, immunization should be recommenced. Any vaccine history prior to Rituximab therapy should be disregarded and complete re-immunization should be initiated. Inactivated vaccines, except the inactivated influenza vaccine, should be administered after 6 months of completion of therapy and live attenuated vaccines at least 12 months later.

Q10. What are the recommendations regarding vaccination of children on chemotherapy for malignancies?

Ans. Children on chemotherapy and radiotherapy for malignancy should avoid all live vaccines during therapy and for at least 3 months after stopping treatment.

Since varicella is a devastating illness in the immunocompromised, varicella vaccine can be administered to children with acute lymphatic leukemia on maintenance therapy provided:
- The child is in remission for more than 1 year
- The platelet count is more than 100,000
- The lymphocyte count is more than 700/mm^3.

Chemotherapy should be withheld for 1 week before and after vaccination.

Q11. Are there any special considerations for vaccination of children on chemotherapy for acute lymphatic leukemia?

Ans. All children who have completed a course of "standard dose" chemotherapy should receive a booster dose of all age eligible vaccines. These can be administered as follows:
- After 3–6 months—IIV
- After 6 months—diphtheria, tetanus, acellular pertussis, IPV, Hib-conjugate, PCV13, MCV4-CV, HepA, HepB
- After 12 months—MMR, children 10 years and older should receive Tdap and HPV vaccines.
- Following highly immunosuppressive chemotherapy, revaccination should be done for all age appropriate vaccines, as is done following HSCT.

Q12. Are there any concerns regarding immunization in infants born of mothers who received biologic response modifiers in pregnancy?

Ans. These infants can have detectable drug concentrations for many months following delivery, resulting in concern for immunosuppression among infants in the 12 months after the last maternal dose during pregnancy. It would be prudent to avoid all live vaccines till 12 months of age.

Q13. What are the recommendations regarding vaccination of children before HSCT?

Ans. In general, transplant recipients should receive all recommended immunizations, prior to transplantation and on accelerated schedules if indicated, provided the ongoing immunosuppression regimen dose not contraindicate vaccinations. Live vaccines should be administered at least 4 weeks prior to immunosuppression and inactivated vaccine 2 weeks prior. This is done with the hope that some protection will persist in the months after transplant.

The donor should be current with routinely recommended vaccines, but if not up to date, vaccination of the donor for benefit of the recipient is not recommended.

Q14. What are the recommendations regarding vaccination of children after HSCT?

Ans. HSCT recipients should be viewed as "immunization naive" and require reimmunization after transplant because the ablation of hematopoietic cells in the bone marrow prior to the HSCT, and immunosuppressant drugs used subsequent to transplant, further depletes the immune response, and eliminates most or all immune memory cells.

All routine inactivated vaccines should be given (or repeated) for HSCT recipients generally beginning 6–12 months post-transplant **(Table 1)**:

- Pneumococcal polysaccharide vaccine should be administered as a single dose, 12–18 months post-HSCT if no GVHD (8 weeks after the last dose of PCV 13).
- If GVHD, give 4th dose of PCV 13 and delay polysaccharide until GVHD is resolved.
- HPV vaccine is recommended if indicated by age. 3 doses beginning 6–12 months post-HSCT.

Table 1: Recommendations for vaccination after hematopoietic stem cell transplantation (HSCT) in children.

When*	Vaccine	Comments
3–6 months post-HSCT	Influenza (2 doses may be considered if given this early)	24 months if GVHD
6 to 12 months post-HSCT	Three doses of IPV, Hib, Hep B, PCV, DPT, 2 doses of inactivated Hep A, Three doses of HPV (9–26 years old), age appropriate doses of conjugate meningococcal vaccine	>7 years: Tdap-Td-Td Hep B: additional doses if postimmunization titer is less than 10 IU/L PCV and Hib: 3 doses regardless of age
24 months post-HSCT	MMR, Varicella RZV Zoster vaccine (> 50 years)	2 doses 2–6 months apart

(GVHD: graft-versus-host disease)
*Pneumococcal conjugate vaccine and Hib vaccine should be given regardless of age.

- Meningococcal conjugate vaccine (MCV), Meningococcal B and C conjugate vaccines, Japanese encephalitis vaccines, and the oral cholera vaccines can be administered, if indicated, beginning 6 months post-HSCT.
- Pre-exposure prophylaxis for Rabies can be administered beginning 6–12 months post-HSCT. 4 doses are recommended for postexposure prophylaxis and postimmunization serology is recommended. Intradermal rabies vaccination is not recommended. Category 2 bites should also be managed as category 3 exposure with RIG/Mab and 4 doses of vaccine.
- Live vaccines: BCG, live Influenza, live Zoster, Rotavirus, MMR vaccine and live typhoid vaccines are contraindicated.
- Recombinant Zoster vaccine can be administered if indicated.
- Univalent Varicella vaccine is recommended in a 2 dose schedule beginning 24 months post-HSCT. Serology recommended after 2nd dose.
- MMR vaccine is recommended in a 2-dose schedule beginning 24 months post-HSCT. Serology is recommended after 2nd dose.
- Yellow fever vaccine can be given, if indicated, beginning 24 months post-HSCT.

Q15. What are the recommendations regarding vaccination of children for solid organ transplants (SOT)?

Ans.

Pre-SOT

Subjects due for solid organ transplantation candidates should be immunized with all age appropriate vaccines, prior to transplantation and as early in the course of disease as possible because vaccine response may be reduced in people with organ failure pretransplant. Schedules of inactivated vaccines should be completed at least 2 weeks before transplant and live vaccines 4 weeks before transplant. MMR and varicella vaccine may be given to infants 6–11 months of age if transplantation is expected to occur before age 12 months. Antibody response should be determined by serology for those vaccines with an antibody correlate of immunity available.

Post-SOT

Solid organ recipients generally receive lifelong immunosuppression, which varies substantially depending on the organ transplanted. Recommended inactivated vaccines that were not given pretransplant and recommended booster doses should be given.

Vaccination with inactivated vaccines can recommence 6 months post-transplant when immunosuppression has been lowered.

IIV can be given as early as 1–2 months post-transplant, during community outbreaks. Boosters for inactivated vaccines should be given as per schedule/when antibody levels wane (Hepatitis A and B) starting 6 months after transplant. No live vaccines can be administered, post-transplant.

Q16. What are the vaccine recommendations for children with asplenia or children scheduled for splenectomy?

Ans. Asplenia, congenital or following splenectomy, is associated with an increased risk of fulminant septicemia, especially associated with encapsulated bacteria, which is associated with a high mortality rate. Hence, vaccination with pneumococcal (both conjugate and polysaccharide), Hib, meningococcal, and typhoid conjugate vaccine is indicated in addition to all routine vaccines. The vaccination schedules should be completed at least 2 weeks prior to splenectomy. In those who have undergone emergency splenectomy, superior functional antibody responses are obtained when the vaccination are done 2 weeks after splenectomy. All live vaccines may be safely given.

A special mention is to be made of Pneumococcal vaccines. Pneumococcal conjugate and polysaccharide vaccines are vital for all children with asplenia.

For those <2 years, with no PCV 13 administration or an incomplete schedule, the age appropriate schedule of PCV 13 is to be completed at least 2 weeks prior to splenectomy.

For those between 2 and 5 years, who have received 4 previous doses of PCV13 before 24 month of age, 1 dose of PPSV23 vaccine is recommended at 24 month of age, ≥8 week after last dose of PCV13.

For those between 2 and 5 years, who have received 3 previous doses of PCV13 before 24 months of age, 1 dose of PCV13 is recommended ≥8 week after the last dose of PCV13 and 1 dose of PPSV23 vaccine, ≥8 week after the last dose of PCV13.

For those between 2 and 5 years, who have received <3 previous doses of PCV13 before 24 month of age, 2 doses of PCV13 is recommended, ≥8 week after last dose of PCV13 (if applicable), at an interval of 8 weeks between doses and 1 dose of PPSV23 vaccine, ≥8 week after the last dose of PCV13.

For children 6 through 18 years of age who have not received PCV13, 1 supplemental dose of PCV13 should be administered. When splenectomy is planned for a patient 2 years or older who is PPSV23 naive, PPSV23 should be administered well in advance and at least 8 weeks after indicated dose(s) of PCV13 and at least 2 weeks before surgery.

Q17. What are the peculiarities of vaccinating children with HIV?

Ans. Children infected by human immunodeficiency virus (HIV) are vulnerable to severe, recurrent, or unusual infections by vaccine preventable pathogens. Risk of infection and response to vaccines are dependent on the degree of immune suppression which can be assessed by a recent CD4 count or CD4 cell percentage. Vaccination is usually safe and effective early in infancy before HIV infection causes severe immune suppression. The duration of protection may be compromised as there is impairment of memory response with immune attrition **(Table 2)**.

Table 2: Recommendation for immunization in HIV infected children.

Vaccine	Asymptomatic	Symptomatic
BCG	Yes (at birth)*	No
DTwP/DTaP/TT/Td/Tdap	Yes, at 6, 10, 14 weeks, 18 months, 5 years and 10 years	
Polio vaccines	IPV at 6, 10, 14 weeks, 16–18 months, and 5 years. Preferable to avoid OPV	
MR/MMR	Yes, at 9 months. Repeat at 15 month and 4–5 years	Yes, if CD4+ count >15%
Hib	Yes, at 6, 10, 14 weeks, 18 months	
Hepatitis B	Yes. Birth, 6-10-14 weeks	Yes, regular schedule, check for seroconversion and additional doses if necessary. Give regular boosters
Pneumococcal vaccines PCV	Yes, as per routine schedule at 6, 10, 14 weeks, and 12–15 months	
Pneumococcal vaccines PPSV23	If > 2 years; one dose 8 weeks after PCV, 2nd dose 5 years after first dose (not more than two doses)	
Influenza vaccine	Yes. Only inactivated vaccines. Beginning at 6 months, revaccination every year	
Rotavirus vaccine	Yes. Routine use	No
Hepatitis A vaccine	Yes, inactivated	Yes, check for seroconversion, boosters if needed
Varicella vaccine	Yes. Children ≥12 months of age: 2 doses 3–6 months apart. If not significantly immunocompromised	Yes, if CD4 count ≥15% in children <5 years for a duration ≥6 months, In those > 5 years, CD4 count >200/mm^3 for ≥6 months. Two doses 4–12 weeks apart
HPV vaccine	Yes (females only), as per routine schedule of 3 doses at 0, 1–2 and 6 months starting at 10 years of age	
Yellow fever vaccine	May be considered if CD4 count greater than 200 × 10^6/L (or if age 9 months-5 years and asymptomatic with CD4 ≥15%)	

* In asymptomatic babies born to HIV positive mothers, BCG vaccination may be deferred till virological studies establish that the baby is uninfected.

All inactivated vaccines can be administered when indicated. The immune response may be suboptimal. Serological documentation of response and repeated boosters and double doses (for hepatitis B vaccine) may be necessary. Live vaccines are generally contraindicated in the severely immunocompromised. Those with CD4 counts <15% or <200/mm^3 are considered as severely immunocompromised.

Q18. A 5 year boy with hemophilia is brought for vaccinations. What are the special considerations?

Ans. Children with bleeding disorders may be more prone to hematoma formation following intramuscular (IM) injections. When an IM route of administration is essential, it is preferable to schedule it after administration of replacement therapy. A 23G or thinner needle is to be used, firm pressure is to be given on injection site after the injection and the site should not be rubbed. Alternately, vaccines recommended by the IM route may be administered by the subcutaneous route, if the immune response and clinical reaction to these vaccines are expected to be comparable by either route of injection, such as Hepatitis A vaccine, Hib conjugate vaccine, IPV, pneumococcal polysaccharide vaccine, etc. Children with mild to moderate thrombocytopenia and platelet function defects, can be safely vaccinated with above precautions.

Q19. Why are children with chronic diseases considered as a special group for purposes of vaccination?

Ans. Chronic diseases may increase a person's risk of infection or increase a person's risk of more severe disease should infection occur. Frequent outpatient visits and hospitalizations render these children to an increased risk of nosocomial exposure to vaccine preventable diseases. Hence, the necessity that children with chronic diseases who are immunocompetent be immunized with both live and inactivated vaccines, according to routine immunization schedules. Vaccines may be less immunogenic in this population. Hence additional doses, or higher dosages of vaccines may be required to provide adequate protection. Ideally, vaccination is best accomplished early in the disease when the response is likely to be similar to other persons of a similar age with no chronic medical condition.

The necessity of hepatitis A vaccine in patients with liver disease and pertussis booster in those with stable neurologic disease is to be emphasized. Children with severe cardiac and pulmonary diseases should receive pneumococcal and annual influenza vaccines. In general, individuals with chronic disease are at higher risk of invasive pneumococcal disease (IPD), influenza and influenza-related complications, and should be immunized using the recommended vaccine and schedule.

Q20. What are the vaccine requirements for children scheduled for a cochlear implant?

Ans. Children with cochlear implants are more prone to bacterial meningitis than people without cochlear implants. Children due for cochlear implants may have anatomic factors that may increase their risk for meningitis. *Streptococcus pneumoniae* causes most cases of meningitis in children with cochlear implants.

People with cochlear implants or those who are receiving cochlear implants should receive all age appropriate vaccinations, including PCV, Hib and influenza vaccines. Children 24 months and older and adults should also receive a single dose of PPSV23 vaccine, 8 weeks after the last dose of PCV. The schedule should be completed at least 2 weeks prior to the implant. Children with CSF leaks also have similar vaccine requirements.

Q21. Why is vaccination of pregnant women so important?

Ans. The altered immune responses associated with pregnancy may result in an increased risk of infection and an increased risk of severe outcomes once infected. The fetus, neonate and young infant can also be affected by infections that can result in congenital abnormalities, impaired fetal growth or severe neonatal illness.

Inactivated vaccines are considered to be safe when administered in pregnancy.

Vaccines recommended for the protection of all pregnant women include: the inactivated influenza vaccine, at any time in pregnancy and the Tdap vaccine between 28 and 36 weeks of pregnancy. Other inactivated vaccines may be administered based on indications.

Live vaccines are contraindicated in pregnancy due to the theoretical risks to the developing fetus.

Q22. What is the course of action if a pregnant lady is inadvertently administered the MMR vaccine in the 1st trimester?

Ans. Smallpox vaccine is the only live vaccine with demonstrated teratogenicity. To date, there is no evidence demonstrating a teratogenic or other adverse effect from MMR or Varicella vaccine given during pregnancy. Inadvertent immunization with these vaccines is therefore not a reason for pregnancy termination.

Q23. Which are the vaccines contraindicated in a breastfeeding woman?

Ans. Yellow fever (YF) vaccine is the only vaccine contraindicated in a breast feeding woman. There have been three reported cases of probable transmission of YF vaccine strain virus from mothers to their infants through breastfeeding, resulting in meningoencephalitis in the infants.

Q24. Are there any special considerations in the vaccination of preterm and low birth weight babies?

Ans. Premature (<37 weeks GA) and low birth weight infants (<2 kg) in stable clinical condition, should be immunized with age-appropriate doses of vaccine at the same chronological age and according to the same schedule as full-term infants, with some exceptions.

All stable newborns can receive BCG. OPV should preferably be administered at discharge.

The immune response to hepatitis B (HB) vaccine may be diminished in infants with birth weight less than 2 kg. Routine HB immunization of infants should be delayed until 4 weeks of age, at which time it can be administered, irrespective of the weight at 4 weeks. In situations where the mother is HBsAg positive or where the birth dose is a routine, infants <2 kg can receive the birth dose, which should be considered as an invalid dose and the infant should receive 3 more doses of a HB containing vaccine.

Premature infants, especially those weighing less than 1,500 g at birth, are at higher risk of apnea and bradycardia following vaccination compared to full-term infants. Any increase or recurrence of apnea and bradycardia following vaccination of a premature infant is generally self-limited, subsides within 48 hours, and does not alter the infant's overall clinical progress. Hospitalized premature infants should have continuous cardiac and respiratory monitoring for 48 hours after their first immunization.

Q25. A 6 week preterm infant is still in the NICU for ongoing care. Can the infant receive all the vaccines due at 6 weeks?

Ans. In medically stable infants, all inactivated vaccines required at 6 weeks of age can be administered simultaneously to preterm or low birth weight infants, except for oral rotavirus vaccine, as this is a transmissible vaccine and can pose a risk to other sick newborns in the NICU. While rotavirus vaccine is to be deferred till discharge, IPV should be preferred over OPV.

■ SUGGESTED READING

1. AAP Committee on Infectious Diseases. Red Book. 2018–2021, 31st edition. Illinois: American Academy of Pediatrics; 2018.
2. Balasubramanian S. IAP Guidebook on Immunization 2018–2019, 3rd edition. Advisory Committee on Vaccines and Immunization Practices, Indian Academy of Pediatrics. New Delhi: Jaypee Brothers Medical Publishers (P) Ltd.; 2020.
3. Levin MJ. Varicella vaccination of immunocompromised children. J Infect Dis. 2008;197:S200-6.
4. Medical Advisory Committee of the Immune Deficiency Foundation. Recommendations for live viral and bacterial vaccines in immunodeficient patients and their close-contacts. J Allergy Clin Immunol. 2014;133(4):961-6.
5. Principi N, Esposito S. Vaccine use in primary immunodeficiency disorders. Vaccine. 2014;32:3725-31.
6. Rubin LG, Levin MJ, Ljungman P, Davies EG, Avery R, Tomblyn M, et al. 2013 IDSA Clinical practice guideline for vaccination of the immunocompromised host. Clin Infect Dis. 2014;58(3):309-18.

CHAPTER 9

Vaccine Safety

Srinivas G Kasi

Q1. What is vaccine safety?

Ans. It is the process of ensuring and monitoring all aspects of immunization safety from the conception of the vaccine till the administration to the individual and beyond.

Q2. Why is vaccine safety important?

Ans. Vaccines are generally given to healthy populations to prevent disease. Hence, higher standard of safety is generally expected of vaccines than of other medical interventions including other drugs. Public are intolerant to even minor adverse reactions related to products given to healthy people, especially healthy babies. An erroneous association or attributable risk can undermine confidence in a vaccine and have disastrous consequences for vaccine acceptance, vaccination programs and disease incidence.

There are three important reasons for continued assessment of vaccine safety:

1. The most important reason is to detect rare reactions that happen rarely and cannot be detected in phase 3 studies. If serious reactions are found when the vaccine is in widespread use, the vaccine may be withdrawn.
2. To assure safety in special groups, such as the elderly, those with chronic medical conditions, and pregnant women. Vaccine trials may deliberately exclude members of these groups.
3. Monitoring vaccine safety also helps to maintain public confidence needed to keep enough people vaccinated to prevent disease outbreaks.

Q3. What is the vaccine safety paradox?

Ans. Vaccines have become the victims of their own success. With progressively increased coverage of vaccinations, especially against the life-threatening diseases, society is no longer exposed to these devastating illnesses. On the other hand, adverse effects due to vaccines get highlighted, widely disseminated and leads to loss of confidence in vaccine. The antivaccine lobbies utilize these events to compound the opposition to vaccines. All this leads to a reduction of uptake of vaccines and the consequent increase in the diseases that they prevent. In the recent past, opposition to whole cell pertussis vaccines in Japan and Sweden led to a massive resurgence of these diseases. More recently, opposition to measles/MMR vaccines has led to a massive resurgence of Measles in Europe and USA. The question often raised is, "If there is no discernible risk from the infectious disease concerned, why should one take the risk of being vaccinated against it in the first place?"

Q4. Are there instances where vaccine safety was an issue?

Ans. Yes. There are instances wherein the issues with vaccine quality led to tragedies. Pasteur's Rabies vaccine caused neurological adverse effect in 1 in 230 recipients.

In 1942, hundreds of thousands of American servicemen were injected with a yellow fever vaccine to which human serum was added as a stabilizer which was unknowingly infected with hepatitis B virus. As a consequence, 330,000 soldiers were infected, severe hepatitis developed in 50,000, and 62 died.

The Cutter Tragedy, in which inadequately inactivated IPV was administered in 1955. In 40,000, mild polio developed, 200 were permanently paralyzed, and 10 were killed.

Q5. How is vaccine safety assured during development of the vaccine and later?

Ans. Vaccine safety is assessed rigorously in all stages of development to ensure quality, safety and efficacy:
- First, computers are used to predict how the vaccine will interact with the immune system. Then researchers test the vaccine on animals including mice, guinea pigs, rabbits, and monkeys, predominantly to assess safety. After the vaccine completes these laboratory tests successfully, it is given the permission for its use in clinical studies on human subjects. It now progresses to phase 1 studies in humans.
- *Phase I/1*: Assess the safety and obtain limited immunogenicity and dosing data. This is done in a small number of healthy adults, n = 10–50. Data obtained in this stage determines the progress to phase 2.
- *Phase II/2*: Assess common reactions and obtain immunogenicity data in infants and other age groups. The number of subjects is more (100–200). Favorable data from phase 2 determines progress to phase 3.
- *Phase III/3*: Assess protective efficacy, identify laboratory correlates of protection, assess rarer reactions. The number of subjects is determined by the targeted disease. In the phase 3 studies of the rotavirus vaccines, the subject numbers exceeded 60,000.

Following these clinical trials, permission is sought from the National Regulatory Authorities (NRA) for licensure and marketing of the vaccine. The NRA re-examines all the data, asks for clarifications and if satisfied, licensure is granted. Two types of licensures are necessary—product licensure and process (manufacturing) licensure.

Q6. How is safety assured during the manufacturing process?

Ans. Numerous regulations ensure the safety and quality of vaccines. They include the precise identification (characterization) of starting materials, compliance with the principles of good manufacturing practices, the use of detailed control procedures, and the independent release of vaccines on a lot-by-lot basis by national regulatory authorities. Responsibility for quality and safety rests with the national regulatory authority (NRA) in the country of manufacture and, where exported, with the NRAs of the receiving countries. In India, the NRA is the Drug Controller General of India (DCGI).

Q7. What are the implications of World Health Organization (WHO) prequalification?

Ans. WHO prequalification of vaccines is a comprehensive assessment that takes place through a standardized procedure aimed at determining whether the product meets requirements for safety and efficacy in immunization programs. The full prequalification assessment process includes the following components:
- Review of production process and quality control procedures.
- Laboratory testing.
- WHO site audit of manufacturing facilities with the responsible NRA.

Once a vaccine is prequalified and introduced to the market, WHO ensures it continues to meet standards through:
- Reassessments at regular intervals.
- Targeted testing of lots supplied through UN agencies.
- Investigating any complaints from the field and reports of adverse events following immunization (AEFI).

Q8. Does safety assessment end with vaccine licensure?

Ans. No. Safety assessment does not end with licensure of a vaccine as phase 3 studies cannot detect rare adverse effects or AE occurring a few years after vaccination. Rare side effects and delayed reactions may not be evident until the vaccine is administered to millions of people.

Q9. What are the objectives of postlicensure surveillance?

Ans.
- Identify rare reactions which were not detected in phase 3 studies
- Identify increases in known adverse reactions
- Identify occurrence of new adverse reactions, e.g., intussusception after rotavirus vaccination
- Identify preexisting illnesses that may increase incidence of adverse reactions
- Identify defective vaccine lots.

Q10. How is postlicensure surveillance done?

Ans. After a vaccine is licensed for public use, its safety is monitored continually. The NRA requires all manufacturers to submit samples from each vaccine lot prior to its release. In addition, the manufacturers must provide the NRA with their test results for vaccine safety, potency, and purity. Each lot must be tested because vaccines are sensitive to environmental factors like temperature, and can be contaminated during production.

Robust vaccine adverse event reporting systems exist in most of the developed countries which monitor AEs by active or passive surveillance systems. When an AE is reported, studies are done to establish causality by internationally accepted protocols and monetary compensation is offered to the victim/family. This results in confidence in the vaccination program. Recognizing the fact that vaccines may have AEs, which may lead to loss of confidence in immunization programs, the WHO in 2003, initiated the Vaccine Safety Network (VSN). As part of this network, the global advisory committee on vaccine safety (GACVS) was formed with a mandate to respond immediately when AE occurs with a new vaccine introduction in the NIPs.

The WHO and the Government of India have published guidelines for surveillance and response to AEFIs.

Q11. Who is responsible for assurance of vaccine safety?

Ans. Almost all national immunization programs in developed countries have a system for reporting adverse events. The United States Vaccine Adverse Event Reporting System (VAERS), the Canadian Adverse Events following Immunization Surveillance System (CAEFISS) and the Yellow card system in UK, are examples. In most developing countries, the NRA in conjunction with Global Advisory Committee on Vaccine Safety (GACVS) of the WHO are responsible for vaccine safety **(Fig. 1)**.

The GACVS was set up in 1999 to provide the WHO with independent advice on vaccine safety issues. The role of the GACVS is both to analyze and to interpret reports of the adverse effects of vaccines that impact on global vaccination programs and strategies, and to foster the development of improved surveillance systems to detect any adverse effects of vaccines, particularly in low- and middle-income countries. It also monitors the development of new vaccines during clinical testing and advises on the safe use of vaccines in immunization programs.

Q12. What are the types of post-marketing surveillance?

Ans.
These are of two types:
1. *Active*: This includes phase 4 studies by the manufacturers. In USA, large linked databases and tertiary clinical centers conduct active surveillance.

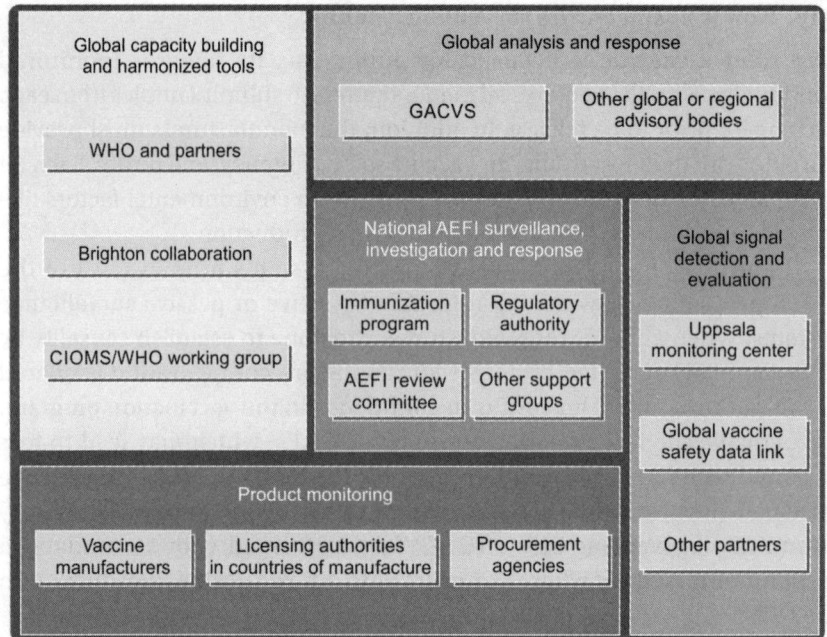

Fig. 1: Components of a 21st century global vaccine safety monitoring, investigation and response system.
Source: Global Advisory Committee on Vaccine Safety (GACVS); WHO secretariat. Global safety of vaccines: strengthening systems for monitoring, management and the role of GACVS. Expert Rev. Vaccines. 2009;8(6):705-16.

2. *Passive*: This is a spontaneous reporting system which is relatively easier to implement, and has the ability to capture unexpected events. The system depends on reporting by the patients, caregivers and health care professionals (HCPs). Only data collection and integration are done. No causality assessment is done, e.g., Vaccine Adverse Event Reporting System (VAERS) in USA.

Q13. What is the role of the pediatrician in assuring vaccine safety in office practice?

Ans.
- Use approved vaccines with peer-reviewed, published immunogenicity/efficacy studies
- Anticipatory guidance should be provided to parents and vaccinees about common side effects such as fever, pain, fainting, etc.
- Use the right vaccines at the right age
- Administer vaccine at appropriate site, route, and position
- Observe valid precautions and contraindications
- Observe the proper cold chain maintenance protocol and expiry dates
- Follow safe injection practices

- Maintain records
- Observe every vaccinated child for 15 min following vaccination
- Be ready for emergencies: Adrenaline, O_2, steroids, IV apparatus
- Have a plan of action ready for any eventuality.

■ SUGGESTED READING

1. Global Advisory Committee on Vaccine Safety (GACVS); WHO secretariat. Global safety of vaccines: strengthening systems for monitoring, management and the role of GACVS. Expert Rev. Vaccines. 2009;8(6):705-16.
2. National Academy of Sciences. Adverse Effects of Vaccines: Evidence and Causality. [online] Available from: http://www.nap.edu/catalog.php?record_id=13164. [Last Accessed October, 2020].
3. WHO. Vaccine safety in immunization programs. [online] Available from: http://vaccine-safety-training.org/vaccine-safety-in-immunization-programmes.html. [Last Accessed October, 2020].

CHAPTER 10: Setting Up a Vaccination Clinic

Vijay Kumar Guduru, Srinivas G Kasi

Q1. What is the importance of vaccination clinics?

Ans. Vaccination service is an important and integral part of any pediatric service, whether hospital based or office practice based. The children availing these services are generally healthy and should not get exposed to infections during the vaccination procedure. While exclusive vaccination areas may not be feasible in office practice, it should be the norm in hospitals.

Q2. How do vaccination clinics work in public sector?

Ans. Exclusive vaccination clinic is conducted in every Primary Health Centre, throughout the country on Wednesdays. Trained staff in specified area, conduct the vaccination session for identified well babies.

Q3. What are some of the special prerequisites of vaccination clinics?

Ans. The needs of children availing vaccination services are different from the needs of sick children who avail of these services. Some of these issues are: segregating vaccination areas from infected areas, appropriate prevaccination screening, following all safe immunization practices during vaccination, observing for reactions, counseling for further doses. All this is to be done with minimum possible waiting and inconvenience.

Q4. What is the suggested layout of a vaccination clinic in a hospital setting?

Ans. The location should be in an accessible part of the hospital but separate from the general OPDs, where sick children are attended to. It should be setup as unidirectional flow. The attendees begin at the waiting area (prevaccination eligibility and medical screening, counseling about the vaccines to be administered) → vaccination area → postvaccination observation area → exit at a location distant from the entrance (*see* suggested layout plan in **Figure 1**).

Q5. What are the requirements of the waiting area?

Ans. The waiting area should be large enough to provide comfortable seating for at least five children, each with two caregivers. It should have handouts and information material about vaccinations and general health

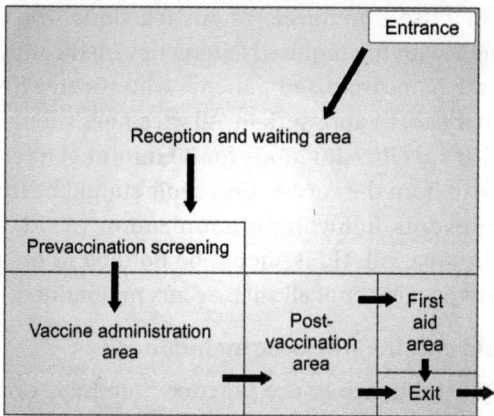

Fig. 1: Layout of a vaccination clinic.

perspectives for children. It should be preferably staffed with a receptionist and 1–2 counselors, who will conduct the prevaccination eligibility, medical screening and counsel about the vaccines to be administered. The waiting area should have clean toilets and drinking water availability. Hand sanitizer, fixed in a no-touch stand and surgical masks should be available.

Q6. What are the requirements of the vaccination area?

Ans. The vaccination area should have adequate lighting, ventilation, hand washing sink and an examination table/couch for administering the vaccine. The refrigerator/ice lined refrigerator should be placed in a corner away from doors and windows and not exposed directly to sunlight. The refrigerator/ice-lined refrigerator (ILR) should be placed at least 10 cm away from the walls to permit adequate circulation of air around it. This should be an exclusive vaccine fridge and nothing else should be stored in it. Back-up power facilities should be available (*see* chapter on Cold Chain). A cupboard should be available to store syringes, needles, swabs and other equipment necessary for the vaccine administration process. This cupboard may also store vaccination cards, record keeping register and information material. This cupboard should be close to the vaccine preparation area, which in turn should be in a location not easily visualized by the child, due for the vaccination. The exit from this room should open into the postvaccination observation area. All efforts should be made to keep records in electronic form. It not only saves space, but it also helps in sending vaccine reminders easily, helps in easy maintenance of inventory and gives an indication if a vaccine is nearing expiry.

Q7. What are the requirements of the postvaccination observation area?

Ans. This should be adjacent to the vaccination area, with seating area, a transparent screen to observe children, from the vaccination area, where the medical staff will be present. A shielded corner should be made to render first aid to those who develop some reactions. The corner should be stocked adequately with the required emergency medications and an oxygen cylinder. Medically compromised patients who receive first aid should be referred for further care as appropriate. All vaccinees should be made to wait for 15 minutes (in specific situations for 30 minutes) after the vaccination procedure. The exit from the vaccination clinic should be from this area.

The adverse events following immunization (AEFI) form should be completed in this area. All AEFIs should be notified to the concerned DIO/SMO and a record or register of all such events maintained.

Q8. How should vaccine stocks be maintained?

Ans. Depending on the size of the practice, purchase orders for different vaccines should be made. Purchase vouchers with details of quantity of vaccines indented, manufacturer, date of expiry should be filed and maintained in a stock register. Syringes, needles (22–25 gauge in various lengths), alcohol wipes, spot and rectangular Band-Aids, gauze or cotton balls, are among the needed basic supplies. Date-wise vaccination session details are maintained in a second register. A third vaccine expenditure register is maintained in addition to stock register. All stock returned to the retailer and reason for return should be entered in the stock register. It is advisable not to stock more than a month's vaccine requirements.

Q9. What are the emergency drugs and medical equipment that should be available in the first-aid area?

Ans. All health facilities, including exclusive pediatric clinics which offer vaccinations, should keep ready the emergency resuscitation kit in case of a rare anaphylaxis or other adverse events in the clinic itself immediately.

The kit contains:
- Inj. Epinephrine (adrenaline), Inj. Chlorpheniramine maleate vial, and Inj. Hydrocortisone (expiry dates should be checked regularly)
- Syringes 1 mL, 2 mL, 5 mL and 20 mL
- Normal saline for infusion, IV cannula, tape and splint
- Self-inflating (Ambu) bag, infant, child and adult sizes, face masks—infant, child and adult, laryngeal mask airway (LMA).
- Airways, small, medium and large, laryngoscope with different size blades, pulse-oximeter, Stethoscope, Sphygmomanometer with infant, child and large cuffs
- Portable oxygen cylinder in a good working condition
- Agreement with transport facility (licensed ambulance service) to shift a child if needed to the nearest hospital.

Q10. How are these guidelines to be adapted in office practice?

Ans. Vaccination in office practice has two main drawbacks: (1) lack of adequate space, (2) mixing of healthy and sick children in the common waiting area. These drawbacks can be overcome by having exclusive vaccination timings, generally the 1st hour in each session, to avoid mixing of healthy and sick children in the common waiting area. Separate areas for vaccination and postvaccination observation may not be possible. This can be overcome by insisting that the child wait in the reception area for 15–30 minutes after vaccination and report immediately any untoward happening.

Every pediatrician who runs a vaccination clinic should be well-versed with current immunization recommendations, clear understanding of all individual and combination vaccines, age and route of administration of different vaccines, vaccines to be used in special situations within the scope of his practice, special precautions and contraindications, availability/scarcity of a brand, interchangeability of different brands, purchase and maintain supplies, follow vaccine storage protocols, temperature monitoring and recording, ensure competence of his/her support staff, identifying back-up person trained in all skills and experience to run this clinic.

■ SUGGESTED READING

1. Carr C, Durrheim D, Eastwood K, Massey P, Jaggers D, Caelli, M, et al. Australia's first pandemic influenza mass vaccination clinic exercise. Aus J Emerg Manag. 2011;26(1):47-53.
2. Centers for Disease Control and Prevention. Resources for Hosting a Vaccination Clinic. [online] Available from: https://www.cdc.gov/flu/business/hosting-vaccination-clinic.htm. [Last Accessed October, 2020].
3. Department of State Health Services. Starting a Vaccination Clinic. [online] Available from: https://dshs.texas.gov/immunize/nurse/default.shtm. [Last Accessed October, 2020].
4. Immunization Action Coalition. Setting Up for Vaccination Service. [online] Available from: https://www.immunize.org/guide/pdfs/vacc-adults-step2.pdf. [Last Accessed October, 2020].
5. Immunization Action Coalition. Setting Up for Vaccination Services: Vaccinating Adults: A Step-by-Step Guide. [online] Available from: www.immunize.org and www.vaccineinformation.org. [Last Accessed October, 2020].

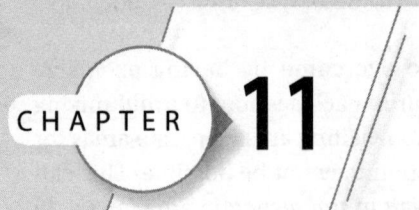

CHAPTER 11: Combination Vaccines

P Sivaraman

Q1. What is a combination vaccine?

Ans. A combination vaccine consists of two or more separate immunogens that have been physically combined in a single preparation.

Q2. Which was the first combination vaccine?

Ans. The first combination vaccine licensed was trivalent influenza vaccine approved in 1945 and the second was the hexavalent polysaccharide pneumococcal vaccine in 1947. Diphtheria and tetanus toxoids and whole-cell pertussis vaccine (DTwP) was licensed in 1948.

Q3. What are the advantages and disadvantages of combination vaccines?

Ans. The advantages to the consumer are reduced number of injections, reduced healthcare visits, reduced parental anxiety and easy record keeping. The advantages to health planner are reduced burden on shipping, handlings and cold storage space, decreased possibility of errors, increased compliance, increased coverage and reduced paper work. The disadvantages are adverse events that might occur more frequently, reduced immunogenicity of one or more components, and a shorter shelf life than the individual component vaccines.

Q4. Does reduced immunogenicity of some combination vaccines result in reduced efficacy?

Ans. Even if the antibody concentrations induced by the combination vaccine are lower than those induced by the monocomponent vaccines, a protective antibody level is attained. There is no need for an efficacy trial for a combination vaccine that has proven efficacy when administered individually. Instead only a demonstration of adequate immunogenicity is required.

Q5. What are the other factors to be considered while producing combination vaccines?

Ans. The immune response to vaccine may be altered by chemical or physical interactions among the vaccine components being combined. Other components including adjuvants, preservatives, buffers, stabilizers and excipients included in one vaccine may interfere with the components of another vaccine (e.g., thimerosal inactivates IPV or combination of an adjuvanted component may interfere with the potency of an unadjuvanted component).

When combining different live-attenuated viral vaccine strains, competition between the viruses may interfere with immunogenicity of some components. This can be overcome by increasing the content of the virus which induces a suboptimal response, e.g., OPV, MMRV.

Q6. What is carrier-induced epitope modification?

Ans. Carrier-induced epitope-specific modification (suppression or enhancement) of the immune response is a phenomenon in which the antibody responses to the epitopes on a carrier protein are modified by prior administration of the same carrier protein. Concurrent administration of two conjugate vaccines using the same carrier may also lead to interference and reduced immunogenicity of the vaccine administered second. Thus, administration of pneumococcal conjugate vaccines and quadrivalent meningococcal vaccines in asplenic children simultaneously may result in reduced immunogenicity of some pneumococcal conjugate vaccine (PCV) serotypes. In this situation, PCV should be administered first followed by quadrivalent-meningococcal conjugate vaccine (Q-MCV) 4 weeks later.

Q7. What do the symbols + , / and // indicate while using combination vaccine?

Ans.

Plus (+): The vaccines linked by plus sign are administered at separate sites during a single vaccination session. *Example*: DTaP + Hib two separate vaccines given separately but at the same visit.

Single (/): The vaccines linked by a single virgule are premixed from the manufacturer and are administered in a single injection. *Example*: DTaP / Hib; the two vaccines are shipped by the manufacture mixed together in a single container.

Double (//): The liquid vaccine(s) preceding the double virgule are used to reconstitute the dry vaccine following the double virgule. *Example*: DTaP // Hib; the manufacturer ships together a container of liquid DTaP and container of Powder Hib, with the DTaP used to reconstitute the Hib and the resulting mixture administered as a single injection.

Q8. What are the currently available combination vaccines licensed in India?

Ans.
- DTwP / Hib
- DTWP / Hib / HepB

- DTwP / Hib / HepB / IPV
- MMR
- MMRV
- DTaP / Hib / IPV
- DTaP / Hib / HepB / IPV

Strictly speaking, even DPT, OPV, IPV, PCV, Q-MCV, influenza vaccines are all combination vaccines.

Q9. What are the types of combination vaccine?

Ans. Combination vaccines are either single pathogen or multiple pathogen vaccines. Single pathogen vaccines contain various antigens or serotypes of a pathogen, e.g., OPV, IPV, Rota virus, HPV, PCV. Multiple pathogen vaccines contain various antigens or serotypes from multiple pathogens, e.g., DPwT, DTaP, DTa/P/Hib/IPV/MMR.

Q10. Can we interchange the different brands of combination vaccines?

Ans. Certain vaccines such as Hib, HepB, HepA and quadrivalent MCV can be interchanged within their respective series. For DTaP vaccine alone it is recommended not to change the brand as there are no data on the interchangeability of the products. But if brand is not available or not known then any licensed appropriate brand can be used.

Q11. What is a second shot or companion combination?

Ans. A DTaP-based combination that incorporates a conjugate meningococcal antigen or a pneumococcal is a second shot vaccine.

Q12. What is a simultaneous/concurrent vaccination?

Ans. Simultaneous/concurrent vaccination implies vaccines that are administered at the same time but at separate sites or separate routes.

Q13. A baby has been administered a dose of Hepatitis B at birth. Can you give 3 dose of the combined vaccine containing hepatitis B, thereby giving four doses?

Ans. When a patient has a recommended immunization for some of the components in a combination vaccine, administering the extra antigen(s) in the combination vaccine is permissible, if the extra antigen is not contraindicated and its administration will not result in increased reactogenicity.

Some antigens, e.g., diphtheria toxoid and tetanus toxoid, are associated with increased adverse effects if administered too frequently.

Q14. What is an ad-hoc combination?

Ans. Ad-hoc combination is a combination vaccine wherein the healthcare provider creates their own combination by mixing separate vaccine in the same syringe without establishing the stability, safety and immunogenicity of the resultant combination as reflected in the package inserts. This is not permitted.

Q15. Does giving too many vaccines cause immune overload?

Ans. There is no evidence to support such an assertion and there is evidence to refute it. A concern that infant immune system may be overwhelmed by simultaneous exposures to several antigens is difficult to entertain when one considers the thousands of antigens to which a newborn is naturally exposed in the first few months of life. Moreover although many vaccines are administered today, fewer antigens are delivered than in the past, when DTwP was used routinely.

Q16. Are combination vaccines safe?

Ans. Systemic adverse events are increased only modestly, after concurrent administration of multiple vaccines compared with events after the administration of the most reactogenic vaccine alone. Local adverse events often are somewhat more common and more severe at the combination vaccine site. No combination vaccine has elicited a new type of reaction not previously seen with its separate components. Combination vaccines do not cause type 1 diabetes or asthma.

Q17. Can we switch back and forth from separate vaccines at one visit to combination vaccines at another visit?

Ans. Switching between combination and single antigen vaccines poses no problem as long as you maintain the recommended minimum intervals for all vaccines and the vaccines are licensed for the age of the patient.

Q18. How should we record combination vaccines on paper records (e.g., parent-maintained records, non-computerized office system)?

Ans. You should records the generic abbreviation for the type of vaccine given (e.g., DTaP/IPV/Hep B) in each of the sections that correspond to the separate antigens listed on the record (e.g., DTaP section, Polio section, hepatitis B section). If possible avoid using trade names, since trade names could be misinterpreted or discontinued.

■ SUGGESTED READING

1. American Academy of Pediatrics. Red book, 2018–2021, 31st edition. Illinois: AAP; 2018.
2. CDC. National Center for Immunization and Respiratory Diseases general recommendations of the Advisory Committee on Immunization Practices (ACIP). MMWR Recomm Rep. 2011;60:1-64.

3. Decker MD, Edwards KM, Bogaerts II. Combination vaccines. In: Plotkin SA, Orenstein WA, Offit PA (Eds). Vaccines, 4th edition. Philadelphia: WB Saunder; 2004. pp. 825-61.
4. Halsey NA. Safety of combination vaccines: perception versus reality. Pediatr Infect Dis J. 2001;20(Suppl) S40-S318.
5. Marin M, Broder KR, Temte JL, Snider DE, Seward JF, Centers for Disease Control and Prevention. Use of combination measles, mumps, rubella, and varicella vaccine: recommendation of the Advisory Committee on Immunization Practices (ACIP). MMWR Recomm Rep. 2010;59(RR-3):1-12.
6. National Center for Immunization and Respiratory Diseases general recommendations of the Advisory Committee on Immunization Practices (ACIP). MMWR Recomm Rep. 2011;60:1-64.
7. Plotkin S, Orenstein W, Offit P, Edwards KM. Combination vaccines. In: Plotkin's Vaccines, 7th edition. Gurugram: Elsevier India Limited; 2017.
8. Singhal T, Amdekar YK, Agrawal RK. IAP Guidebook on Immunization. New Delhi: Jaypee Brothers Medical Publishers (P) Ltd.; 2009.

CHAPTER 12

Immunoglobulins for Passive Protection against Vaccine-Preventable Diseases

Raju C Shah, Pratima Shah

Q1. What are Immunoglobulins?

Ans. Immunoglobulins are pooled preformed antibodies which are derived from either human (homologous) or animal, usually horses (heterologous) sources. They are used to provide passive protection against certain infectious diseases. This protection is temporary as the antibodies will degrade over a period of time (a few weeks as the half-life of human immunoglobulins is usually 10–21 days) and the recipient will no longer be protected thereafter.

Initially the use was limited to intramuscular (IM) use as untreated immunoglobulins when administered intravenously (IV) evoke severe reactions. The IM route restricts the quantity of immune globulins that can be injected, which was suboptimal in treating many conditions including primary immune deficiency (PID). With the advent of purification and better treatment processes, intravenous immunoglobulin G (IVIG) was first ever licensed in 1981 by FDA which helped the clinicians to administer large doses of immunoglobulin G in treating various conditions.

Various products of immunoglobulins available can be categorized as follows:
- Standard immunoglobulins (IG) for intramuscular administration (IMIG)
- Subcutaneous immunoglobulins (SCIG)
- *Hyperimmune globulins*: Most of them are for intramuscular use, few are available for IV use. Some of these preparations are of animal origin also.
- Intravenous immunoglobulins G (IGIV)
- Anti-D immune globulins
- Monoclonal antibodies (mAbs).

Q2. How are intravenous immunoglobulins prepared?

Ans. Pooled plasma of minimum 1,000 donors undergoes cold alcohol fractionation for isolating immunoglobulin containing fraction. Further purification techniques and additional precipitation steps are applied to remove non-immunoglobulin G proteins. It undergoes ion exchange chromatography to further separate and purify IgG. Following further purification steps, the final product contains almost 96% of immunoglobulin G and small quantities of IgM and IgA. All the donors are screened for the markers of certain viruses such as Hepatitis B, Hepatitis C, HIV 1 and 2, West Nile virus, HTLV 1 and 2 and parasites *Treponema pallidum* and *T. cruzi*. Several brands use certain other steps including low pH treatment, solvent detergent treatment, fatty acid/alcohol treatment and/or pasteurization taken during process so as to minimize transmission of most of the likely pathogens. To remove potential prions these products also undergo nanofiltration or depth filtration.

Q3. What are the indications for use of immunoglobulins?

Ans. Indications for use of immunoglobulins can be grouped into three categories:
1. Protection against infections—especially in immunodeficiency or antibody deficiency and hypogammaglobulinemic states. It works by replacement mechanism.
2. Suppression of autoimmune or inflammatory process—by several immunomodulatory and anti-inflammatory mechanisms.
3. Alloimmunization especially in setting of RhD-negative mother with potentially RhD positive fetus. It works by elimination of circulating Rh-positive fetal cells from maternal circulation preventing maternal Rh-sensitization.

Q4. How does it protect against infections?

Ans. Immune globulins: In children having immunodeficiency states, antibody deficiency disorders or hypogammaglobulinemic state IVIG or other immune globulin products will provide adequate concentration of antibodies against a broad range of pathogens to protect them until sometime.

Hyperimmune globulins: These products are generated from individuals having high-titer antibodies against certain organisms or antigens and are used in a setting of a known or expected exposure to that organism.

The mechanisms of action of Ig not only involve the blockade of Fc receptors of phagocytes, but also control complement pathways, idiotype-anti-idiotype dimer formation, blockage of superantigen binding to T cells, inhibition of dendritic cells and stimulation of regulatory T cells (Tregs).

Q5. What are the indications for the use of intravenous immune globulins?

Ans.
- Immunodeficiency states:
  - Primary immunodeficiencies—congenital/hereditary
  - Pre- or posthematopoietic cell transplantation (HCT)
  - Therapies that suppress immunoglobulin production—secondary immunodeficiency induced by biologic products
  - Chronic lymphocytic leukemia
- Multiple myloma

- *Severe protein loss*: GI loss or renal loss
- Infections:
  - Measles postexposure prophylaxis
  - Chronic parvovirus infection with severe anemia
  - Chronic lymphocytic leukemia with recurrent infections
  - Toxic shock syndrome as adjunct therapy
  - Severe sepsis in premature newborns as adjunct therapy
  - Some enteroviral infections
  - Varicella infection in immune compromised host if specific immunoglobulins not available
  - Active EBV infection
  - Active CMV infection if specific immunoglobulins not available
- Autoimmune or inflammatory conditions:
  - Kawasaki disease
  - Immune thrombocytopenia
  - Neonatal alloimmune thrombocytopenia
  - Guillain-Barré syndrome
  - Autoimmune hemolytic anemia
  - ADEM
  - NNDM encephalitis
  - Myasthenia gravis
  - Multifocal motor neuropathy
  - Autoimmune neutropenia
  - Autoimmune lymphoproliferative disorder (ALPS)
  - Hemophagocytic lymphohistiocytosis (HLH)
  - Macrophage activation syndrome (MAS) in systemic vascular inflammatory diseases such as rheumatoid arthritis (RA) or systemic lupus erythematosus (SLE)
- Autoimmune processes:
  - Hemolytic disease of fetus and newborn
  - Post-transfusion purpura
  - Antibody-mediated organ transplant rejection
  - Hyperhemolytic crisis
  - Platelet alloimmunization with bleeding.

Q6. What are the uses of hyperimmune globulins?

Ans. Hyperimmune globulins are recommended when a child is exposed to certain pathogens and the child is either not vaccinated and is at high risk for complications or vaccines are not available for that infection and the infection carries significant morbidity and mortality. These are available for use by intravenous or intramuscular route.

Some infection prophylaxis and/or therapy are as follows:
- Hepatitis b immunoglobulin (HBIG)—for use in infants born to hepatitis B infected mother, nonvaccinated child exposed to HBV, HBV infected

child undergoing liver transplant, postexposure prophylaxis to non-responders to hepatitis B vaccine
- Varicella Zoster immunoglobulin (VariZIG)—postexposure prophylaxis and specifically to HCT recipient not yet reimmunized
- Rabies immunoglobulins—human and equine for postexposure prophylaxis. Now monoclonal antibodies are available for this indication
- Tetanus immunoglobulins—for treatment of tetanus as well as postexposure prophylaxis in a child with puncture or road traffic wound
- Diphtheria immunoglobulins—for management of diphtheria—human or animal IG
- Cytomegalovirus immune globulins (CMVIG) as postexposure prophylaxis
- Botulism immunoglobulin—for treatment of botulism in infants less than 1 year
- Vaccinia immune globulins—for selected cases of inadvertent inoculation or complication of vaccinia.

Q7. What are the doses of IVIG?

Ans. Doses differ as per the indication of the condition for which it is prescribed.

Immune deficiencies: For replacement therapy IVIG is usually used in doses of 400–800 mg/kg/month. They are given as slow infusions every 3–4 weeks. If subcutaneous immunoglobulin therapy is used as replacement, lower weekly doses are used in range of 100–150 mg/kg/week.

Inflammatory/Autoimmune disorders: In children needing anti-inflammatory or immune modulatory effect of IVIG, high doses of IVIG are usually recommended. Patients of Kawasaki disease requires dose of 2 g/kg as a single dose. In other conditions and in older patients who are predisposed to thrombosis or other complications, needing therapeutic doses of IVIG of larger than 1 g/kg, it is recommended to give in multiple increments divided over several consecutive days so as not to give more than 500 mg/kg in a 24-hour period.

Q8. What are the doses for prophylaxis and management in certain infective conditions?

Ans. Hyperimmune globulins are used in the setting of specific exposures. These products can be administered intravenously or intramuscularly.

Specific infection prophylaxis and therapy include the following:

Hepatitis B: To prevent perinatal transmission

As soon as possible and within 12 hours after birth, infants born to women who are HBsAg-positive or women whose prenatal HBsAg results are not available at the time of delivery but who have other evidence of maternal HBV infection—HBIG 0.5 mL IM.

For exposure to hepatitis B beyond the newborn period, HBIG is indicated in the nonimmune subject at a dose of HBIG 0.06 mL/kg IM once.

Hepatitis A, prophylaxis
Infants, children, and adolescents: Consider splitting doses <10 mL based on patient size.

Pre-exposure prophylaxis upon travel into endemic areas (CDC 2017):
For those younger than 6 months:
1. Anticipated duration of risk ≤1 month: IM: 0.1 mL/kg/dose as a single dose
   Anticipated duration of risk 1-2 months: IM: 0.2 mL/kg/dose
   Anticipated duration of risk ≥2 months: IM: 0.2 mL/kg/dose every 2 months

For those 6-11 months of age:
1. Dose of inactivated Hep A vaccine. This dose should not be counted toward the routine 2-dose series, which should be initiated at age 12 months.
Postexposure prophylaxis: Younger than 6 months: IM: 0.1 mL/kg/dose as a single dose given within 14 days of exposure and prior to manifestation of disease.

Varicella-zoster, postexposure prophylaxis (independent of HIV-status)
Who needs passive protection?
- Immunocompromised child
- Pregnant women
- Newborn, whose mother has developed varicella within 5 days before and 48 hours after delivery.
- Hospitalized preterm infants (>28 weeks GA), mother has no immunity against varicella
- Hospitalized preterm infants (<28 weeks GA) or birth weight <1,000 g, irrespective of maternal immunity status.

VZIG-IM (if available): 125 U/10 kg body weight to a maximum of 625 U. 62.5 U if <2 kg.

IVIG: *Note:* Use only if varicella-zoster immune globulin is unavailable.

IV: 400 mg/kg as a single infusion as soon as possible and within 10 days of exposure; ideally within 96 hours of exposure.

IM: 0.6-1.2 mL/kg/dose as a single dose within 72 hours of exposure (in pediatric patients, consider splitting doses <10 mL based on patient size).

Measles, prophylaxis
Pre-exposure prophylaxis *(e.g., during an outbreak, travel to endemic area):*
In those ineligible to receive vaccine

IV: 400 mg/kg/dose within 3 weeks before anticipated exposure.

Subcutaneous: 200 mg/kg/dose once weekly for 2 consecutive weeks prior to anticipated exposure

Postexposure prophylaxis

Measles vaccine, if administered within 72 hours after exposure, to susceptible individuals, may prevent or modify the disease and is the intervention of choice for postexposure prophylaxis in immunocompetent hosts.

For those ineligible to receive the vaccine:

IM: 0.5 mL/kg/dose; maximum dose: 15 mL within 6 days of exposure; in adults, doses >10 mL should be split into multiple injections and administered at different sites; in pediatric patients, may also split doses <10 mL based on patient size.

IVIG is recommended in a dose of 400 mg/kg/dose, IV within 6 days of exposure. This intervention is recommended in pregnant women without evidence of measles immunity and for severely immunocompromised hosts, regardless of immunologic or vaccination status.

Tetanus

Therapeutic use: HTIG is the preparation of choice. A dose of 3,000–6,000 units intramuscularly should be given as soon as the diagnosis of tetanus is considered, with part of the dose infiltrated around the wound. HTIG should be administered at different sites than tetanus toxoid.

HTIG is also indicated for postexposure prophylaxis in individuals with tetanus prone wounds and nonimmunized, partially immunized or not received a tetanus toxoid containing vaccine in past 5 years.

The use of pooled intravenous immune globulin (IVIG), in a dose of 200–400 mg/kg, can be considered when HTIG is unavailable.

Diphtheria

Prophylactic use: DAT (Diphtheria Antitoxin - immunoglobulin antigen-binding fragments) is used prophylactically only under very exceptional circumstances. Eligibility for prophylactic use of DAT will be limited to the following situations:
- An individual who:
  - Has had known exposure to toxigenic *C. diphtheriae* (or possibly other toxigenic *Corynebacterium*)
  - And is not up-to-date for vaccination against diphtheria
  - And cannot be kept under surveillance for the development of clinical symptoms or is not available for follow-up of results of culturing for the diphtheria organism.
- An individual who has suspected or known injection of diphtheria toxin (e.g., laboratorians). Needle sticks do not qualify as injections.

Therapeutic use:
- Perform sensitivity tests, and desensitization if necessary.

- Give the entire treatment dose of DAT IV (or IM) in a single administration (except for series of injections needed for desensitization).
- The recommended DAT treatment dosage ranges are:

Diphtheria clinical presentation	DAT dose (units)
Pharyngeal or laryngeal disease of 2 days duration	20,000–40,000
Nasopharyngeal disease	40,000–60,000
Extensive disease of 3 or more days duration, Or any patient with diffuse swelling of neck	80,000–100,000
Skin lesions only (rare case where treatment is indicated)	20,000–40,000

- Give children the same dose as adults.
- Repeated doses of DAT after an appropriate initial dose are not recommended and may increase the risk of adverse reactions.

Rubella
Postexposure administration of IG following exposure to rubella will not prevent infection or viremia. Therefore, IG is not recommended for routine postexposure prophylaxis of rubella in early pregnancy or any other circumstance.

Rabies
The recommended dose of HRIG is 20 international units/kg in all age groups. If ERIG is used the dose is 40 international units/kg body weight. RIG can partially suppress antibody production, so no more than the single recommended dose should be administered and not later than 7 days after the 1st dose of vaccine.

Maximum quantity of RIG should be infiltrated in the area around and in the wounds.

HIV infection in infants and children
Primary prophylaxis for serious bacterial infection in patients with hypogammaglobulinemia (IgG <400 mg/dL): IV: 400 mg/kg/dose every 2-4 weeks.

Secondary prophylaxis for invasive bacterial infections: Should only be used if subsequent infections are frequent severe infections (>2 infections during a 1-year period): IV: 400 mg/kg/dose every 2-4 weeks.

Colitis due to *Clostridioides* (formerly *Clostridium*) difficile, chronic
Limited data available: Infants and Children—IV: 400 mg/kg/dose every 3 weeks resulted in resolution of colitis symptoms during treatment; duration of therapy was unclear (n = 5; age range: 6-37 months).

Hematopoietic cell transplantation (HCT) with hypogammaglobulinemia (IgG < 400 mg/dL), prevention of bacterial infection
Note: Increase dose or frequency to maintain IgG concentration >400 mg/dL.

Within first 100 days after HCT:
Infants and children (Allogeneic HCT recipients): IV: 400 mg/kg/dose once monthly.

Adolescents: IV: 500 mg/kg/dose once weekly.

>100 days after HCT: Infants, children, and adolescents: IV: 500 mg/kg/dose every 3–4 weeks.

Q9. Do we need to do any pretreatment testing?

Ans. We need to do pretreatment laboratory testing according to the underlying indication for which IVIG is recommended. This is done to look for evidence of viral infections as well as autoantibodies.

For almost all patients following tests are recommended:
- Complete blood count (CBC)
- Serum glucose
- Serum creatinine
- Hepatic transaminases
- Urine analysis.

Q10. What are adverse events?

Ans. They are immediate, delayed or late reactions.

Immediate Reactions
- *Anaphylaxis resembling reaction:* It is usually rate related and in most cases occurs midway through infusion. Patients may develop tachycardia, flushing, urticaria, wheezing, dyspnea, chest tightness, pain in chest, hypertension, nausea and/or vomiting and sudden anxiety. These reactions become milder with subsequent infusions. These are non-IgE-mediated reactions. Exact mechanism is unknown.

Management: Interrupt the infusion and treat the symptoms. In most cases interruption or temporary stopping the infusion will take care of the most of the symptoms.

Transfusion related acute lung injury (TRALI): It is characterized by the sudden onset of hypoxemic respiratory insufficiency during or shortly after transfusion. Mechanism is likely involvement of activation and/or agglutination of neutrophils by antileukocyte antibodies in the IVIG or rapid complement activation.
- *Transfusion-associated circulatory overload (TACO):* It is a syndrome of pulmonary edema due to either volume or salt overload. It is more likely to occur when high volume of IVIG is used in patients with inflammation or autoimmune disorders. It causes tachycardia, hypertension, dyspnea, orthopnea and headache.

CHAPTER 12: Immunoglobulins for Passive Protection against...

Table 1: Guidelines for intervals between administration of immunoglobulin preparations and measles- or varicella-containing vaccine.

Product/Indication	Dose, including mg immunoglobulin G (IgG)/kg body weight	Recommended interval before measles or varicella-containing vaccine administration
Botulinum Immune Globulin Intravenous (Human)	1.5 mL/kg (75 mg IgG/kg) IV	5 months
Tetanus IG (TIG)	250 units (10 mg IgG/kg) IM	3 months
Hepatitis A IG – Contact prophylaxis – International travel	0.02 mL/kg (3.3 mg IgG/kg) IM 0.06 mL/kg (10 mg IgG/kg) IM	3 months 3 months
Hepatitis B IG (HBIG)	0.06 mL/kg (10 mg IgG/kg) IM	3 months
Rabies IG (RIG)	20 IU/kg (22 mg IgG/kg) IM	4 months
Varicella IG	125 units/10 kg (60–200 mg IgG/kg) IM, maximum 625 units	5 months
Measles prophylaxis IG – Standard (i.e., nonimmunocompromised) contact – Immunocompromised contact	0.25 mL/kg (40 mg IgG/kg) IM 0.5 mL/kg (80 mg IgG/kg) IM	5 months 6 months
Blood transfusion – Red blood cells (RBCs), washed – RBCs, adenine-saline added – Packed RBCs (hematocrit 65%)[2] – Whole blood (hematocrit 35%–50%) – Plasma/platelet products	10 mL/kg (negligible IgG/kg) IV 10 mL/kg (10 mg IgG/kg) IV 10 mL/kg (60 mg IgG/kg) IV 10 mL/kg (80–100 mg IgG/kg) IV 10 mL/kg (160 mg IgG/kg) IV	None 3 months 6 months 6 months 7 months
Cytomegalovirus IGIV	150 mg/kg maximum	6 months
IGIV – Replacement therapy for immune deficiencies – Immune thrombocytopenic purpura treatment – Immune thrombocytopenic purpura treatment – Kawasaki disease – Postexposure varicella prophylaxis	300–400 mg/kg IV 400 mg/kg IV 1,000 mg/kg IV 2 g/kg IV 400 mg/kg IV	8 months 8 months 10 months 11 months 8 months
Monoclonal antibody to respiratory syncytial virus F protein (Synagis™)	15 mg/kg (IM)	None

Delayed Reactions

These reactions occur usually after few days of infusion. Almost 40% of all reactions are delayed reactions. These include thromboembolic reaction, central nervous system effects of which headache is the most common, renal complications which include acute renal failure, hyponatremia, osmotic nephrosis and renal dysfunction, hemolytic anemia and neutropenia.

Late Reactions

They may occur weeks to months after IVIG therapy. It includes dermatological reactions such as palmoplantar eczema, erythema multiforme and alopecia; noninfectious hepatitis, serum sickness with arthritis and impaired vaccination response.

Q11. What should be recommendations for vaccination following IVIG?

Ans. Preformed antibodies in the IG preparation will interfere with the immune response to vaccines especially the live-attenuated vaccines.

One may follow recommendations for advising vaccines, which are given in **Table 1**.

■ SUGGESTED READING

1. Perez EE, Orange JS, Bonilla F, Chinen J, Chinn IK, Dorsey M, et al. Update on the use of immunoglobulin in human disease: a review of evidence. J Allergy Clin Immunol. 2017;139(3S):S1.
2. Singh-Grewal D, Kemp A, Wong M. A prospective study of the immediate and delayed adverse events following intravenous immunoglobulin infusions. Arch Dis Child. 2006;91(8):651.
3. Stiehm ER. Adverse effects of human immunoglobulin therapy. Transfus Med Rev. 2013;27(3):171-8.
4. Update: Recommendations of the Advisory Committee on Immunization Practices for Use of Hepatitis A Vaccine for Postexposure Prophylaxis and for Preexposure Prophylaxis for International Travel. MMWR. 2018;67(43):1212-20.
5. UpToDate. Overview of intravenous immune globulin (IVIG) therapy (Ballow M, Shehata N). [online] Available from https://www.uptodate.com/contents/overview-of-intravenous-immune-globulin-ivig-therapy?search=ivig&source=search_result&selectedTitle=2~148&usage_type=default&display_rank=1. [Last accessed, November, 2020].
6. World Health Organization. Requirements for the collection, processing, and quality control of blood, blood components, and plasma derivatives (WHO technical Report Series No. 786, Annexure 4). Geneva: WHO; 1986.

SECTION 2

Individual Vaccines

- **BCG Vaccine**
  Baldev S Prajapati

- **Polio Vaccines**
  Srinivas G Kasi

- **Diphtheria, Pertussis, and Tetanus Vaccines**
  S Balasubramanium, Silky Mittal

- **Haemophilus Influenzae Type b Vaccine**
  Sumitha Nayak

- **Hepatitis B Vaccines**
  S Shivananda, Arun Wadhwa

- **Rotavirus Vaccines**
  Abhay K Shah, Aashay Abhay Shah

- **Pneumococcal Conjugate Vaccines**
  Sanjay Srirampur

- **Influenza Vaccines**
  Nitin Shah

- **Measles, Mumps and Rubella Vaccines MR/MMR/MMRV Vaccines**
  Rohit Agrawal

- **Typhoid Vaccines**
  Vijay Yewale

- **Hepatitis A Vaccines**
  Jaydeep Choudhury

- **Varicella Vaccines**
  Tanu Singhal

- **Human Papillomavirus (HPV) Vaccines**
  Sanjay Marathe

- **Rabies Vaccines**
  Arun Wadhwa

- **Meningococcal Vaccines**
  M Surendranath

- **Japanese Encephalitis Vaccines**
  Pravin Mehta

- **Cholera Vaccines**
  Arun Kumar Manglik

- **Yellow Fever Vaccine**
  Rupesh Masand

- **Zoster Vaccines**
  Srinivas G Kasi

CHAPTER 13

BCG Vaccine

Baldev S Prajapati

Q1. What is the magnitude of tuberculosis in children in India?

Ans. As per Global Tuberculosis Report, 2018, an estimated 220,000 children become ill with tuberculosis (TB) each year in India, accounting for 22% of global tuberculosis burden. Pulmonary TB is the most common form in children but extrapulmonary TB also forms a larger proportion of cases. About 10% of the cases reported to Revised National TB Control Program (RNTCP) are from children under the age of 14 years.

Q2. Describe the BCG vaccine. How is it prepared and stored?

Ans. BCG vaccine is a live bacterial vaccine. It is derived from bovine tuberculosis strain and was first developed in 1921 by French microbiologist, Albert Calmette and the veterinary surgeon, Camille Guérin, who performed 231 repeated subcultures over 13 years. In India, BCG vaccine laboratory was started in Chennai in 1948 for the production of Bacilli-Calmette-Guérin (BCG) vaccine for use in India and also for supply to some neighboring countries. Since 1966, Danish strain 1331 is being used for preparation of both the liquid vaccine (no more available world over) and freeze-dried vaccine.

For preparing the liquid and freeze dried BCG vaccine, the BCG Laboratory in Chennai used the method followed at the Staten Serum Institute, Copenhagen, using Sauton potato medium for maintaining the BCG strain.

BCG vaccine is now available only as the freeze-dried vaccine world over. The attenuated Calmette Guérin strain of bovine *Mycobacterium tuberculosis* is present in a concentration of 0.1–0.4 million colony forming unit (CFU) per dose of 0.05 mL of the vaccine [2×10^6 and 8×10^6 Colony Forming Units (CFU) per mL after reconstitution]. The WHO recommended the "Danish 1331" strain for the production of BCG vaccine, which has been used by the BCG Laboratory, Guindy, Chennai since 1966. Quality control is ensured by the International Reference Center at Copenhagen.

Due to repeated passages under different conditions in different laboratories worldwide, more than 10 manufacturing strains are in use worldwide.

Currently, five main strains account for more than 90% of the vaccines in use worldwide. These include the Pasteur 1173 P2, the Danish 1331, the Glaxo 1077 (derived from the Danish strain), the Tokyo 172-1, the Russian BCG-I, and the Moreau RDJ strains.

Q3. How is the BCG vaccine reconstituted?

Ans. The BCG vaccine is supplied as lyophilized (freeze-dried) preparation in vacuum sealed, dark colored multidose vial with normal saline as diluent. The ampoules of freeze-dried BCG vaccine are long and sealed under vacuum. They have to be opened carefully by gradually filling at the junction of neck and the body of the ampoule so that air does not rush in, causing spillage. The vaccine is reconstituted by dissolving it in normal saline and not the distilled water which is quite an irritant. The diluents should always be kept with the vaccine in the main compartment of the refrigerator to maintain its temperature at the time of reconstitution. Reconstituted BCG vaccine should be used within 6 hours which is the typical duration of an immunization session in public health. It should be stored at 2–8°C and protected from light and discarded within 6 hours of reconstitution. As the vaccine does not contain preservatives or antibiotics, bacterial contamination may lead to toxic shock syndrome, if it is kept for long time after reconstitution.

Q4. What is the dosage of BCG vaccine?

Ans. The standard dose of BCG vaccine is 0.1 mL volume. Dosage does not depend up on the age or weight of the baby.

Some experts recommend a dose of 0.05 mL to newborns aged less than 4 weeks as they consider a higher incidence of regional lymphadenitis on full dose administration. In controlled trials the incidence of lymphadenitis observed was 1.3% with 0.1 mL as compared to 1% with 0.05 mL. However, doubts on the efficacy of the lower dose still remain. Therefore, 0.1 mg (0.1 mL) should be given universally at all ages.

However, IAP Advisory Committee Vaccines and Immunization Practices (IAP-ACVIP) recommends using 0.05 mL for newborns <4 weeks of age and 0.1 mL thereafter and the WHO recommend dose of 0.05 mL for infants less than 1 year of age and 0.1 mL thereafter.

Q5. What are the routes and the techniques of administration of BCG vaccine?

Ans. BCG is given by intradermal route by BCG syringe or tuberculin syringe. The rounded, convex aspect of left shoulder at the level of deltoid insertion is the site of BCG vaccination. It is the site with optimum lymphatic drainage and ease for visualization of the BCG scar. The site is cleaned using sterile water and not any antiseptic agent. A wheal of 5 mm with Peau d' orange (multiple dimples seen in the skin resembling an orange, due to pitting by hair follicles) appearance indicates successful intradermal administration of the vaccine. The parents should be explained not to press it or apply anything at injection site.

Q6. What is classical BCG reaction?

Ans. The wheal following intradermal administration of BCG, subsides within 30 minutes and it does not show visible change for several days. Subsequently, a papule develops after 2–3 weeks, increases in size up to 4–8 mm by the end of 5–6 weeks. This papule gets converted into pustule which bursts open. It may get sealed off and again bursts open which may repeat several times and ultimately a scab is formed. In due course of time, the scab dries up and falls off with formation of a superficial, very tiny scar. Nothing should be applied over the site during this process. This classical BCG reaction may not be observed in all babies, in some it may be papule or ulceration and finally a scar is seen. Both the types of reactions are equally immunogenic. Healing is usually completed by 10–12 weeks and the site is marked by a small scar of 5–7 mm in size.

Q7. What are the complications of BCG vaccination?

Ans. Local lymphadenitis is the most common complication of BCG vaccination. Mild BCG lymphadenitis is defined as swelling of the ipsilateral regional lymph nodes (usually axillary but may also be cervical and/or supraclavicular). The lymph nodes remain small (<1.5 cm), are firm in consistency and do not adhere to overlying skin. This does not need any treatment except a follow-up. Severe lymphadenitis is defined as nodes which have become fluctuant, adherent to overlying skin with or without rupture or a sinus formation.

Repeated aspiration is the treatment of first choice for fluctuant nodes. Failed multiple aspirations will need surgical excision. When aspiration is done, the fluid may be AFB positive, but growth will reveal *M. bovis*. There is no indication for antituberculous chemotherapy. Common local reactions include subcutaneous abscesses, keloids and rarely lupus vulgaris.

Q8. What are the severe complications of BCG?

Ans. Osteitis and osteomyelitis are rare and severe complications of BCG vaccination. If BCG lymphadenitis is also contralateral and/or multiple or disseminated, one should suspect defects of cell-mediated immunity (CMI). Disseminated BCG disease is a serious complication with an incidence of <5 per 1 million vaccines in non-HIV infected individuals. In HIV-infected infants, the incidence is 1,100–4,170 per 1 million vaccinees. Disseminated BCG disease is usually seen in children having defects in CMI. The conditions associated with disseminated BCG disease include Severe combined immunodeficiency (SCID), Common Variable Immunodeficiency (CVID), Human Immunodeficiency (HIV) infection and Mendelian Susceptibility to Mycobacterial Disease (MSMD).

Q9. What are the contraindications of BCG vaccination?

Ans. BCG vaccine should not be given to children with immune suppressive conditions such as primary immunodeficiency, HIV, leukemia, lymphoma, etc. The BCG vaccine should be withheld in children who are on immunosuppressants or radiation therapy.

It is best to avoid BCG for a period of 4–6 weeks following viral infections such as measles, chicken pox, hepatitis B, etc.

Q10. What are the reasons for the variable efficacy of BCG? In spite of this variable efficacy, why does the WHO recommend universal BCG vaccination?

Ans. The following reasons are considered for the lack of efficacy in both low tuberculosis burden such as United States and high tuberculosis burden countries such as India:

- It has been hypothesized that in areas with high levels of background exposures to tuberculosis, every susceptible person is already exposed and has got natural immunizing effect. In such a person, BCG can hardly offer any more protection.
- There is genetic variation in the BCG strains used in different trials which explains variable efficacy in different trials.
- Different genetic makeup of different populations may explain difference in efficacy.
- Exposure to environmental mycobacteria, especially *Mycobacterium avium, Mycobacterium marinum* and *Mycobacterium intracellulare*, results in nonspecific immune response against mycobacteria. Administering BCG to someone who already had a nonspecific immune response against mycobacteria hardly augments the response that is already there. BCG may not be efficacious in these people.
- Concurrent parasitic infection may change immune response to BCG making it less efficacious. T helper (Th_1) cell response is required for an effective immune response to BCG. Concurrent parasitic infections produce a simultaneous Th_2 response which may built the effect of BCG.

In spite of variable efficacy of BCG, BCG vaccination is recommended by WHO as BCG is known to prevent severe forms of tuberculosis such as tuberculous meningitis, miliary tuberculosis and other disseminated varieties in infants and young children. BCG vaccination remains the effective measure for prevention of these forms of tuberculosis in most countries. It is inexpensive and rarely causes serious complications.

Q11. Is there any correlation of BCG scar with induction of cell-mediated immune response (CMIR)?

Ans. It has been observed in many studies that after BCG vaccination, almost 12–15% of neonates do not develop scar but have positive CMIR. The absence of scar is more conspicuous among those who were given BCG immediately after delivery. The frequency of tuberculin reactions do not vary in children with and without a scar.

Q12. A newborn brought for routine check up on 7th day of life and BCG was not given at birth. When can we give BCG to this infant?

Ans. BCG vaccine can be given any time till the 2 weeks of age, so that there is a gap of 4 weeks until next immunization at 6 weeks of age. If BCG is not given during neonatal period, it can be given at 6 weeks along with other vaccines.

BCG is preferably given at birth to provide protection from tuberculosis in the early years when infection can often lead to disseminated diseases such as miliary tuberculosis and tuberculous meningitis. This is specifically important for countries such as ours with high prevalence of disease and chance of being infected in very early life is high.

Catch up vaccination with BCG is recommended till 5 years of age and routine tuberculous skin testing (TST) is not required prior to vaccination.

Q13. What is the recommendation of BCG vaccination at birth, in HIV infected/exposed children?

Ans. Both, the IAP and the UIP, recommend BCG vaccination of all asymptomatic newborns of HIV +ve mothers. Considering the high incidence of disseminated BCG disease in infants of HIV +ve mothers, who become symptomatic later in the first year, the WHO in 2007, published revised guidelines.

The guidelines stated that National and local decision-making on the revision and application of BCG immunization will ultimately be based on a range of locally determined factors, which include prevalence of TB in the general population, potential for infant exposure to TB, prevalence of HIV infection, coverage and efficacy of interventions to prevent MTCT of HIV; rates of exclusive and mixed breastfeeding; capacity to conduct follow up of immunized children; capacity to perform early virological infant diagnosis (in the first months of life).

All infants born to women of unknown HIV status should be immunized. For infants, whose HIV infection status is unknown and who demonstrate no signs or reported symptoms suggestive of HIV infection but who are born to known HIV-infected women, BCG may be deferred till a virological diagnosis is established.

Infants who are known to be HIV infected with or without signs or reported symptoms of HIV infection should not be immunized.

Infants whose HIV infection status is unknown but who have signs or reported symptoms suggestive of HIV infection and who are born to HIV-infected mothers should not be immunized.

Q14. Should the children be revaccinated with BCG?

Ans. It has been observed that both natural and BCG induced tuberculin sensitivity tend to wane in the course of time. It could also be associated with some degree of protection against exogenous super infection. It has been observed that only 26% children were Mantoux positive after 3–6 years of BCG vaccination compared to 35% in less than 3 year group. Theoretically, these observations would favor revaccination in children at a later age. However, WHO discourages BCG revaccination on the basis of lack of evidence for additional protection to that from a first vaccination.

Q15. Are there any other uses of BCG?

Ans. BCG vaccine is also being tried for prevention of leprosy. It has also been used as an immunomodulating agent in diseases such as nephrotic syndrome and bladder cancer.

Q16. Why is the reactivation of BCG scar in Kawasaki Disease ?

Ans. The reactivation of BCG scar in Kawasaki Disease is possibly due to cross reactivity between Mycobacterial & Human Homologue Heat Shock Protein. It occurs in 30 to 50% cases of Kawasaki Disease with a higher prevalence than cervical lymphadenopathy & rash.

Q17. Is there any role of BCG vaccination to reduce the impact of coronavirus disease (COVID-19)?

Ans. Early on during COVID 2019 era an ecological study Miller A et al. compared COVID-19 infection and mortality rates in countries that have childhood BCG in their national immunization program (NIP) and compared it with rates in those that do not have BCG in NIP. They showed that the COVID-19 infection rates were 4–5 times less and mortality rates nearly 20 times less in countries having BCG in NIP. However the study had its own drawback, the major one being that countries having BCG in NIP were low income countries which were not testing enough in the initial phase of COVID-19. This was then followed by an article published in the Lancet journal that stated following points:

1. In addition to its specific effect against tuberculosis, the BCG vaccine has beneficial nonspecific effects on immune system that protect against wide range of other infections.
2. Severe acute respiratory syndrome coronavirus 2 (SARS-COV-2) is a single stranded positive sense RNA virus, and the BCG vaccine has been shown to reduce severity of infections by other viruses with that structure in controlled trials. For example, the BCG vaccine reduced yellow fever vaccine viremia by 71% in volunteers in the Netherlands, and it markedly reduced the severity of Mengo virus (encephalomyocarditis virus) infection in two studies in mice.

3. The BCG vaccine and some other live vaccines induce metabolic epigenetic changes that enhance the innate immune response to subsequent infections, a process termed trained immunity. The BCG vaccine might therefore reduce viremia after SARS-COV-2 exposure, with consequent less severe COVID-19 and more rapid recovery.

However, a recent article published from Israel does not support the idea that BCG vaccination in childhood has a protective effect against COVID-19 in adulthood. Trials are underway to understand if BCG vaccine may offer protection against COVID-19. One trial in Australia is recruiting medicos to receive BCG (either first time or revaccination if they have received it during childhood) versus no BCG. Results will be out in next 3 months that may answer whether BCG has any role in preventing COVID-19 infection or its severity. Similar studies are also going on in Boston, USA and the Netherland. Before drawing the conclusion regarding role of BCG vaccination in COVID-19, we will have to wait till clear evidences are available. Till then use of BCG for prevention of COVID-19 should be only in the trial set up.

■ SUGGESTED READING

1. Aaron M, Reandelar MJ, Fasciglione K, Roumenova V, Li Y, Otazu GH. Correlation between universal BCG vaccination policy and reduced morbidity and mortality for COVID-19: an epidemiological study. medRxiv. 2020.
2. Abubakar I, Pimpin L, Ariti C, Beynon R, Mangtani P, Sterne JA, et al. Systemic review and meta-analysis of the current evidence on the duration of protection by bacillus Calmette – Guerin vaccination against tuberculosis. Health Technol Assess. 2013;17(37):1-372.
3. Balasubramanian S. IAP Guidebook on Immunization 2018-2019. In: S. Balasubramanian S, Shashtri DD, Shah AK (Eds). ACVIP – IAP, 3rd edition. New Delhi: Jaypee Brothers Medical Publishers (P) Ltd.; 2020. pp. 93-101.
4. Hamiel U, Kozer E, Youngster I. SRS-CoV-2 rates in BCG-vaccinated and unvaccinated young adults. JAMA. 2020;323(22):2340-1.
5. Mangtani P, Abubakar I, Ariti C, Beynon R, Pimpin L, Fine PE, et al. Protection by BCG vaccine against tuberculosis: a systematic review of randomized controlled trails. Clin Infect Dis. 2014;58(4):470-80.
6. Marais BJ, Gie RP, Schaaf HS, Hesseling AC, Obihara CC, Nelson LJ, et al. The clinical epidemiology of childhood pulmonary tuberculosis: a critical review of literature from the prechemotherapy era. Int J Tuberc Lung Dis. 2004;8(3):278-85.
7. Nissen TN Birk, NM, Kjærgaard J, Thøstesen LM, Pihl GT, Hoffmann T, et al. Adverse reactions to the Bacillus Calmetter – Guerin (BCG) vaccine in new born infants – an evaluation of the Danish strain 1331 SSI in a randomized clinical trial. Vaccine. 2016;34(22):2477-82.
8. Plotkin S, Orenstein W, Offit P, Edwards KM. Tuberculosis (and Leprosy). In: Plotkin's Vaccines, 7th edition. New York: Elsevier; 2017.
9. World Health Organization (WHO). (2018). Evidence to recommendation table: BCG efficacy against TB. [online] Available from: http://www.who.int/entity/immunization/policy/position_papers/bcg_efficacy_tb.pdf. [Last Accessed November, 2019].
10. World Health Organization (WHO) (2018). Evidence to recommendation table: Need for vaccination at birth vs at 6 weeks. [online] Available from: http://www.who.int/immunization/policy/position_papers/bcg_vaccination_birth_vs_6weeks.pdf. [Last Accessed November, 2019].

CHAPTER 14

Polio Vaccines

Srinivas G Kasi

Q1. What is the present status of polio in the world?

Ans. As of 17 November 2020, there were 135 cases of wild polio virus (WPV) and 688 cases of circulating vaccine derived virus (cVDPV) (17 of type 1 and 655 of type 2). Polio remains endemic in two countries, Pakistan and Afghanistan. Type 1 PV remains the only endemis circulating strain.

Q2. What is the present status of polio in India?

Ans. In 2009, India contributed to 60% of polio cases in the world. The last reported cases of wild polio in India were in West Bengal on January 13th, 2011. On March 27th 2014, the World Health Organization (WHO) declared India a polio free country, since no cases of wild polio were reported for 3 years.

Q3. Which are the vaccines available against polio?

Ans. Two vaccines are in use against polio: Oral polio vaccine (OPV) and injectable polio vaccine (IPV).

Q4. What are the characteristics of OPV? Which are the different types of OPV?

Ans. OPV is a live attenuated vaccine derived from parent WPV strains by passage in nonhuman cells. Attenuation of the virus in cell culture greatly reduces its neurovirulence and transmissibility.

The licensed formulations of OPV are: (1) monovalent OPVs against type 1 (mOPV1), type 2 (mOPV2) or type 3 (mOPV3); (2) bivalent OPV (bOPV) containing types 1 and 3. Trivalent OPV is no longer in use since April 2016.

The type 2 strain of OPV is immunodominant and in formulating tOPV, the amount of type 2 virus is reduced compared with the other viruses. This feature of the vaccine has led to the disappearance of WPV in 1999.

OPV is administered orally, as 2 drops (~0.1 mL) dose. OPV is a highly heat-sensitive vaccine and has a VVM2. Any vaccine which has reached discard point on the VVM, should not be used.

In high-income countries, seroconversion rates in children following administration of 3 doses of tOPV approach 100% for all 3 poliovirus types. However, in developing countries, tOPV has been found to be less immunogenic with an average of 73, 90 and 70% of children seroconverting to types 1, 2 and 3, respectively after three tOPV doses.

OPV induces high levels of intestinal immunity, thus preventing virus shedding (and therefore transmission) and resulting in population protection.

Q5. What is bivalent OPV?

Ans. Following the switch in April 2016, globally, tOPV was replaced with the bivalent oral poliovirus vaccine (bOPV) in routine immunization around the world. bOPV contains only serotypes 1 and 3. bOPV elicits a better immune response against poliovirus types 1 and 3 than tOPV, but does not give immunity against serotype 2.

Q6. What is monovalent OPV?

Ans. Monovalent oral polio vaccines (mOPV) confer immunity to just one of the three serotypes of OPV. They elicit a superior immune response to the serotype targeted than tOPV, but do not provide protection to the other two types.

Monovalent OPVs for type 1 (mOPV1) and type 3 (mOPV3) poliovirus were relicensed in 2005. They elicit the best immune response against the serotype they target of all the vaccines. Monovalent OPV type 2 (mOPV2) has been stockpiled in the event of a cVDPV2 outbreak.

Q7. Why was OPV chosen for polio eradication?

Ans. OPV was preferred over IPV for several reasons: OPV costs substantially less than IPV; primary immunization with OPV induces superior intestinal immunity compared with IPV and thus has the potential to better prevent transmission of wild viruses; OPV confers contact immunity through passive immunization of unvaccinated persons from viruses shed by vaccines; and OPV is administered in oral drops, which is easier to administer than IPV injections.

Q8. What are the major drawbacks of OPV?

Ans. Two major drawbacks of OPV are VAPP and VDPV:

Vaccine-associated paralytic polio (VAPP): OPV is associated with vaccine-associated paralytic polio (VAPP) in approximately 1 in 2.7 million doses of OPV. VAPP is caused by a strain of poliovirus that has mutated from the original attenuated vaccine strain contained in OPV. It can occur in the recipient of OPV or can occur in a close unvaccinated or nonimmune contact of the vaccine recipient who is excreting the mutated virus.

The risk of VAPP varies by dose and by setting. In developed countries, the risk is greatest with the first dose. This is because the first does results in seroconversion. In developing countries, the risk of VAPP is higher from subsequent doses than following the first dose probably because of delayed intake of OPV.

As the virus causing VAPP is not transmissible, there are no outbreaks associated with VAPP. Thus, VAPP is a risk to an individual and not to the community.

Vaccine derived poliovirus (VDPV): A VDPV is a strain of poliovirus which has mutated from the original strain contained in OPV. This strain may regain neurovirulence and transmissibility. The latter is known as a circulating VPDV (cVDPV). cVDPV is associated with sustained person-to-person transmission and is circulating in the environment. "Persistent cVDPVs" refer to cVDPVs known to have circulated for more than 6 months. cVDPVs occur when routine immunization or supplementary immunization activities (SIAs) are poorly conducted and a significant proportion of the population is left susceptible to poliovirus.

There are three types of VDPV:
1. cVDPV (circulating vaccine derived polio virus): As mentioned earlier.
2. iVDPV (immunodeficiency-related vaccine derived polio virus) reported in immunodeficient patients who have prolonged infections after exposure to OPV.
3. aVDPV (ambiguous vaccine derived polio virus) currently have unclassified source (i.e., a single isolate from a healthy or non-immunodeficient person; environmental isolates without an associated AFP case).

Q9. What is the magnitude of VAPP in India?

Ans. It has been estimated in developed countries that VAPP cases occur at a frequency of 2–4 cases/million birth cohort per year in countries using OPV, 40% of which is caused by OPV2. Using the above incidence rate, about 50–100 children are estimated to suffer from VAPP every year in India. Though India and other developing counties lack reliable data on VAPP, some reports in previous years suggest that cases could be much higher in India. In 1999, with 199 cases of VAPP, overall risk in India was estimated to be 1 case per 4.6 million OPV doses. The risk of first-dose recipient VAPP (1 case per 2.8 million doses) was higher than the risk of subsequent-dose recipient VAPP (1 case per 13.9 million doses).

Q10. What is the data on VDPV in India?

Ans. The last case of cVDPV 2 was reported in October 2009. Between January 2015 and May 2016, a total of 14 sewage samples collected from different parts of the country tested positive for VDPVs. All of these have been responded to urgently and appropriately with polio vaccination campaigns. So far, none of these VDPVs detected in the sewage have infected any children. The last detection of cVDPV in sewage sample was from Telangana on May 17th, 2016.

This was countered by immunization with 1 dose of IPV to more than 300,000 in the area. No children have been found to be affected by the detected VDPV isolate in the nearby areas.

Q11. Why was tOPV replaced by bOPV?

Ans. The last case of type 2 WPV was reported in 1999. Since 2009, 97% of cVDPV cases and 40% of VAPP are due to type 2. Hence, type 2 was dropped from tOPV with the purpose of reducing risks of VAPP and cVDPV associated with type 2 in the OPV.

Q12. What was the polio endgame strategy adopted between 2013 and 2018?

Ans. This was a three-pronged strategy:
- *Step 1*: Introduction of IPV into routine immunization by October 2015, at least 6 months before the switch from tOPV to bOPV.
- *Step 2*: tOPV-bOPV switch by April 2016.
- *Step 3*: Withdrawal of routine OPV use—Initially planned for the eventual withdrawal of all OPV in routine use by 2019–2020.

Q13. What is the data about IPV in India?

Ans. IPV has been shown to be highly effective in eliciting humoral antibody responses to poliovirus in both high-income and low-income settings. IPV shows a similar effect to OPV in inducing pharyngeal immunity, but has limited effect in inducing primary intestinal immunity when administered alone. Correlates of protection for IPV containing vaccines require neutralizing antibody levels at or above a 1:8 dilution threshold.

In a study published in 1983, the overall seroconversion rates to polio virus types 1, 2, and 3 were 99%, 89%, and 91%, respectively. The seroconversion rates in infants without maternal antibody, who were given three doses of IPV at 8-week intervals, were 100%, 100%, and 96.21% to poliovirus types 1, 2, and 3 respectively. In another study published in 2006 with a DTaP-IPV/Hib vaccine, in a 6-10-14 weeks schedule, seroconversion rates of 100%, 99.1% and 100% were observed for types 1, 2 and 3 respectively.

Studies in India have shown that IPV given to OPV primed children boosts the mucosal intestinal immunity and this boosting is superior to that observed after a booster of OPV in OPV primed children.

IPV is a very safe vaccine in humans, whether used alone or in combination vaccines. No serious adverse events have been reported, only minor side effects. IPV does not cause VAPP or cVDPV. Minor local reactions, such as redness and tenderness, may occur following IPV. IPV can be safely administered to children with immunodeficiencies. IPV has VVM 7.

Q14. What was the purpose of IPV introduction in the national immunization program (NIP)?

Ans. There are three main reasons for introducing IPV in the NIP:
1. The primary purpose of introducing IPV into routine immunization (RI) is to boost population immunity against type 2 poliovirus during and after the planned global withdrawal of OPV2 and switch from tOPV to bOPV.
2. To boost both humoral and mucosal immunity against poliovirus types 1 and 3, which may also hasten the eradication of these WPVs.
3. Priming with type 2 in IPV would enhance the immune response on subsequent exposure to type 2, either through the environment or mOPV2.

What should be noted is that the purpose of introduction of IPV in the NIP is as a risk mitigation strategy associated with the withdrawal of type 2 from OPV. It is not meant for protection against PV in the absence of OPV.

Until polio is eradicated globally, OPV is still the main preventative measure against polio. IPV is recommended in addition to OPV and does not replace OPV.

Q15. What is an ideal IPV schedule for an individual?

Ans. Overall, studies show that the persistence of poliovirus-neutralizing antibodies is well-established at least until school-entry age (4–6 years) by the 3+1, 2+1, and 3+0 schedules, with slightly higher titers in favor of the most complete schedule (3+1).

Q16. What is the importance of the birth dose of OPV (OPV-0)?

Ans. Since 1985, the WHO has recommended administration of one dose of OPV at birth in countries at risk for polio, where the serological response to 3 doses of OPV, in the primary immunization schedule, was found to be sub-optimal.

The birth dose should be administered at birth, or as soon as possible after birth. Although data on birth dose seroconversion rates show great variability - low rates in India (~10–15%), this OPV-0 increases the seroconversion rates of subsequent doses and induces mucosal protection before enteric pathogens may interfere with the immune response. Administration of OPV-0 under cover of maternally derived antibodies may theoretically be protective against VAPP. Presently, in India, OPV-0 is advised even with an all IPV schedule.

Q17. What are the recommendations regarding IM-IPV at 14 weeks?

Ans. IPV administration is recommended at 14 weeks of age because it provides the optimal balance between vaccine efficacy and early protection. At this age, the maternal antibodies have diminished and immunogenicity is significantly higher.

Postponing this dose to a later to elicit a higher antibody response is not recommended as it leaves children unprotected against type 2 for a longer period of time.

Q18. What is fIPV?

Ans. The tOPV to bOPV switch, with the recommendation for IPV in the NIP in all OPV using countries and the challenges in scaling up bulk production by the two main IPV producers has led to a severe global shortage of IPV.

There is conclusive evidence that two fractional doses administered via the intradermal (ID) route offer higher immunogenicity compared to one full intramuscular (IM) dose of IPV. As a result, a two-dose fIPV schedule has been strongly recommended to countries by the WHO Strategic Advisory Group of Experts on Immunization (SAGE), and in the WHO Position Paper on polio vaccines.

A fractional dose is one-fifth (1/5, 0.1 mL) of a full dose of IPV, injected via the intradermal (ID) route. It is given on the left arm, at the insertion of the deltoid muscle.

Q19. What is the duration of protection following vaccination with OPV and IPV?

Ans.
- IPV: Studies have shown that the persistence of poliovirus-neutralizing antibodies is well-established at least until school-entry age (5–6 years) by the 3+1, 2+1, and 3+0 schedules. No studies have yet evaluated persistence of poliovirus-neutralizing antibodies beyond childhood following complete primary immunization.
- OPV: Data from population-based studies of antibody seroprevalence conducted among army recruits and school-age children in the United States and in Gambia demonstrate that poliovirus antibodies induced by OPV persist for many years. The intestinal immunity induced by OPV does not persist beyond a year.

Q20. What are the IAP recommended IPV schedules?

Ans. The preferred schedule is bOPV at birth followed by IPV at 6–10–14 week solo or as part of DTwP/DTaP combos and boosters at 15–18 months and 4–6 years. In the IAP schedule, IPV is the main preventive measure against polio.

An alternate schedule is two doses of intramuscular IPV instead of three for primary series if started at 8 weeks, with an interval of 8 weeks between two doses is an alternative.

All IPV immunized children should receive OPV on all SIA days till 5 years of age. In case IPV is not available or feasible, the child should be offered three doses of bOPV. In such cases, the child should be referred for two fractional doses of IPV at a government facility at 6 and 14 weeks or at least one dose of intramuscular IPV, either standalone or as a combination vaccine, at 14 weeks of age.

Q21. What is the risk administering only bOPV and not administering any IPV?

Ans. Two main risks are:
1. Immediate time-limited risk of cVDPV2 emergence; and
2. Medium and long-term risks of poliovirus reintroduction from a vaccine manufacturing site, research facility or diagnostic laboratory.

While all countries face a time-limited (1–2 years) risk of cVDPV2 outbreak during OPV type 2 withdrawal if they do not introduce a dose of IPV, certain countries are at higher risk than others. India is a high-risk country and is placed in Tier 1 category.

Q22. What if type 2 cVDPV outbreak occurs? Will mOPV2 be used or IPV to curtail the outbreak?

Ans. The recommendation is to utilize mOPV2 as the vaccine of choice. Close contacts of immunodeficiency-related vaccine-derived poliovirus (i-VDPV) cases should be vaccinated with IPV.

The SAGE Working Group has recommended that current supply constraints require prioritization of IPV use to provide protection to the general population through RI in countries at risk of VDPV2 emergence and spread rather than in response to outbreaks where the impact is less pronounced. At this time, the risk of ongoing transmission outweighs the risk of seeding additional VDPVs from using mOPV2.

Q23. In children who have received an all-IPV schedule, should an outbreak of cVDPV occur, do they need to take additional OPV doses?

Ans. Mucosal immunity following OPV or IPV wanes rapidly and does not last longer than 1 year. In the above situation, the child should receive additional doses of OPV to boost intestinal immunity. Such an outbreak could be rapidly interrupted through mOPV type 2.

Q24. What is nOPV?

Ans. Novel OPV2 (nOPV) are candidate vaccines designed to stabilize the poliovirus genome and minimize the acquisition of neurovirulence, to provide safer alternatives for outbreak control of cVDPVs in the era following OPV2 cessation. Two such vaccines are in phase 2 trials. Codon deoptimization of the capsid region, combined with stabilization of known attenuation determinants in the Sabin 5′ untranslated region (UTR), has been utilized to engineer a nOPV2 strain that is genetically stable.

Preclinical analysis of both candidates provided strong evidence of increased genetic stability of the viral genome, with a lower risk of reversion to neurovirulence relative to Sabin OPV2. In a phase 1 study done in 60 adults, who had received only IPV in past, both novel OPV2 candidates were immunogenic and 100% of participants were seroprotected after vaccination. Reversion to neurovirulence, assessed as paralysis of transgenic mice, was low in isolates from those vaccinated with both candidates, and sequencing of shed virus indicated that there was no loss of attenuation in domain V of the 5'-untranslated region, the primary site of reversion in Sabin OPV.

Q25. What is the status of Sabin-IPV (sIPV)?

Ans. In the final phase of polio eradication, OPV has to be stopped and replaced by an all-IPV schedule. IPV is expensive, requires Biosafety level (BSL) IV for production facilities, which is available only in the developed countries.

The goal of research in the area of sIPV is to enable low-income countries to produce IPV, as production of sIPV does not need BSL IV requirements. A range of manufacturers and research institutes have active programs at various stages of development, including the Netherlands Vaccine Institute, Panacea and JPRI/Takeda.

The first Sabin strain IPV (sIPV) was developed in the United States in the 1980s but was not licensed for use. Improvements in manufacturing technology resulting in enhanced yields prior to inactivation have now made sIPV commercially feasible and further encouraged sIPV development. sIPV combined with tetanus and diphtheria toxoids and acellular pertussis vaccine was introduced in Japan in 2012, and 2 standalone sIPVs have recently been licensed for distribution in China.

■ SUGGESTED READING

1. Bandyopadhyay AS, Garon J, Seib K, Orenstein WA. Polio vaccination: past, present and future. Future Microbiol. 2015;10(5):791-808.
2. Damme PV, De Coster I, Bandyopadhyay AS, Revets H, Withanage K, De Smedt P, et al. The safety and immunogenicity of two novel live attenuated monovalent (serotype 2) oral poliovirus vaccines in healthy adults: a double-blind, single-centre phase 1 study. Lancet. 2019;394:148-58.
3. Global Polio Eradication Initiative. Polio this week. [online] Available from: http://polioeradication.org/polio-today/polio-now/this-week/. [Last Accessed November, 2020].
4. Global Polio Eradication Initiative. Strategic Plan 2013-2018. [online] Available from: http://polioeradication.org/who-we-are/strategic-plan-2013-2018/[Last Accessed November, 2020].
5. Global Polio Eradication Initiative. The Vaccines. [online] Available from: http://polioeradication.org/polio-today/polio-prevention/the-vaccines/. [Last Accessed November, 2020].

6. John TJ. The golden jubilee of vaccination against poliomyelitis. Indian J Med Res. 2004;119(1): 1-17.
7. Krishnan R, Jadhav M, John TJ. Efficacy of inactivated polio vaccine in India. Bull World Health Organ. 1983;61(4): 689-92.
8. Nafi OA, Ramadan B. Sabin vaccine in poliomyelitis eradication: achievements and risks. J Pure Appl Microbiol. 2019;13(1):413-8.
9. Parker EP, Molodecky NA, Pons-Salort M, O'Reilly KM, Grassly NC. Impact of inactivated poliovirus vaccine on mucosal immunity: implications for the polio eradication endgame. Exp Rev Vaccines. 2015;14(8):1113-23.
10. WHO (2016). Polio vaccines: WHO position paper No 12. [online] Available from: https://www.who.int/immunization/policy/position_papers/polio/en/. [Last Accessed November, 2020].
11. WHO. Planning for IPV introduction: Frequently asked questions (FAQs). [online] Available from: https://www.who.int/immunization/diseases/poliomyelitis/inactivated_polio_vaccine/ipv_general_faq_04mar2014.pdf. [Last Accessed November, 2020].

CHAPTER 15

Diphtheria, Pertussis, and Tetanus Vaccines

S Balasubramanium, Silky Mittal

Q1. What is the burden of diphtheria, pertussis, and tetanus?

Ans. Incidence of diphtheria has globally declined in the past 20 years due to increasing vaccine coverage, but it is high in India accounting for about half of all cases reported globally. As per the national level health survey in India, the coverage is about 80% for primary immunization, though no such information exists for booster doses. Due to waning vaccine-induced immunity among school-going children and adolescents, majority of outbreaks and cases are observed in this age group **(Table 1)**.

Similar to diphtheria, the incidence of pertussis has increased probably due to improved surveillance and diagnostic methods polymerase chain reaction (PCR). The World Health Organization (WHO) reported true resurgence of incidence in countries using acellular pertussis (aP) vaccine instead of whole-cell pertussis (wP).

In May 2015, it was declared that neonatal maternal tetanus was eliminated in India based on figures of incidence of <1 case per 1,000 live births in all districts of the country for 2 consecutive years. This is mainly attributed to good maternal immunization coverage and increased institutional deliveries. Tetanus still exists among children and adults especially male population, due to increased occurrence of tetanus prone injuries and poor immunization coverage.

Q2. What are the various available vaccines for diphtheria, pertussis, and tetanus together?

Ans. The combination vaccines are composed of toxoids of diphtheria, tetanus, and pertussis in the form of whole-cell inactivated component (wP)

Table 1: Age distribution of cases in states of India with case-based surveillance 2016.

State	Total cases	Under 5 years	5–10 years	Over 10 years
Bihar	71	41%	34%	25%
Haryana	59	27%	53%	20%
Kerala	556	8%	18%	74%
Uttar Pradesh	844	25%	53%	22%
Total	**1,530**	**20%**	**39%**	**41%**

or as acellular pertussis vaccine containing variable amount of inactivated bacterial components [pertussis toxin (PT), filamentous hemagglutinin (FHA), pertactin (PRN), and fimbrial hemagglutinin]. The small alphabets "d" and "p" correspond to reduced content of diphtheria and acellular pertussis component respectively.

- Diphtheria, Tetanus toxoids, and whole-cell Pertussis (DTwP)
- Diphtheria, Tetanus, and acellular Pertussis (DTaP)
- Tetanus, Diphtheria, and acellular Pertussis (Tdap)
- Tetanus and Diphtheria (Td)
- Diphtheria and Tetanus (DT)

Q3. What is the role of adjuvants in DPT vaccine?

Ans. Adjuvants are molecules with immunomodulatory properties which enhance host antigen-specific immune responses compared to those given without adjuvants. Inactivated whole-cell pertussis bacilli adsorbed on insoluble aluminum salts acts as an adjuvant in diphtheria, pertussis, and tetanus (DPT) vaccines. Adjuvants help antigen to elicit an early, high, and long-lasting immune response with fewer antigens, thus saving on vaccine production costs. Aluminum salts (aluminum phosphate or aluminum hydroxide) are commonly used as adjuvants.

Q4. How is DPT containing vaccine stored?

Ans. All available forms should be stored at 2–8°C in the lower compartment of the refrigerator and should never be frozen. Freezing causes agglomeration and sedimentation of antigen adjuvant particles. This results in loss of antigen and thus loss of immunogenicity. Such damaged flocculation is more painful and can cause sterile abscesses.

Q5. What are the adverse reactions encountered with DPT containing vaccines?

Ans. Minor adverse effects—local site pain, swelling, and redness; minor systemic side effects such as fever, fussiness, anorexia, and vomiting occur in almost half the vaccinees. Serious adverse events are infrequent and include persistent inconsolable crying, hypotonic hyporesponsive episodes (HHE), seizures, and encephalopathy.

Q6. What are the absolute contraindications for DTwP/DTaP vaccines?

Ans.
- Severe allergic reaction to vaccine component or following a prior dose
- Progressive or evolving neurological disease
- Encephalopathy not due to another identifiable cause occurring within 7 days after vaccination. Neurological side effects are attributed to pertussis component and occurrence of encephalopathy warrants further immunization with only DT component.

Q7. What are the precautions for administering these vaccines?

Ans.
- Moderate or severe acute illness
- Temperature 105°F (40.5°C) or higher within 48 hours with no other identifiable cause
- Collapse or shock-like state (hypotonic-hyporesponsive episode) within 48 hours
- Persistent inconsolable crying lasting 3 hours or longer, occurring within 48 hours
- Convulsions with or without fever occurring within 3 days

The above-mentioned points are situations where we can consider administration during outbreak.

Q8. What about giving paracetamol after DPT vaccination for fever and pain?

Ans. Prophylactic paracetamol should not be given routinely but should be withheld until symptoms of vaccine-related fever and discomfort develop. It is recommended to administer syrup paracetamol to the child in case of fever (axillary temperature of 38°C/100.4°F/feels hot to touch) following DPT vaccination as per recent Indian guidelines. However, there is concern that administration of paracetamol might bring down the immune response.

Q9. What is the efficacy of DPT vaccine?

Ans. Diphtheria toxoid has been estimated to have a clinical efficacy of 97%. Efficacy of pertussis is very variable. It ranges from 65 to 98% for different serotypes. A complete tetanus toxoid series has a clinical efficacy of virtually 100%; cases of tetanus occurring in fully immunized persons whose last dose was within the last 10 years are extremely rare.

Q10. What is the recommended schedule for DTwP/DTaP as of now?

Ans. The primary series consist of three primary doses at 6, 10, and 14 weeks of age followed by booster doses at 18 months and 5 years. The catch-up immunization consists of three doses at 0, 1, and 6 months with DTwP or DTaP. This can be given up to 7 years of age.

For children beyond 7 years and in adults, reduced component vaccine (Tdap or Td) is recommended to reduce reactogenicity. The primary series is three doses: 0, 1, and 6–12 months. The first two doses should be separated by at least 4 weeks, and the third dose should be given 6–12 months after the second dose. It is preferable that one of these doses (preferably the first) should be administered as Tdap. A booster dose of Td should be given every 10 years. Persons who have never received Tdap should be given a dose of Tdap as one of these boosters.

Q11. What is the prime difference between acellular pertussis and whole-cell pertussis vaccine?

Ans. Acellular pertussis-containing vaccines are less reactogenic leading to better acceptance; however, efficacy and immunological memory is superior for whole-cell pertussis (wP).

Q12. What are the issues regarding DTaP and DTwP?

Ans. Since 2009, large outbreaks of pertussis are regularly reported from both acellular pertussis (aP) and whole-cell pertussis (wP) using countries but majorly from the aP using countries. The shorter duration of protection and probable lower impact of aP vaccines on transmission are considered as major factors. Baboon studies have shown a superior effect of wP vaccines on disease transmission and quality of the immune response, predominantly Th1 and Th17 versus Th2 and Th17 of the aP vaccines. Superior priming has been indirectly demonstrated from attack rates of pertussis during outbreaks in countries where there is a heterogeneity of childhood pertussis vaccines received. Hence, there is sufficient proof that wP vaccines are superior to aP vaccines in the prevention of pertussis.

Q13. Why has the world not changed to wP vaccines?

Ans. Whole-cell pertussis (wP) vaccines were given up due to the reactogenicity profile and not because of superior efficacy of aP vaccines. The industrialized world would not take the risk of reverting to wP vaccines considering the low acceptance of these vaccines by the public in the past. Moreover, the wP vaccines have not been used in developed countries for >30 years. Manufacturing capacity will have to be reinstalled and re-licensure will have to be done.

Q14. Does the occurrence of hypotensive-hyporesponsive episodes, simple febrile seizures or hyperpyrexia contraindicate further doses of wP vaccines?

Ans. No. These conditions are precautions and not contraindications. These episodes may not occur with subsequent doses, may be milder following subsequent doses, and may occur even with aP vaccines albeit at a much lesser frequency. The incidence of these reactions is 75–90% lesser with aP vaccines. Parents should be counseled and helped to make a choice. Dropping further doses of pertussis vaccines should not be a choice.

Q15. What are the differences between DTwP and DTaP?

Ans. The differences between DTwP and DTaP have been described in **Table 2**.

Table 2: Differences between DTwP and DTaP.

Characteristics	Whole-cell pertussis (wP)	Acellular pertussis (aP)
Mechanism of action	Th-1 bias + Th-17	Th-2 bias
Correlate of protection	Not known	Not known
Animal model (for potency)	Known	Not known
Immunogenicity data (India)	Available	Available
Efficacy (Global)	Variable data	Robust data
Efficacy (India)	No trial	No trial
Effectiveness (Global)	Well established	Not established universally
Effectiveness (India)	Established	No data
Priming	Superior	Inferior
Duration of protection/waning	Longer	Shorter
Herd effect	Documented	No herd effect
Minor adverse event	1 episode in 2–10 injections	Equal to control
Serious adverse event	Very rare	Very rare (at par with wP)
Acceptance (global)	Poor	Good
Acceptance (India)	Good (no documentation of resistance)	Good

Q16. What are different components in aP vaccine?

Ans. The acellular pertussis vaccine contains one or more of the separately purified antigens—pertussis toxin (PT), filamentous hemagglutinin (FHA), pertactin (PRN), and fimbrial hemagglutinin (FHA types 1, 2, and 3).

Q17. What is the relation between number of components of DTaP and efficacy?

Ans. Two systematic reviews concluded that acellular pertussis vaccines with three or more components are more efficacious than the single- or two-component vaccines. However, use of two component acellular pertussis vaccines in Sweden and Japan and a single component vaccine in Denmark showed high effectiveness in prevention of pertussis. Thus, the higher efficacy for the multicomponent vaccine as demonstrated in the trials should be cautiously interpreted, and at present the evidence is insufficient to conclude categorically that the effectiveness of the aP vaccines is related to the number of components alone.

Q18. What are the various acellular pertussis vaccines currently available in India?

Ans. The acellular pertussis vaccines available in India are **(Table 3)**:
- Infanrix® (DTaP, IPV, Hib, and hepatitis B)

Table 3: Availability of various acellular pertussis vaccines in India.

	Tetanus toxoid (TT)	Diphtheria toxoid (DT)	Pertussis toxin (PT)	Acellular pertussis Filamentous hemagglutinin (FHA)	Pertactin (PRN)
Infanrix hexa™	40 IU	30 IU	25 mcg	25 mcg	8 mcg
Hexaxim®	40 IU	20 IU	25 mcg	25 mcg	xx
Pentaxim®	40 IU	30 IU	25 mcg	25 mcg	xx
Tetraxim®	40 IU	30 IU	25 mcg	25 mcg	xx
Boostrix®	20 IU	2 IU	8 mcg	8 mcg	2.5 mcg

Adacel® has TT 5 Lf, DT 2 Lf, PT 2.5 mcg, FHA 5 mcg, PRN 3 mcg, and fimbriae 2 and 3: 5 mcg.

- Hexaxim® (DTaP, IPV, Hib, and Hepatitis B)
- Pentaxim® (DTaP, IPV, and Hib)
- Tetraxim® (DTaP and IPV)
- Boostrix® and Adacel® (Tdap)

Q19. Are the DTaP brands interchangeable?

Ans. The available brands of DTaP vary in number of components, quantity of components, and method of inactivation of the components. Hence, interchangeability should be avoided as far as possible. However, in the event of nonavailability of the same brand, interchangeability is permitted.

Q20. How early can the first booster be administered?

Ans. First booster can be the earliest administered 6 months after the last dose of the primary schedule.

Q21. After how long can I give the second booster (dose 5) after first booster (dose 4)?

Ans. The minimal interval between dose 4 and 5 is 6 months but remember that the second booster cannot be given before 4 years of age.

Q22. How many doses of DTaP/DTwP can a child receive in early childhood?

Ans. The Advisory Committee on Immunization Practices (ACIP) and the American Academy of Pediatrics (AAP) recommend that no child should receive >6 doses of DTaP/DTwP before the 7th birthday due to concerns of reactogenicity.

Q23. Is it necessary to immunize individual who experienced natural infection for diphtheria, tetanus, or pertussis?

Ans. Yes, because natural infection does not confer adequate protection.

CHAPTER 15: Diphtheria, Pertussis, and Tetanus Vaccines

Q24. Why is the content of diphtheria and pertussis antigen reduced in Tdap, while tetanus remains unchanged?

Ans. The reactogenicity of diphtheria and pertussis antigen is related to the dose of the antigen, while the reactogenicity of tetanus is related to the number of doses.

Q25. Can Tdap be given as second booster at 5 years of age?

Ans. Although Tdap is licensed for use above 4 years of age it is best avoided as a second booster. Full dose DTwP or DTaP should be preferred. If Tdap has been given, there is no need to repeat the dose but ensure that the child gets the 10 years Tdap booster.

Q26. A pediatrician gave Tdap as third primary dose as the infant had febrile convulsion last time. Is the dose valid?

Ans. No. Low dose diphtheria and pertussis containing vaccine cannot be taken as valid dose in primary series. The dose has to be repeated by giving DTwP or DTaP.

Q27. If a child has received Tdap at 8 years as a delayed 4-6 years booster dose or for any other reason, when should the adolescent Tdap be administered?

Ans. For persons age 7–10 years who receive a dose of Tdap as part of the catch-up series, an adolescent Tdap vaccine dose should be administered at age 11–12 years.

This recommendation is as per the latest CDC/ACIP guidelines.

Q28. What are the recommendations for tetanus prophylaxis following an injury?

Ans. The recommendations for tetanus prophylaxis following an injury are mentioned in **Table 4**.

The recommended dose for TIG is 250 IU IM, give as soon as practicable after the injury. If >24 hours have elapsed, 500 IU should be given. Because of its viscosity, TIG should be given slowly using a 23-gauge needle.

Table 4: Recommended dose for tetanus immune globulin (TIG).

	Clean minor wounds		Other wounds	
	TT/Td/Tdap	TIG	TT/Td/Tdap	TIG
≥3 doses	Yes. If >10 years since last booster	No	Yes if >5 years since last booster	No
<3 doses or uncertain or unimmunized	Yes	No	Yes	Yes

Q29. What is the reactogenicity profile of repeated doses of tetanus toxoid?

Ans. Repeated doses of tetanus toxoid result in very high antitoxin levels. In this situation, an additional dose may result in antigen-antibody complex formation, which gets deposited in the skin, glomeruli, etc. This is known as the "Arthus reaction". Also, the fever and local pain is more if repeated doses are given.

Q30. What are the recommendations for immunization of pregnant women with Tdap/Td?

Ans. One dose of Tdap is recommended for pregnant woman between 28 and 37 weeks to protect the newborn and infants from pertussis. The second dose, if required for tetanus, is given as only Td after 4 weeks and at least 2 weeks prior to delivery.

Q31. What is the efficacy of maternal immunization in preventing infant pertussis?

Ans. Pertussis in infants, < 6 months of age has the highest mortality. These infants are too young to be completely immunized and hence needs passive protection by maternal immunization. In a study, mother was the source of infection in 37.3% of infant pertussis cases. In another study assessing the effectiveness of vaccination during pregnancy to prevent infant pertussis and hospitalization, the efficacy of maternal immunization was 91.4% (19.5-99.1) at the end of 2 months and 69% (43.4-82) at the end of 12 months.

Q32. What is cocooning?

Ans. The term "cocooning" means vaccinating anyone who comes in close contact with an infant. It is the practice of immunizing household people and healthcare professionals to prevent transmission to newborn babies. It is practiced for protection of newborn against pertussis. In this strategy, all individuals who would come in regular contact with newborn infant is administered a booster dose of Tdap including antenatal one dose of Tdap to mother.

Q33. If the mother did not receive Tdap in pregnancy, can she receive it after delivery?

Ans. Yes, the mother and close caregivers of the newborn should ideally be given a Tdap dose.

Q34. A 70+ years old couple want to visit their newborn grandchild in the United States of America. They have been told to have Tdap and come. I have heard it is not licensed for 64 years and above. Should I give it off label?

Ans. Of the two Tdap vaccines Adacel® is licensed till 64 years of age but Boostrix® can be given at 65+ years of age also. If availability is an issue, either can be given and is counted as valid.

SUGGESTED READING

1. ACOG/Clinical. (2017). Update on Immunization and Pregnancy: Tetanus, Diphtheria and Pertussis vaccination. [online] Available from: https://www.acog.org/clinical/clinical-guidance/committee-opinion/articles/2017/09/update-on-immunization-and-pregnancy-tetanus-diphtheria-and-pertussis-vaccination [Last accessed October, 2020].
2. Balasubramanian S, Shah A, Pemde HK, Chatterjee P, Shivananda S, Guduru VK, et al. Indian Academy of Pediatrics (IAP) Advisory Committee on Vaccines and Immunization Practices (ACVIP) Recommended Immunization Schedule (2018–19) and Update on Immunization for Children Aged 0 Through 18 Years. Indian Pediatr. 2018;55:1066-74.
3. Centers for Disease Control and Prevention. (2020). Vaccines and Preventable Diseases: About Diphtheria, Tetanus, and Pertussis Vaccines. [online] Available from: https://www.cdc.gov/vaccines/vpd/dtap-tdap-td/hcp/about-vaccine.html [Last accessed October, 2020].
4. Clarke KEN, US Centers For Disease Control and Prevention. (2017). Review of the epidemiology of diphtheria 2000–2016. [online] Available from: https://www.who.int/immunization/sage/meetings/2017/april/1_Final_report_Clarke_april3.pdf [Last accessed October, 2020].
5. Gowda VK, Veerappa BG, Handral A, Benakappa A. Re-emergence of Tetanus: Epidemiological Features, Clinical Profile and Outcome from South India. Indian J Pediatr. 2016;83(9):1015-7.
6. Kole AK, Roy R, Kole DC. Tetanus: still a public health problem in India—observations in an infectious diseases hospital in Kolkata. WHO South-East Asia J Public Health. 2013;2(3–4):184-6.
7. Marulappa VG, Manjunath R, Mahesh Babu N, Maligegowda L. A Ten-Year Retrospective Study on Adult Tetanus at the Epidemic Disease (ED) Hospital, Mysore in Southern India: A Review of 512 Cases. J Clin Diagn Res. 2012;6(8):1377-80.
8. Murhekar M. Epidemiology of Diphtheria in India, 1996–2016: Implications for Prevention and Control. Am J Trop Med Hyg. 2017;97(2):313-8.
9. Rubin LG, Levin MJ, Ljungman P, Davies EG, Avery R, Tomblyn M, et al. 2013 IDSA clinical practice guideline for vaccination of the immunocompromised host. Clin Infect Dis. 2014;58(3):e44-100.
10. Sidhu J, Dewan P, Gupta P. Maternal and Neonatal Tetanus: A Journey into Oblivion. Indian Pediatr. 2016;53:1057-61.
11. World Health Organization. (2015). WHO Pertussis position paper August 2015. [online] Available from: https://www.who.int/wer/2015/wer9035.pdf?ua=1 [Last accessed October, 2020].

CHAPTER 16

Haemophilus Influenzae Type b Vaccines

Sumitha Nayak

Q1. What is *Haemophilus influenzae*?

Ans. *Haemophilus influenzae* is a pleomorphic gram-negative coccobacillus which exists in encapsulated and non-encapsulated forms. The encapsulated organisms, also called the typeable *H. influenzae* are classified from a to f, based on distinct capsular polysaccharide. The non-encapsulated forms are known as nontypeable strains.

Q2. What are the disease syndromes associated with *H. influenzae* infections?

Ans. The *H. influenzae* type b (Hib) is responsible for a variety of diseases including pneumonia, bacteremia, meningitis, epiglottitis, septic arthritis, cellulitis, otitis media and purulent pericarditis, less commonly endocarditis and osteomyelitis.

Nontypeable *Haemophilus influenzae* (NTHi), which is commonly present in the nasopharynx of young children, is a common cause of localized respiratory tract disease, including sinusitis, otitis media, bronchitis, and pneumonia. Invasive disease due to NTHi is generally seen in the elderly and the immunocompromised.

Q3. Is there any change in the mortality rate caused by *H. influenzae* infection?

Ans. According to the World Health Organization, in the year 2000, an estimated 371,000 children died every year from Hib infection, while it was also responsible for 8.13 million serious illnesses in the same year. However, in 2008, the globally deaths due to Hib infection was estimated to be 199,000. In 2008, it was estimated that 19% of deaths in < 5 years age was due to Hib disease of which 20–25% was due to Hib infection. This resulted in 900,000 cases leading to over 48,000 deaths/year.

Q4. What is the case fatality rate from Hib infection?

Ans. Hib infection can result in complications such as meningitis, blindness, deafness, mental retardation, disability and death. About 10–15% of the cases have severe neurologic sequelae, while 15–20% of cases develop permanent deafness. The case fatality rate from Hib meningitis is about 5%.

CHAPTER 16: Haemophilus Influenzae Type b Vaccines

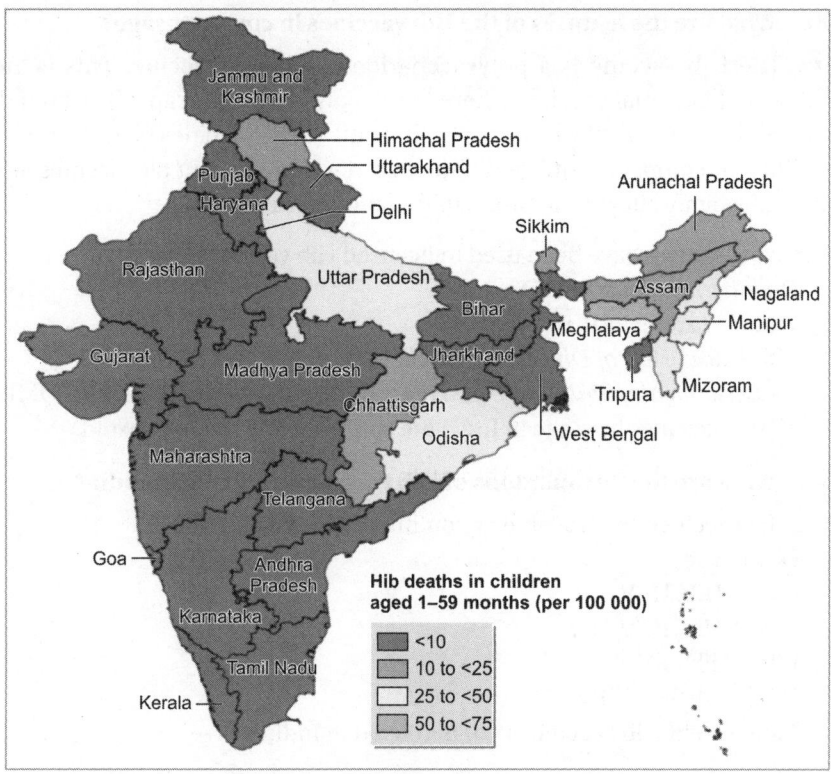

Fig. 1: Disease burden in India.
Source: Wahl B, Sharan A, Knoll MD, Kumar R, Liu L, Chu Y, et al. National, regional and state-level burden of *Streptococcus pneumoniae* and *Haemophilus influenzae* type b disease in India: modelled estimates for 2000-2015. Lancet. 2019;7:e735-47.

Q5. What is the disease burden in India?

Ans. According to current data available (2015), there were an estimated 15,600 (9,800–21,500) deaths in India between 1 and 59 months of age, which were attributed as Hib deaths. In the year 2000, there were 82,600 [uncertainty range (UR) 52,300–112,000] Hib deaths in India. Hence, a decline of 81% of Hib deaths has been observed since the year 2000. Despite this significant reduction, Hib is responsible for 3% of all deaths among children aged 1–59 months in India **(Fig. 1)**.

Being a vast country, regional differences in Hib mortality were noted in 2015. Approximately 65% [10,300 (6,500–14,100)] of Hib deaths were estimated to have been reported from the central region, which actually constitutes only 33% of the child population in that year. 83% of Hib deaths [13,000 (8,100–17,800)] occurred in the 8 Empowered Action Group (EAG states) and Assam, which together accounted for 55% of the <5 years age population. However, the overall Hib mortality declined in all regions, by 57% in the north east and 90% in the central region between the year 2000 and 2015.

Q6. What are the features of the Hib vaccines in current usage?

Ans. The Hib vaccine is a polysaccharide conjugate vaccine. This is an inactivated bacterial vaccine, where in the polysaccharide capsule is bound to a protein carrier by the process of conjugation. The vaccines manufactured by different companies utilize different carrier proteins, but all vaccines are generally highly effective in protecting against disease.

Four carrier types have been used in licensed Hib vaccines:
1. *Diphtheria toxoid*: PRP-D
2. *Tetanus toxoid*: PRP-T
3. *Nontoxic variety of Diphtheria toxoid CRM-197*: PRP-CRM 197
4. *Neisseria meningitidis type b outer membrane protein complex*: PRP-OMP.
All the vaccines in usage in India are conjugated to tetanus toxoid.

Q7. What are the formulations of Hib vaccines available in India?

Ans. Hib vaccines are available as combination vaccines:
- DTwP/Hib
- DTwP/Hib/HBV
- DTwP/Hib/HBV/IPV
- DTaP/Hib/IPV
- DTaP/Hib/HBV/IPV

Monovalent Hib vaccine is not marketed in India.

Q8. Is there any difference in the efficacy of the various formulations available in India?

Ans. As per available data there is no difference in the efficacy of the various Hib conjugate vaccines currently licensed for use. All the licensed vaccines produce the desired antibody levels in the body.

Q9. Are there any specifications regarding the vaccine storage?

Ans. According to the WHO guidelines, all Hib conjugate vaccines must be stored between +2 to + 8°C. As per the guidelines, the liquid Hib vaccines must not be frozen and the lyophilized vaccine may be frozen until reconstitution.

Q10. What is the schedule of administration of Hib vaccine?

Ans. Three primary doses to be administered as early as 6 weeks of age, at an interval of 4 weeks. The primary series must be completed by 6 months of age. A booster dose is given between 15 and 18 months, as per the Advisory Committee on Vaccines and Immunization Practices (ACVIP) guidelines of the Indian Academy of Pediatrics.

Q11. Is there any interference with the administration of other vaccines that are given in the immunization schedule?

Ans. There is no interference and the vaccine can be safely administered along with the other childhood vaccines. In case it is given as a separate vaccine, it can be administered as a separate injection at the same time as the other vaccines, at a different site.

Q12. Can the Hib vaccine be mixed with other vaccines before administration?

Ans. Unless the formulation has been specifically manufactured and licensed to be mixed in the vial or syringe with other vaccines, it should not be mixed with any other vaccine.

Q13. Is there any data pertaining to the correlates of protection and immunogenicity of the Hib vaccines?

Ans. Anti-PRP antibody titers >0.15 µg/mL correlate with short-term protection, while levels of >1.0 µg/mL have been found to correlate with long term protection against invasive Hib disease.

The Hib conjugate vaccines are highly effective in producing immunity to Hib bacteria and over 95% of the infants develop protective antibody levels with the primary series of the vaccine.

Q14. How efficacious is the Hib vaccine? Is the efficacy dose-dependent?

Ans. Meta-analysis data of trials done with conjugate Hib vaccines are available for review. All studies demonstrated high vaccine efficacy against invasive Hib disease with 2 or 3 doses of the vaccine. With one dose of vaccine, the pooled estimate was 59% (95% CI–20 to 86) with low heterogeneity. The pooled vaccine effectiveness from three case control studies was 95% (95% CI 82–99) after three doses and 92% (95% CI 81–97) following two doses. The evidence for confirmed Hib meningitis and Hib pneumonia is less robust because of fewer study reports with smaller sample sizes and pooled estimates.

Q15. What are the side effects that may occur after the Hib vaccine?

Ans. As with any vaccine administered, the injection site reactions may occur in about 20–25% of the vaccines. This usually is in the form of pain and tenderness at the site of injection within 24 hours. These reactions are mild and transient and generally resolve spontaneously within 3 days. About 2% of the vaccinees develop fever which is transient.

Q16. Are there any serious side effects of Hib vaccine?

Ans. Hib vaccine has been shown to be among the safest vaccines available currently. Serious adverse events are uncommon with all types of vaccines. This has been shown in a follow-up study of a large cohort of over 4,000 infants.

Anaphylaxis has not been reported in prelicensing trails. In postmarketing surveillance, causal relationship has not been conclusively proven between Hib vaccine and anaphylaxis.

Q17. Are there any definite contraindications to the administration of Hib vaccine?

Ans. According to the WHO, there are no contraindications to the use of Hib vaccine except in those with previous known allergies to any component of the vaccine.

Q18. What are the various schedules employed for Hib vaccines?

Ans. The WHO recommends any one of the following schedules for Hib vaccination:
- 3 primary doses without a booster (3p)
- 2 primary doses and 1 booster (2p + 1)
- 3 primary doses with one booster (3p + 1).

Q19. How is the number of primary doses decided?

Ans. In countries where the burden of disease is high, it is better to administer 3 doses of the vaccine early in life.

Q20. Does the booster dose provide any added benefit?

Ans. In regions where the disease burden is high and where there is a possibility of incomplete primary series, a booster dose is helpful in increasing the antibody titers. In case the disease burden peaks later in life, the booster is useful. Also, the waning antibody titers can be overcome by an additional booster dose in the 2nd year of life.

Q21. Is there any guideline for interrupted vaccination?

Ans. In case of delayed doses or missed doses of the vaccine, it is required that the remaining doses be completed, as per the recommended schedule, without restarting the schedule again. In case the child is over 12 months of age when the first dose is given, a single dose of the Hib vaccine is sufficient.

Q22. If a child received the 1st dose at 5 months and the 2nd dose at 15 months, is a 3rd dose necessary?

Ans. No. Single dose after 12 months of age is adequate for protection.

Q23. Can the Hib vaccine be administered above the age of 5 years?

Ans. For healthy children over 5 years of age, there is no indication for administering the Hib vaccine.

Q24. Should an unvaccinated child who has recovered from invasive Hib disease be vaccinated with Hib vaccine?

Ans. Yes. Invasive Hib disease below the age of 2 years, may not result in development of protective antibody levels. Vaccination should commence as soon as clinical recovery occurs. Child should receive an age appropriate schedule.

Q25. What is the impact of Hib vaccination in India?

Ans. According to data collected from the meta-analytic studies, there were almost 883,000 (517,000–1,750,000) cases of severe Hib disease in India during the year 2000. However, after the introduction of Hib vaccination in the National Immunization Program (NIP), the number of cases of severe Hib estimated in 2015 had reduced to 236,000 (138,000–468,000) cases. This is a significant reduction of over 75%.

Q26. Has the vaccination impacted the deaths due to Hib?

Ans. Since the introduction of the Hib vaccine as part of the pentavalent vaccine in 2012, there has been an 81% decline in Hib deaths. The estimated numbers were 82,600 (52,300–112,000) in the year 2000, which dropped to 15,600 (9,800–21,500) in the year 2015.

■ SUGGESTED READING

1. Balasubramanian S, Shah A, Pemde HK, Chatterjee P, Shivananda S, Gudurru VK, et al. Indian Academy of Pediatrics (IAP) advisory committee on vaccines and immunization practices recommended immunization schedule (2018-12019) and update on immunization for children for ages 0 through 18 years. Ind Pedaitr. 2018;55:1066-74.
2. CDC. Vaccines and preventable diseases. Hib vaccine recommendations. [online] Available from: https://www.cdc.gov/vaccines/vpd/hib/hcp/recommendations.html. [Last Accessed November, 2020].
3. Center for Disease Control and Prevention. *Haemophilus influenzae* Disease (Including Hib). [online] Available from: www.cdc.gov/hi-disease/clinicians.html. [Last Accessed November, 2020].
4. Center for Disease Control and Prevention. Vaccines and preventable diseases. About Hib Vaccines. [online] Available from: https://www.cdc.gov/vaccines/vpd/hib/hcp/about-vaccine.html. [Last Accessed November, 2020].
5. Griffiths UK, Clark A, Gessner B, Miners A, Sanderson C, Sedyaningsih ER, et al. Dose-specific efficacy of *Haemophilus influenzae* type b conjugate vaccines: a systematic review and meta-analysis of random controlled clinical trials. Epidemiol Infect. 2012;140:1343-55.
6. Jackson C, Mann A, Mangtani P, Fine P. Systematic review of observational data on the effectiveness of *Haemophilus influenzae* b (Hib) vaccines to allow optimization of vaccine schedules. London: London School of hygiene and Tropical Medicine; 2012.
7. Wahl B, Sharan A, Knoll MD, Kumar R, Liu L, Chu Y, et al. National, regional and state-level burden of *Streptococcus pneumoniae* and *Haemophilus influenzae* type b disease in India: modelled estimates for 2000-2015. Lancet. 2019;7:e735-47.
8. WHO. (2013). *Haemophilus influenzae* b vaccination. [online] Available from: https://www.who.int/immunization/position_papers/Hib_summary.pdf?ua=1. [Last Accessed November, 2020].
9. WHO. Contraindications. [online] Available from: Https://Www.Who.Int/Immunization/Policy/Contraindications.Pdf. [Last Accessed November, 2020].
10. WHO. *Haemophilus influenzae* type b, Disease burden. [online] Available from: http://www.emro.who.int/health-topics/haemophilus-influenzae-type-b/disease-burden.html. [Last Accessed November, 2020].
11. WHO. Hib vaccine. Weekly Epidemiolog Record. 2003;88(39):413-28.

CHAPTER 17

Hepatitis B Vaccines

S Shivananda, Arun Wadhwa

Q1. Which are the viruses known to cause hepatitis?

Ans. Hepatitis A, B, C, D, and E viruses are known to cause hepatitis. Hepatitis A and E are waterborne and B, C, and D are bloodborne.

A, E, and B are known to cause acute hepatitis syndromes; B, C, and D are associated with chronicity. Occasionally E also causes chronic hepatitis.

Q2. Is hepatitis B a problem in the world?

Ans. In 1995, it was estimated that nearly 2 billion people in the world had evidence of past or present hepatitis infection, which amounts to almost one in four persons. In 2015, the global prevalence of hepatitis B in the world was about 3.5% and 257 million people were having chronic hepatitis B infection. In 2015, hepatitis B resulted in estimated 887 000 deaths, mostly from cirrhosis and hepatocellular carcinoma (i.e., primary liver cancer).

Q3. How is hepatitis B endemicity classified?

Ans. The endemicity is assessed by the prevalence of surface antigen of the hepatitis B virus (HBsAg) carrier rate in the community. The country is classified as high prevalence if carrier rate is >5%, medium prevalence if 2–4% and low prevalence if <2%. India with a carrier rate of 3.8–4.2% is considered as a medium prevalence country. Tropical Africa with 6.1% carrier rate and Western Pacific countries with 6.2% carrier rate are considered as high prevalence areas.

Q4. Why is hepatitis B virus (HBV) given so much importance?

Ans. Hepatitis B virus is extremely infectious and very little quantities of serum (as low as 0.00001 mL for parenteral transmission) would suffice for transmitting the virus. It is known to cause chronic diseases such as chronic hepatitis, cirrhosis, and hepatocellular carcinoma. Also, the people have a risk of transmitting the infection. In 2015, nearly 9 lakh people died of HBV infection, nearly 3.4 lakh due to HCC, 4.6 lakh due to cirrhosis, and 1 lakh due to acute infection.

Q5. What are all the antigens related to HBV and how are they important in promoting vaccination?

Ans. There are three antigens—c, e, and s (**Fig. 1**):

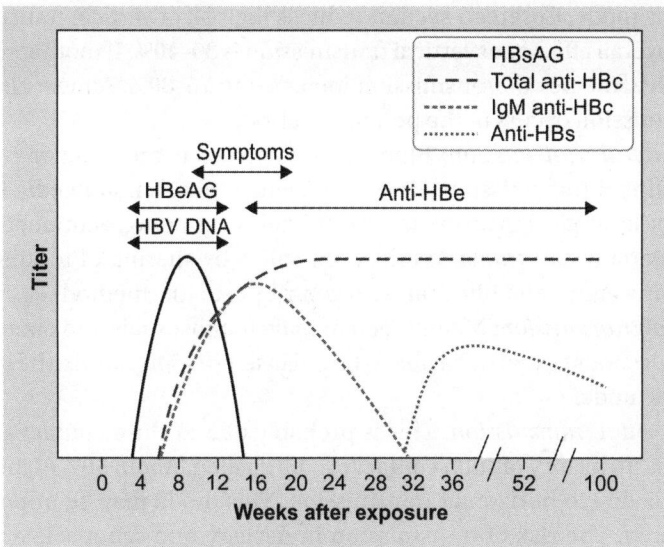

Fig. 1: Antigens related to hepatitis B virus (HBV). (DNA: deoxyribonucleic acid; IgG: immunoglobulin G)

HBcAg is a core antigen and indicates acute infection. Anti-HBcAg antibody is formed in the infection stage in high titers but they are not protective and persist almost for life.

HBeAg is an envelope protein. It indicates that virus is actively multiplying in blood, and other body fluids such as saliva and semen and such a person is highly infectious to others.

HBsAg is a surface antigen. It is a marker of infectivity. Its presence indicates acute or chronic HBV infection. Antibody to this antigen indicates protective immunity as developed either after infection or after successful vaccination or passively acquired as after immunoglobulin preparations.

Q6. What are the consequences of HBV infection?

Ans.
- Acute infection
- Chronic infection which can further lead to:
  - Persistent HBV infection indicated by the presence of detectable HBsAg in the blood with or without the presence of replication of virus or hepatocellular injury referred to as carrier state.
  - High risk of cirrhosis
  - Hepatocellular carcinoma

Q7. How is hepatitis B transmitted?

Ans.
- *Vertical transmission*: From the mother to the fetus or newborn during perinatal period mostly during birth. 50% of the carrier pool is contributed

by this mode. Cesarean section reduces the risk of vertical transmission. The overall efficacy of vertical transmission is 30–40%. If mother is HBeAg positive, the risk of transmission increases to 75–80%. Almost all vertical transmission occurs in the perinatal period.
- *Parenteral transmission*: Blood and its products are a major reason of hepatitis B transmission. Unsterile needles, accidental needle injuries, unsterile surgical instruments, razor blades, tattooing, acupuncture, and ear piercing can transmit infection. Saliva by sharing of toothbrushes, chewing gums, and bites can also contribute to this method.
- *Sexual transmission*: Mainly seen in male homosexuals and couples with promiscuous sexual behavior. Artificial insemination can also be included in this mode.
- *Horizontal transmission*: This is probably due to close contact although in 50% no history of such contact can be elicited. About 50% of the carrier pool is due to horizontal transmission. This mode may be important in children. The risk of transmission in daycare and schools is extremely low, except by bites of HBsAg positive inmates. Kissing, hugging, or oral sex does not result in transmission. Sharing drinking cups, straws, or other eating utensils have not been shown to cause transmission.

Q8. What is the importance of the "Birth dose"?

Ans. Vertical transmission is responsible for >50% of all childhood hepatitis B infection. The risk and development of chronic HBV infection is inversely related to the age of acquiring infection. Newborns usually do not develop acute symptoms but have a high risk of developing chronic carrier state. Approximately 90% of newborns infected at birth become chronic carriers and 25% of these will develop chronic liver disease including cirrhosis or hepatocellular carcinoma (HCC) later in life. That is why it is necessary to give hepatitis B vaccination within 24 hours of birth.

Q9. How long does hepatitis B virus survive in the environment. What infection control measures can be used to prevent spread of infection?

Ans. Humans are the only reservoir of hepatitis B infection. Hepatitis B virus is a heat stable virus can survive for a week and is highly infectious during this time. It is sensitive to solvents and detergents.

Q10. Will there be immunity after the natural infection? Is repeat infection possible?

Ans. Most HBV infections are self-limiting and like any viral infection, natural immunity develops by development of antibodies against HBs and HBc antigens. It takes about 4–6 months. Repeat infection is unlikely. Rarely another infection may occur because of another variant, different subtype, or a mutant HB virus.

Q11. Does co-infection occur with HBV infection?

Ans. 7% of HBV infections has an associated HIV infection. 10–15% of chronic HBV infection has associated HBC infection. About 5% of chronic HBV has HDV infection. HDV infection cannot occur alone, it requires HBsAg to form envelope.

Q12. Can we prevent HBV infection?

Ans. There are two ways of preventing HBV infection and they are mutually inclusive and not exclusive.
1. By taking universal precautions and practicing safe sex
2. Hepatitis B immunization

Q13. What are the hepatitis B vaccines available?

Ans. The older plasma derived vaccine, which consisted of purified inactivated HBsAg particles extracted from healthy chronic carriers of the virus, is no longer available. Since 1986 deoxyribonucleic acid (DNA) recombinant vaccines are available. They are derived from *Saccharomyces cerevisiae*, a type of yeast, and contain aluminum phosphate as adjuvants. Some vaccines utilize a different yeast, known as *Hansenula polymorpha*. Single dose vials contain 10 µg for children and 20 µg for adults. It is also available as multidose vials, 20 µg/mL. Most of the hepatitis B vaccine is now available as combination vaccine.

Q14. How many doses are recommended and what is the schedule?

Ans. Standard pediatric dose contains 10 µg of HBsAg and adult dose contains 20 µg of the antigen. Immune compromised persons and in special groups double dose is used. It is given as a three-dose schedule of 0-1-6 for adults and older children as catch-up schedule. For infants 0, 4–6 weeks, and 14–24 weeks schedule can be used. For programatic reasons, four doses can be given, with the birth dose, followed by 3 doses in a combination vaccine at 6-10-14 weeks. The pediatric formulation is recommended till 12 years of age.

Q15. What is suggested by the National Immunization Program (NIP)?

Ans. A monovalent vaccine should be given within 24 hours of birth, before the mother leaves the health facility followed by three more doses at 6-10-14 weeks as pentavalent vaccine when the infant attends the immunization clinic.

Q16. What does Indian Academy of Pediatrics (IAP) recommend?

Ans. Birth dose within 24 hours as monovalent dose and then at 6-10-14 weeks as a combination vaccine either as pentavalent or hexavalent vaccine. This additional dose does not cause any adverse effects.

Q17. An adolescent comes back for his second dose after 4 months instead of the usual 1 month. Should I restart the schedule? When should I give the third dose?

Ans. The minimal interval is at least 4 weeks between doses 1 and 2, and at least 8 weeks between doses 2 and 3, and at least 16 weeks between doses 1 and 3. It is not necessary to restart the series because of an extended interval between doses, no matter how long.

Q18. What is rapid schedule?

Ans. A rapid schedule of day 0, 1 month, and 2 months with an additional dose at 12 months and a very rapid schedule of day 0, day 7, and day 21 with a booster dose at 12 months have been approved by national regulatory authorities in some countries.

Q19. Is there any two-dose schedule?

Ans. For the two-dose schedule, the adult dose (1.0 mL) is administered to adolescents' age 11 through 15 years with the second dose given 4–6 months after the first dose. In immunogenicity studies, end seroprotection rates were similar between the two-dose and the three-dose schedules of 0.5 mL dose. Adolescents who have begun vaccination with a pediatric (0.5 mL) dose or if it is not clear which dose an adolescent was administered at the start of a series, the series should be completed with the three-dose schedule. However, this two-dose schedule is not a standard schedule.

Q20. What is the route of administration?

Ans. For primary schedule, the vaccine is given alone or along with combination vaccines in anterolateral aspect of the thigh. In adults, it is given intramuscularly (IM) in the arm in the deltoid area. It should never be given in gluteal region due to excess fat there which will interfere with the seroconversion, besides making this site difficult to access and risk of injury to sciatic nerve, especially in children.

Q21. Are the different vaccine brands interchangeable?

Ans. Yes. All brands of hepatitis B vaccines are interchangeable.

Q22. Is it necessary to observe the cold chain to store and transport the HB vaccine? What if cold chain facilities available are not adequate at the peripheral level and the vaccine has been exposed to heat?

Ans. Hepatitis B vaccines should be transported and stored at 2–8°C to maintain potency. Freezing causes dissociation of the antigen from the alum adjuvant resulting in loss of potency and higher reactogenicity. Hence, freezing should be avoided and a frozen vaccine should be discarded.

"Controlled Temperature Chain" (CTC), vaccines are kept at temperatures outside of recommended cold chain of +2°C to +8°C for a limited period of time under monitored and controlled condition. The birth dose of hepatitis B vaccine is authorized for use under the CTC, only in the NIPs.

Q23. What is the correlate? How do we know that the vaccine is immunogenic?

Ans. Hepatitis B vaccines induce immunoglobulin (Ig) antibodies to HBsAg. After the completion of three doses of vaccine, the HBs antibody levels can be assessed 4 weeks after the last dose. An anti-HBs antibody concentration of ≥10 mIU/mL measured 1-2 months after administration of the last dose of the vaccination series is a reliable serological indicator marker of long-term protection against HBV infection. >95% of infants, children, and young adults seroconvert to the three doses of vaccine. Studies have shown that no difference in the proportion of infants who were seroprotected after using different schedules such as 0,1,6, or 0,2,4, or 0,1,2, etc., although the GMT titers may be different. Titers may not matter as HBV infection has a long incubation period allowing anamnestic response to come in play and protect the person.

However, it may not be the same in case of immune compromised individuals such as human immunodeficiency virus (HIV), diabetes, chronic renal failure patients, where the seroprotection may not be optimal. In these conditions, there is a need to use double dose of the vaccine and/or to use extra one to three doses.

Q24. How long does the protection last after the completion of vaccination schedule?

Ans. In 90% of patients a three-dose vaccination schedule prevents all clinically apparent and chronic HBV infection for at least 30 years even in the persons in whom seroprotective levels of anti-HBs antibody is <10 mIU/mL. Most (88%) persons without this seroprotective level of anti-HBs antibody responded with a rapid rise in titer after a booster dose indicating immunologic memory and almost lifelong persistence of protection.

Q25. Is there any need for a booster dose?

Ans. Meta-analysis has documented that even after 30 years of three-dose schedule vaccination, no chronic hepatitis infection even in the presence of transient anti-HBc immunoglobulin M (IgM) antibody. It was concluded that individuals adequately vaccinated in a three-dose or four-dose schedule do not require a booster dose. Also, no evidence of a difference in protection with or without a booster dose administered when anti-HBs antibody concentrations decline to <10 mIU/mL. Vast majority of previously vaccinated people whose anti-HBs antibody concentration decreases to <10 mIU/mL mount an anamnestic response when they receive a booster dose or on natural exposure to HBV showing that they remained protected by memory T-cells.

Q26. Is HBV vaccine safe? What about anaphylaxis after the vaccine?

Ans. Hepatitis B vaccine has excellent safety profile. There may be minimal local reactions such as pain, fever, myalgia within 24 hours after vaccination. They are also rare and milder in children. The estimated incidence of the severe adverse event of anaphylaxis among vaccine recipients is 1.1 per million vaccine doses. Data does not indicate a causal association between hepatitis B vaccine and neurological diseases such as Guillain-Barré syndrome, multiple sclerosis, diabetes chronic renal disease, and arthritis.

Q27. Can the vaccine be given to pregnant women?

Ans. Hepatitis B vaccines are safe and can be given to pregnant women and lactating mothers.

Q28. Are there any contraindications of the vaccine?

Ans. Hepatitis B vaccine is contraindicated only for individuals with a history of serious allergic reactions to any of the vaccine components like yeast or to past doses.

Q29. Can the vaccine be coadministered with other vaccines? Will it not interfere with the immunogenicity of coadministered vaccines?

Ans. Data has shown that HB vaccine will not interfere with the immune response to any other vaccine and vice versa. Combination vaccines are also available and there is no immunological interference. The birth dose of hepatitis B vaccine can be coadministered with Bacillus Calmette–Guérin (BCG) vaccine and/or oral polio vaccine (OPV) within 24 hours of birth. When vaccinating at birth, only monovalent hepatitis B vaccine should be used. Hepatitis B vaccine (monovalent or combined) and other vaccines administered during the same visit should be given at different injection sites.

Q30. Is there any need to take for additional precautions in patients with chronic renal disease?

Ans. The patients with chronic renal disease are at high risk of HBV infection since because of their illness they are frequently exposed to needles, hemodialysis, and lack of adherence to standard infection control precautions. Their seroconversion is suboptimal and they need to be given vaccine containing a higher dose of HBsAg (e.g., double the usual adult dose 40 µg) on each occasion which gives a higher, rapid, and better response and or one to three extra doses. Fendrix, a rDNA vaccine adjuvanted with ASO4, is available in several countries (not in India) for use in those > 15 years of age, with chronic renal failure. It is administered in a 4 dose schedule of 0-1-2-6 months.

Q31. Is there any need of prophylactic vaccination for healthcare workers?

Ans. Yes. The staff working in the health facility and laboratory workers connected to medical facility are of increased risk of HBV infections due to exposure to blood and body fluids, and accidental needle stick injuries. They need to protect themselves by HB vaccination, if they have not received the vaccine before they start of their assignments. If they have received a three-dose series earlier in life, their seroconversion should be documented before joining.

Q32. Is there any specific guideline to be followed in HIV-infected children?

Ans. Immunogenicity and duration of protection depends on immune status of children in case of HIV children.

Severity, stage of the disease, CD4 count, viral load, and highly active antiretroviral therapy (HAART) status determine the response to the vaccination. However, studies have shown that if CD4 count is >1,500 and if the child is on HAART, duration of seroprotection for pediatric dose or adult dose is similar until 5 years after the vaccination.

Q33. What precautions are needed in immunodeficient children?

Ans. In children with immunodeficiency post-vaccination seroconversion should be documented at least 6–8 weeks after the last dose of the series.

Higher doses, greater number of doses should be given and boosters administered, if needed.

Q34. Suppose hepatitis B vaccine is not given in infancy, can we give it in older children, adolescents, and adults?

Ans. By giving the vaccine in older age group, it hastens the development of herd immunity—thereby preventing the spread of hepatitis. It reduces the incidence of acute hepatitis B. By reducing a subsequent chance of carrier state, complications of chronic hepatitis such as cirrhosis and hepatocellular carcinoma are also reduced.

Q35. Who are all eligible for catch-up vaccination?

Ans. Older children, adolescents, adults, and high-risk groups—sex workers, intravenous drug users, transplant recipients, and subjects with chronic diseases like diabetes.

Q36. Is there any role of prevaccination testing?

Ans. Prevaccination serological testing is not necessary routinely as the cost of testing is more than vaccine. It may be recommended for high-risk individuals such as patients with renal disease, HIV, and other immunocompromised conditions where subsequent clinical management depends on knowledge of their immune status.

Q37. Is there any role for postvaccination serology?

Ans. Routine postimmunization testing is not necessary for healthy people. It is recommended in the following groups:
- *Infants of HBsAg positive mothers*: These infants should have postimmunization testing for HBsAg and anti-HBs performed at 9–12 months of age.
- Patients on hemodialysis
- People with HIV infection
- *People at occupational risk of exposure*: Healthcare personnel including dentists, public safety workers
- Other immunocompromised patients (e.g., hematopoietic stem-cell transplant recipients or people receiving chemotherapy); and
- Sexual partners of HBsAg-positive people

Postimmunization testing is to be done 6-8 weeks after the final vaccine dose.

Q38. How should I manage an infant of an HBsAg-positive mother who tests negative for anti-HBs after three properly spaced doses of vaccine?

Ans. HBsAg-negative infants with anti-HBs levels > 10 mIU/mL are protected and need no further medical management. HBsAg-negative infants with anti-HBs < 10 mIU/mL should be revaccinated with a single dose of hepatitis B vaccine and receive postvaccination serologic testing 1–2 months later. Infants whose anti-HBs remains <10 mIU/mL following single dose revaccination should receive two additional doses of hepatitis B vaccine to complete the second series, followed by postvaccination serologic testing 1–2 months after the final dose. If the infant tests negative even after two- to three-dose courses it should be labeled as nonresponder and a third course is not advised.

Q39. Is it safe for an HBsAg-positive mother to breastfeed?

Ans. Yes. An HBsAg-positive mother who wishes to breastfeed should be encouraged to do so immediately after delivery. However, the infant should receive hepatitis B immunoglobulin (HBIG) and hepatitis B vaccine within 12 hours of birth. Although HBsAg can be detected in breast milk, studies have showed that breastfed infants born to HBsAg-positive mothers did not demonstrate an increased rate of perinatal or early childhood HBV infection. More recent studies have shown that, among infants receiving postexposure prophylaxis to prevent perinatal HBV infection, there is no increased risk of infection among breastfed infants. Mothers with cracked/bleeding nipples can also breastfeed. Proper feeding techniques and nipple care should be advised.

Q40. Can hepatitis B vaccine be given to preterm babies and babies less than 2 kg?

Ans. Hepatitis B vaccine is found to have no adverse effects in preterm babies and low birthweight (LBW) infants. Some infants with LBW (<2,000 g) may not respond to the birth dose as well as full term, normal weight infants. By 1 month of chronological age, LBW infants, regardless of their initial weight or gestational age at birth, are likely to respond adequately to three doses.

In babies <2,000 g: (1) If mother HBsAg negative: Dose 1 at 30 days of age, dose 2 and 3 as per schedule adopted for full term infants. (2) If mother HBsAg positive or unknown status: Hepatitis B vaccine + Hepatitis B immunoglobulin (HBIG) (within 12 hours of birth), continue vaccine series with three more doses beginning at 4–6 weeks of age as per schedule for full-term infants. Immunize with four doses, do not count birth dose as part of vaccine series. Check anti-HBs antibody and HBsAg 1 month after completion of vaccine. The WHO recommends that a birth dose of hepatitis B vaccine can be given to low birth weight infants. This birth dose should not be counted and three doses of the standard primary series should be given according to the national vaccination schedule.

Q41. Where else HBIG is used?

Ans. Hepatitis B immunoglobulin (HBIG) induces temporary immunity after exposure in a high-risk situation such as:
- People who have had percutaneous or mucous membrane exposure to HBsAg-positive blood or body fluids.
- Unvaccinated people who have been sexually exposed to an HBsAg-positive person.
- Patients who need protection from recurrent HBV infection following liver transplantation.

Q42. What is the dose of HBIG?

Ans. The dose of HBIG in adults is 0.06 mL/kg and in neonates/infants 0.5 mL.

Q43. There are many situations where healthcare worker gets an accidental needle stick injury. Is there any need of medical care?

Ans. One has to have postexposure prophylaxis measure urgently to prevent hepatitis B. The site of exposure has to be washed with soap and running water thoroughly and not to use disinfectants. The risk of exposure has to be assessed to plan prophylaxis. One has to assess the source of exposure, immunization status of the exposed and also site and severity of the exposure. HBsAg testing should be done on the healthcare personnel (HCP) and the source **(Table 1)**.

Table 1: Exposed individual and HBsAg status of source

Exposed individual	HBsAg status of source		
	HBsAg positive	HBsAg negative	HBsAg unknown
Unimmunized	HBIG (0.06 mL/kg) × 1 and start vaccine series	Start vaccine series	Start vaccine series
Previously immunized			
1. Partially immunized	HBIG × 1 dose and complete vaccine series	Complete schedule	Complete series
2. Response unknown	Test exposed person for anti-HBs • If adequate • no treatment • If inadequate HBIG × 1 and restart three-dose vaccine series	No intervention	Test exposed person for anti-HBs • If adequate • no treatment • If inadequate vaccine booster dose
3. Known nonresponder No revaccination	HBIG × 1 and start revaccination	No treatment; start revaccination for future protection	If known high-risk source, treat as if source were HBsAg positive
4. Known nonresponder to initial and revaccination series	HBIG × 2 doses Second dose 1 month after first dose	No intervention	If known high-risk source, treat as if source were HBsAg positive

(HBsAg: surface antigen of the hepatitis B virus; HBIG: hepatitis B immunoglobulin)

Q44. Are HBV mutants important issues in vaccine failure?

Ans. Hepatitis B virus (HBV) mutations have been found both in acute and chronic patients and in all the four HBV open reading frames (ORFs—preS/S, polymerase, preCore/core, and X). Studies show that 1-14% of hepatitis B infections may be due to mutants. Some mutants may have a role in vaccine failures.

Q45. What is the new adjuvant vaccine Heplisav-B?

Ans. Heplisav-B contains a novel immunostimulatory adjuvant (CpG 1018) that binds to toll-like receptor 9 to stimulate a directed immune response to HBsAg. It is provided in a single dose 0.5 mL vial and given as a two-dose series with doses separated by 1 month. It was found to be more immunogenic than the comparator vaccine, Engerix B™. Local reactions were most commonly reported (injection site pain, redness, and swelling) and were similar in frequency to the recombinant hepatitis B. Heplisav-B was approved by the Food and Drug Administration (FDA) in November 2017 for persons 18 years of age and older.

Q46. Is there any health impact of routine hepatitis B vaccination?

Ans. By the end of 2015, 84% of infants had received three doses of the vaccine across the world. During this period of 1980–2015, after the routine immunization either with standalone or combination vaccination, the prevalence of chronic infection has come down from 4.7 to 1.3%. In Western Pacific countries after the introduction of neonatal immunization, the prevalence of HBV infection has come down from 8 to 1%. It has been estimated that 14.5 million chronic hepatitis infections have been prevented among children under 5 years of age. This emphasizes the importance of this vaccine.

Q47. How many countries have introduced the HBV vaccination in their national immunization program (NIP)?

Ans. Hepatitis B vaccine for infants had been introduced nationwide in 189 countries by the end of 2018, and global coverage with three doses of hepatitis B vaccine was estimated at 84%.

The global coverage with the neonatal dose is 42%.

Q48. What are the goals?

Ans. The United Nations agenda of sustainable development goal (SDG) is to combat hepatitis by 2030. Global health sector strategy 2016 is envisaging to reduce the new hepatitis infections by 30% among under-fives by 2020. That is equivalent to the prevalence of 1% and aim is to achieve a prevalence of 0.1% by the year 2030.

■ SUGGESTED READING

1. Advisory Committee on Vaccines and Immunization Practices, Indian Academy of Pediatrics. IAP Guidebook on Immunization 2018–2019, Third Edition. New Delhi: Jaypee Brothers Medical Publishers; 2019.
2. Centers for Disease Control and Prevention Immunization of Health-Care Personnel: Recommendations of the Advisory Committee on Immunization Practices, MMWR. 2011;60(7):1-4.
3. Centers for Disease Control and Prevention. A Comprehensive Immunization Strategy to Eliminate Transmission of Hepatitis B Virus Infection in the United States: Recommendations of the Advisory Committee on Immunization Practices (ACIP). MMWR. 2005;54:RR16.
4. Damme PV, Ward J, Shouval D, Wiersma S, Zanetti A. Hepatitis B vaccines. In: Plotkin SA, Orenstein WA, Offit PA (Eds). Vaccines, 6th edition, Philadelphia: Saunders Elsevier; 2016.
5. Mast EE, Margolis HS, Fiore AE, Brink EW, Goldstein ST, Wang SA, et al. A Comprehensive Immunization Strategy to Eliminate Transmission of Hepatitis B Virus Infection in the United States: recommendations of the Advisory Committee on Immunization Practices (ACIP) part 1: immunization of infants, children, and adolescents. MMWR Recomm Rep. 2005;54(RR-16):1-31.
6. World Health Organization, Geneva. (2017). Global Hepatitis Report,. (2017). [online] Available from http://apps.who.int/iris/bitstream/10665/255016/1/ 9789241565455-eng. pdf?ua=1 [Last accessed November, 2020].
7. World Health Organization. Hepatitis B vaccines. WHO Position Paper. Weekly Epidemiol Record, No 27. 2017.

CHAPTER 18

Rotavirus Vaccines

Abhay K Shah, Aashay Abhay Shah

Q1. What is the importance of rotavirus (RV) disease in children?

Ans. Diarrheal diseases are the second leading cause of deaths among children under the age of 5 years and accounts for 1 in 10 child deaths worldwide. Rotavirus infections are the most common causes of severe gastroenteritis in children below 5 years of age worldwide and account for 5% of all deaths among children in this age group. Mortality and hospitalization rates are higher in malnourished children and children from poor socioeconomic class. Fortunately, it is a vaccine preventable disease.

Q2. Which are important characteristics related to rotavirus infections? What is the mode of transmission?

Ans. Rotavirus is often called "the democratic virus" because every child in every country, rich or poor, regardless of access to safe water and sanitation, is at a risk of infection; however, the outcome differs depending on the access to healthcare and parent health-seeking behavior. Rotavirus gastroenteritis is associated with severe vomiting and high fever at the onset which leads to failure of oral rehydration solution (ORS) therapy and need for unscheduled intravenous (IV) fluids which will need availability of appropriate healthcare facility for hospitalization or emergency care visit. The most common mode of transmission for rotavirus (RV) is through fecal-oral spread, either from person-to-person or contact with contaminated environmental surfaces. Transmission through respiratory droplets has also been suggested. A seasonal pattern is seen in temperate climates, where the disease is more pronounced during drier and cooler months. No specific seasonal trend is observed in tropical climates. RV infection is generally more severe in children aged 3–35 months, especially malnourished, with the first infection being the most severe. Viral shedding is the highest during the first 2–5 days of illness. Chances of spread of infection within families, daycare centers, and hospitals are high. Nosocomial infections are also common and are a major cause of diarrhea in newborns and infants.

Q3. What is the global burden of RV diseases?

Ans. Rotavirus (RV) infection is the most common cause of severe gastroenteritis in children under 5 years of age in both developed and developing countries. World Health Organization (WHO) estimates (April 2016) that globally 215,000 (197,000–233,000) child deaths occurred during 2013 due to rotavirus infection compared to 528,000 (465,000–591,000) in 2000.

Four countries (India, Nigeria, Pakistan, and the Democratic Republic of the Congo) accounted approximately half (49%) of all RV deaths under the age of 5 years in 2013. Rotavirus has a case-fatality rate (CFR) of approximately 2.5% among children in developing countries who present to health facilities. This CFR is higher in areas without good access to health care.

Q4. What is the burden of rotavirus disease in India?

Ans. It is estimated that by the age of 5 years in India, 1:2 child develops rotavirus (RV) diarrhea, 1:8 needs outpatient treatment, 1:31 inpatient treatment, and 1:345 dies (annually 78,500 deaths effectively) of it. Rotavirus causes an estimated 11.37 million episodes of acute gastroenteritis (AGE) in children <5 years annually in India, requiring 3.27 million outpatient visits and 872,000 inpatient admissions resulting in total direct costs of Indian rupees (INR) 10.37 billion/year. India contributes nearly 22% of rotavirus-related global deaths.

Q5. Does the natural rotavirus infection provide any protection to subsequent episodes?

Ans. Most rotavirus infections occur between 3 months and 2 years of age and are more likely to be severe in this age group. In a cohort study done in Mexico, it was shown that protection rates after a single natural rotaviral infection against a subsequent infection with rotavirus is 40%, against diarrhea caused by a subsequent rotavirus infection is 75%, and against subsequent severe rotavirus diarrhea 88%. No child with two previous infections subsequently developed severe rotavirus diarrhea. A longitudinal study in Mexico showed that the first natural infection protects against subsequent symptomatic disease (irrespective of the serotype) regardless of whether the first infection was symptomatic or asymptomatic indicating that rotavirus vaccines induce heterotypic protection. In a study done in India, protection against moderate or severe disease increased with the order of infection but was only 79% after three infections.

Q6. What are the different strains of rotavirus which are prevalent to cause rotavirus diarrhea?

Ans. The Indian Rotavirus Strain Surveillance Network (IRSN) (November 2005–June 2009) has shown a significant rotavirus disease burden and strain diversity in different geographic regions of the country. During 2005–2009, G1P[8], G2P[4], G3P[8], G4P[8], and G9P[8] were the most common rotavirus strains circulating worldwide. G1P[8] rotavirus strains showed the highest prevalence, except in the year 2009 where G9P[8] was the predominant strain, followed by G2P[4] as the second most predominant strain in other regions of India. Data from the extended-IRSSN (2012–14) showed a changing trend with G1P[8] accounting for 62.7% of isolates, G2P[4] 7.6%, G1P[4] 4.2%, G12P[6] 3.7%, G9P[8] 3.5%, G1P[6] 2.4%, G12P[8] 2.2%, and the rest being other G-P combinations and untypeable strains. In a recently published data G1P[8] (56.3%), G2P[4](9.1%), G9P[4](7.6%), G9P[8](4.2%), and G12P[6](3.7%) were the common genotypes in southern India and G1P[8](36%), G9P[4](11.4%), G2P[4](11.2%), G12P[6](8.4%), and G3P[8](5.9%) in northern India. Recently G9P4 strain is an emerging strain and claimed to be associated with more severe disease.

Q7. Which are the different rotavirus (RV) vaccines available in the market?

Ans. Monovalent and polyvalent RV vaccines available in Indian market are as follows:

Monovalent vaccines:
- Rotarix® (produced by GlaxoSmithKline biologicals) is a live-attenuated monovalent vaccine that contains one strain of live-attenuated human strain 89-12 [type G1P1A(8)] rotavirus strain.
- Indian neonatal rotavirus live vaccine, 116E. This vaccine developed by Bharat Biotech of India is a live vaccine, containing naturally-attenuated monovalent, bovine-human reassortant strain characterized as G9P[11], with the VP4 of bovine rotavirus origin, and all other segments of human rotavirus origin. It is marketed as Rotavac® by BBIL and Rotasure® by Abbott vaccines.

Polyvalent vaccines:
- RotaTeq® is a pentavalent bovine–human, reassortant vaccine (produced by Merck and Company). It contains five reassortant rotaviruses developed from human and bovine parent rotavirus strains that express human rotavirus outer capsid proteins of five common circulating strains [G1, G2, G3, G4, and P8 (subgroup P1A].
- Bovine rotavirus pentavalent vaccine (BRV-PV) (Rotasiil™) is a pentavalent rotavirus vaccine developed from five bovine (UK) X human rotavirus reassortant strains (serotypes G1, G2, G3, G4, and G9) received from the US National Institutes of Health (NIH) and further developed by the Serum Institute of India.

Q8. How does rotavirus (RV) 1, in spite of being monovalent, give protection to other RV strains?

Ans. Development of the RV vaccines currently in use was based on the observation that natural infection can protect against subsequent episodes of severe RV-induced gastroenteritis (RVGE). Cohort studies carried out in Mexico showed that recurrent episodes of RV disease were less severe than the first episode; one episode of RV infection had a protective efficacy of 77% against RV-induced diarrhea. Two infections, either symptomatic or asymptomatic, protected 100% against subsequent moderate to severe disease of any serotype. In Vellore, protection after one episode of RV infection was 43% against RVGE, and it took three infections to induce 79% protection against moderate or severe RVGE. These studies indicate that the protection against subsequent episodes of SRVGE is predominantly heterotypic in nature. This forms the basis of the observed efficacy of monovalent rotavirus vaccines. The results of recent efficacy studies in Africa and Asia, where a high diversity of RV genotypes circulates and infection with multiple serotypes are common, have proved heterotypic protection following use of RV1.

Q9. How will you rate all the available rotavirus vaccines according to their efficacy and effectiveness?

Ans. All the vaccines prevent effectively severe rotavirus gastroenteritis (RVGE) but are less efficacious against mild RVGE or rotavirus infection.

Studies with *RV1 and RV5* have shown that efficacy of these vaccines in Europe and the USA against severe RVGE has been above 90% and in Latin America around 80%. Trials in Africa have yielded efficacy rates between 50 and 80%. In Malawi, the effectiveness of RV1 was 49% compared to about 77% in South Africa. However, since the incidence of severe rotavirus disease is significantly higher in high child mortality settings, the numbers of severe disease cases and deaths averted by vaccines in these settings are likely to be higher than in low mortality settings, despite the lower vaccine efficacy. Hence, despite this lower efficacy in low- and middle-income countries the number of hospitalizations and deaths averted are significantly higher compared with South Africa, Europe, and Latin America. Malawi is the leading country in terms of severe RVGE episodes prevented.

Indian Neonatal Rotavirus Live Vaccine, 116E

Vaccine efficacy against severe rotavirus gastroenteritis was overall, 53.6% (95% CI: 35.0–66.9; $p = 0.0013$), 56.4% (36.6–70.1; $p < 0.0001$) in the first year of life and 48.9% (95% CI: 17.4–68.4; $p = 0.0056$) in the second year of life. Vaccine efficacy against severe gastroenteritis of any cause was overall 18.6% (1.9–32.3, $p = 0.0305$), 24.1% (5.8–38.7, $p = 0.0123$) at the end of the first year of life and 36.2% (20.5–48.7, $p < 0.0001$) in the second year.

Bovine Rotavirus Pentavalent Vaccine

Vaccine efficacy against SRVGE in India at the time of the primary endpoint was 36% (95% CI: 11.7, 53.6, $p = 0.0067$) in the per protocol (PP) analysis and 39.5% (95% CI: 26.7, 50, $p < 0.0001$) in the PP analysis over the entire follow-up period (until children reached 2 years of age). Vaccine efficacy against the very severe rotavirus gastroenteritis cases (VSRVGE) was 60.5% (95% CI: 17.7, 81, p = 0.0131) at the time of the primary analysis and 54.7% (95% CI: 29.7, 70.8, p = 0.0004) for the complete follow-period in the PP population. Vaccine efficacy against severe gastroenteritis of any etiology was negligible at 7.5% (−4.9–18.5, p = 0.2221).

In the study done in Niger, the efficacy of three doses of vaccine as compared with placebo against a first episode of laboratory-confirmed severe rotavirus gastroenteritis beginning 28 days after dose 3 was 66.7% (49.9–7.9).

Q10. What is the impact of rotavirus (RV) vaccines in terms of effectiveness in various set ups?

Ans. A systematic review of 48 peer-reviewed articles with postlicensure data from 24 countries over the first decade of global postlicensure (2006–2016) showed a greater vaccine effectiveness (VE) in low mortality countries (LMCs) and a lower vaccine effectiveness in high mortality countries (HMCs) for both RV1 and RV5 as shown in **Table 1**. VE tended to decline in the second year of life, particularly in medium- and high-mortality settings, and tended to be greater against more severe rotavirus disease.

Q11. What is the effectiveness and seroconversion rate after first dose and second dose of rotavirus vaccine?

Ans. Not much data is available. All the efficacy data are applicable to completed schedules. For RV5, the efficacy of one dose against RVGE hospitalization and ED visits was 88% and two-dose efficacy was 94%. Similar data does not exist for the other RV vaccines. Similarly, for human rotavirus 1 (HRV-1) data shows that vaccine efficacy after dose one up to before dose two (median duration of follow-up), 61 days (IQR 51–64) was 89.8% (95% CI: 8.9–99.8) against any episodes of rotavirus gastroenteritis.

Q12. What is the latest Advisory Committee on Vaccines and Immunization Practices (ACVIP) schedule for RV vaccines?

Ans. Minimum age: 6 weeks for all available brands

Table 1: Vaccine effectiveness of RV1 and RV5 in Low mortality countries (LMCs) and High mortality countries (HMCs).

	RV1		RV5	
VE	LMC	HMC	LMC	HMC
Overall VE	84% (19–97)	57% (18–64)	90% (63–100)	45 (43–92)
RV hospitalization	88 (70–95)		94% (83–100)	
ED visits	80% (78–86)		81% (74–91)	
VSRVGE		64% (−114–83)		72% (58–80)

(ED: emergency department; VSRVGE: very severe rotavirus gastroenteritis)

Only two doses of RV-1 are recommended.
- *Rotavirus (RV)-5, RV-116E, RV-BRV-PV*: Three doses at 4 weeks interval, beginning at 6 weeks (not later than 15 weeks), to be completed by 32 weeks (BRV-5 last dose can be given up to 52 weeks as per product insert).
- *Rotavirus 1*: Two doses beginning at 6 weeks (not later than 15 weeks) with 4 weeks between doses, to be completed by 32 weeks (as per the World Health Organization) (24 weeks as per product insert).
- If any dose in series was RV-5 or RV-116E or BRV-5, or if vaccine product is unknown for any dose in the series, a total of three doses of RV vaccine should be administered.

Catch-up Vaccination

- The maximum age for the first dose in the series is 14 weeks and 6 days.
- Vaccination should not be initiated for infants aged 15 weeks, 0 day or older.
- The maximum age for the final dose in the series is 32 weeks 0 day (BRV-5 last dose can be given up to 52 weeks as per product insert).

Q13. What is the upper limit of age at which it is absolutely contraindicated to give rotavirus vaccine? Why?

Ans. Vaccination should not be initiated for infants aged 15 weeks 0 day or older because there are insufficient data on the safety of dose one in older infants. The maximum age for the last dose of rotavirus vaccine is 32 weeks and 0 day (BRV-5 last dose can be given up to 52 weeks as per product insert).

Q14. What are the guidelines of giving rotavirus vaccine after rotaviral diarrhea?

Ans. Infants who have had rotavirus gastroenteritis before receiving the full series of rotavirus vaccination should still start or complete the schedule according to the age and interval recommendations because the initial rotavirus infection might provide only partial protection against subsequent rotavirus disease.

Q15. What is the risk of intussusception following RV vaccination?

Ans. The available new generations of rotavirus vaccines are considered quite safe and the risk of acute intussusception is very small in comparison to previous vaccine. Rotashield (Wyeth Lederle), the first available rotavirus vaccine, was voluntarily withdrawn by the manufacturer after using for just one season in the United States of America in 1999 due to an increased frequency of intussusception in the first 2 weeks after vaccination. Based on the evidence of efficacy and safety outside India, both the RV1 and RV5 are licensed and are being used in India.

The overall estimate of relative risk (RR) of intussusception during the 7 days post dose 1 is 5.4 (95% CI: 3.9–7.4, three studies) for RV1 and 5.5

(3.3–9.3, three studies) for RV5. The overall estimate of relative risk of intussusception during the 7 days post dose 2 was 1.8 (1.3–2.5, four studies) for RV1 and 1.7 (-1.1–2.6, three studies) for RV5.

Rotavac™: In the pivotal study, six cases of intussusception were recorded in the vaccine (subjects enrolled were double that of placebo arm) group and two in the placebo group, all of which happened after the third dose. The minimum interval between dosing and intussusception was 112 days in the vaccine group and 36 days in the placebo group. 25 (<1%) infants in the vaccine group and 17 (<1%) in the placebo group died; no death was regarded as related to the study product.

Rotasiil™: In the Indian study, 13 cases of intussusception were diagnosed; 6 occurred in the BRV-PV arm, and 7 in the placebo arm. None occurred within 28 days of receiving a dose of BRV-PV or placebo.

Q16. In which states in India has the rotavirus vaccine been included in National Immunization Program (NIP)?

Ans. Government of India, in March 2016, introduced the rotavirus vaccine (116E) in the Universal Immunization Program (UIP) in four states namely Haryana, Himachal Pradesh, Andhra Pradesh, and Odisha. In phase 2, in February 2017, the available Indian vaccines have been expanded to five more states of Assam, Tripura, Madhya Pradesh, Rajasthan, and Tamil Nadu. Additional states included are Jharkhand and Uttar Pradesh. By September 2019, RV vaccines have been introduced in all the states of India.

Q17. Why the age restriction for RV vaccination has not been suggested by the World Health Organization?

Ans. Initially, the WHO recommended upper age limits for vaccination to minimize excess cases of intussusception. These recommendations were changed in 2009 after models demonstrated very encouraging results in terms of number of rotavirus deaths prevented by rotavirus vaccination using an unrestricted schedule, concomitantly with diphtheria,tetanus toxoid and pertusis vaccine up to the age of 2 years. As per WHO paper (2013) the model estimated that a restricted schedule would prevent 155,800 rotavirus deaths (5th–95th centiles, 83,300–217,700) while causing 253 intussusception deaths (76–689). Vaccination without age restrictions would prevent 203000 rotavirus deaths (102,000–281,500) while causing 547 intussusception deaths (237–1160). Thus, the model predicted that removing the age restrictions would avert an additional 47,200 rotavirus deaths (18,700–63,000) and cause an additional 294 (161–471) intussusception deaths for an incremental benefit-risk ratio of 154 deaths averted for every death caused by the vaccine. These additional deaths prevented under an unrestricted versus restricted schedule reflect an additional 21–25% children who would potentially be eligible for rotavirus vaccine. In low- and middle-income countries, the additional lives saved by removing age restrictions for rotavirus vaccination would outnumber the excess vaccine-associated intussusception deaths.

Q18. What is the government schedule for RV vaccine in universal immunization program?

Ans. The rotavirus vaccine is to be administered in three doses at 6, 10, and 14 weeks along with the first dose of the pentavalent (DTwP-HepB-Hib) UIP vaccines. The maximum upper age limit for giving first dose of rotavirus vaccine is 1 year. If the child has received first dose of rotavirus vaccine by 12 months of age, two more doses of the vaccine should be given with an interval of 4 weeks between two doses to complete the course in the second year.

Q19. Can the above schedule be followed in private practice?

Ans. No. In private practice, the manufacturer's recommendations or Indian Academy of Pediatrics (IAP) recommendations should be followed.

Q20. What about regurgitation/vomiting of RV vaccine dose?

Ans. While the product insert of RV5 does not recommend repeating the dose, the product of RV1 and 116E recommend repeating the dose. Readministration need not be done to an infant who regurgitates, spits out, or vomits during or after administration of vaccine as subsequent doses are going to take care of the same. However, the manufacturers of RV1 recommend that the dose may be repeated at the same visit, if the infant spits out or regurgitates the entire vaccine dose. The infant should receive the remaining recommended doses of rotavirus vaccine following the routine schedule (with a 4-week minimum interval between doses).

Q21. Can the RV vaccine be given with oral poliovirus vaccine (OPV)?

Ans. Rotavirus vaccine and OPV when administered simultaneously showed no statistical difference in their mutual immunogenicity and safety. Hence, they can be administered simultaneously.

Q22. What about interaction between RV vaccine and breastfeeding?

Ans. Breastfeeding does not seem to significantly impair the response to the rotavirus vaccines.

Q23. Describe the contraindications and precautions for the use of RV vaccine.

Ans. Rotavirus vaccine should not be administered to infants who have a history of a severe allergic reaction (e.g. anaphylaxis) after a previous dose of rotavirus vaccine or to a vaccine component. History of intussusception in the past is also an absolute contraindication for rotavirus vaccines administration. Latex rubber is contained in the RV1 oral applicator, so infants with a severe (anaphylactic) allergy to latex should not receive RV1 vaccine. Severe combined immunodeficiency (SCID) and history of intussusception are contraindications for use of both rotavirus vaccines.

Precautions for administration of rotavirus vaccine include manifestations of altered immunocompetence (other than SCID, which is a contraindication); moderate to severe illness, including gastroenteritis (vaccination to be postponed); preexisting chronic intestinal tract disease.

Q24. What about immunization with RV vaccine if the child is immunocompromised? What about their contacts?

Ans. Children and adults who are immunocompromised sometimes experience severe or prolonged rotavirus gastroenteritis. However, few safety or efficacy data are available for the administration of rotavirus vaccine to infants who are immunocompromised or potentially immunocompromised, including (1) infants with primary and acquired immunodeficiency, cellular immunodeficiency, and hypogammaglobulinemia and dysgammaglobulinemia; (2) infants with blood dyscrasias, leukemia, lymphomas, or other malignant neoplasms affecting the bone marrow or lymphatic system; (3) infants on immunosuppressive therapy (including high-dose systemic corticosteroids); and (4) infants who are human immunodeficiency virus (HIV)-exposed or infected.

There is no safety or efficacy data related to the administration of rotavirus vaccine to infants who are potentially immunocompromised, including those who are HIV-infected. However, two considerations support vaccination of HIV-exposed or -infected infants: first, the HIV diagnosis may not be established in infants born to HIV-infected mothers before the age of the first rotavirus vaccine dose; and second, vaccine strains of rotavirus are considerably attenuated. As per the safety data available from ACIP, RV is found safe in clinically asymptomatic or mildly symptomatic HIV infected cases. So RV vaccine should be avoided in symptomatic HIV cases with severely compromised states.

Immunocompromised contacts should be advised to avoid contact with stool from the immunized child if possible, particularly after the first vaccine dose for at least 14 days.

Q25. Can preterm infants receive rotavirus vaccine?

Ans. If the infant's chronological age meets the age requirements for rotavirus vaccine (for example, age 6 weeks to 14 weeks 6 days for dose 1), and the infant is clinically stable, vaccine is strongly recommended at the time of discharge from the hospital or after discharge from the hospital. For RV5, there is data in preterms where they did subset analysis for preterms from the original REST (Rotavirus Efficacy and Safety Trial) trial cohort and the results showed that the safety and efficacy were not different in preterms compared to full term babies.

Q26. What about interchanging a brand?

Ans. Ideally, the rotavirus vaccine series should be completed with the same product. However, vaccination should not be deferred because the product used for previous doses is unknown or unavailable. In such cases, the series should be continued with the product that is available. If any dose in the series was RV5/116E/BRV-PV, or if the product is unknown for any dose in the series, a total of three doses should be administered.

Q27. If the first dose of rotavirus vaccine is inadvertently given to a child aged 15 weeks 0 day or older, should the series be continued?

Ans. Infants for whom the first dose of rotavirus vaccine was inadvertently administered at the age of 15 weeks or older should receive the remaining doses of the series at the routinely recommended intervals. Timing of the first dose should not affect the safety and efficacy of the remaining doses. Rotavirus vaccine should not be given after the age of 32 weeks 0 day even if the series is incomplete.

Q28. Can rotavirus vaccine be administered to an infant who has received intravenous immunoglobulin (IVIG) in the neonatal period?

Ans. Yes. Rotavirus vaccine may be administered at any time before, concurrent with, or after administration of any blood product, including antibody-containing blood products. The effectiveness concerns with antibody-containing blood products (ACBP) do not apply to rotavirus vaccine, since it is administered orally and replication of the vaccine virus occurs in the gastrointestinal (GI) tract, "separate" from the site of the ACBP.

Q29. Describe storage and thermostability of available rotavirus vaccines.

Ans. **Table 2** describes storage and thermostability of available rotavirus vaccines along with their efficacy and route of administration.

Recently, two new formulations are available:
1. Serum Institute of India has launched in a single dose tube, Rotasiil™-liquid which can be directly administered in 2 mL dose orally, thus saving time as well as cold-chain space. Rotasiil™-liquid can be stored at 2-8°C for up to 24 months.
2. Bharat Biotech International Limited launched a new variant of rotavirus vaccine (ROTAVAC®) ROTAVAC 5D®, which is the world's first and only liquid formulation with lowest dosage form and can be stored at 2–8°C.

Table 2: Comparative analysis of storage and thermostability of available rotavirus vaccines.

	Rotavac	*Rotasiil*	*Rotarix*	*Rotateq*
Efficacy against very severe disease	India – 54.4	Niger – 66.8% India – 60.5%	Finland – 85% Asia – 48.3%	USA and Finland – 98% Africa – 39.3%
Route	Oral	Oral	Oral	Oral
Presentation	Liquid in frozen form	Lyophilized-reconstituted	Lyophilized-reconstituted	Ready-to-use liquid
Volume	0.5 mL	2.5 mL	1.0 mL	2.0 mL
Storage	Store at 20°C. It can be stored at 2–8°C at any time during shelf life until the expiry of VVV2	Below + 25°C	*Lyophilized vaccine in vials*: Store refrigerator at 2°–8°C *Diluent in oral applicators*: Store refrigerator at 2°–8°C or at a controlled room temperature up to 25°C	Storage and transport refrigerated at 2–8°C
Presentation	Single dose: 0.5 mL vial provided with an oral dropper	1 dose vial + 1 diluent vial (2.5 mL), 1 adapter and sterile disposable syringe	Single-dose vials of lyophilized vaccine, accompanied by a prefilled syringes of diluent (1 mL), and a transfer adapter for reconstitution	Single prefilled 2 mL unit dose in a 4-mL squeezable plastic oral dosing tube with twist-off cap. The dosing tube is contained in a pouch
Shelf life	60 months	30 months	36 months	24 months

SUGGESTED READING

1. Advisory Committee on Vaccines and Immunization Practices (ACVIP): Indian Academy of Pediatrics. (2014). IAP Guidebook on Immunization 2013-14, 2018-19. [online] Available from http://iapcalicut.org/uploads/archive/Guidebook.pdf. [Last accessed November, 2020].
2. Balasubramanian S, Shah A, Pemde HK, Chatterjee P, Shivananda S, Guduru VK, et al. Indian Academy of Pediatrics (IAP) Advisory Committee on Vaccines and Immunization Practices (ACVIP) Recommended Immunization Schedule (2018-19) and Update on Immunization for Children Aged 0 Through 18 Years. Indian Pediatr. 2018;55(12):1066-74.
3. Bhandari N, Rongsen-Chandola T, Bavdekar A, John J, Antony K, Taneja S, et al. Efficacy of a monovalent human-bovine (116E) rotavirus vaccine in Indian infants: A randomised, double-blind, placebo-controlled trial. Lancet. 2014;383:2136-43.

4. Giri S, Nair NP, Mathew A, Manohar B, Simon A, Singh T, et al. Rotavirus gastroenteritis in Indian children < 5 years hospitalized for diarrhoea, 2012 to 2016. BMC Public Health. 2019;19(1):69.
5. Indian Pediatrics. (2016). Rotavirus Disease India; The Present and Future Indian Pediatrics: Special issue on RV diseases, volume 53(7). [online] Available from https://indianpediatrics.net/july2016/current.htm [Last accessed November, 2020].
6. John J, Kawade A, Rongsen-Chandola T, Bavdekar A, Bhandari N, Taneja S, et al. Active surveillance for intussusception in a phase III efficacy trial of an oral monovalent rotavirus vaccine in India. Vaccine. 2014;32:A104-9.
7. John J, Sarkar R, Muliyil J, Bhandari N, Bhan MK, Kang G. Rotavirus gastroenteritis in India, 2011–2013: Revised estimates of disease burden and potential impact of vaccines. Vaccines. 2014;32S:A5-A9.
8. Kulkarni PS, Desai S, Tewari T, Kawade A, Goyal N, Garg BS, et al. A randomized Phase III clinical trial to assess the efficacy of a bovine-human reassortant pentavalent rotavirus vaccine in Indian infants. Vaccine. 2017;35:6228-37.
9. Margaret M Cortese, MD, Penina Haber, MPH. Chapter 19 Rotavirus CDC Pink book.
10. Patel MM, Clark AD, Sanderson CF, Tate J, Parashar UD. Removing the Age Restrictions for Rotavirus Vaccination: A Benefit-Risk Modeling Analysis. PLoS Med. 2012;9(10):e1001330.
11. Rosillon D, Buyse H, Friedland LR, Ng SP, Velázquez FR, Breuer T. Risk of Intussusception After Rotavirus Vaccination: Meta-analysis of Postlicensure Studies. Pediatr Infect Dis J. 2015;34:763-8.
12. Troeger C, Khalil IA, Rao PC, Cao S, Blacker BF, Ahmed T, et al. Rotavirus Vaccination and the Global Burden of Rotavirus Diarrhea Among Children Younger Than 5 Years. JAMA Pediatr. 2018;172(10):958-65.
13. Velázquez FR, Matson DO, Calva JJ, Guerrero L, Morrow AL, Carter-Campbell S, et al. Rotavirus Infection in Infants as Protection against Subsequent Infections. N Engl J Med. 1996;335:1022-8.
14. World Health Organization. (2008). Age restrictions for rotavirus vaccination: evidence-based analysis of rotavirus mortality reduction versus risk of fatal intussusception by mortality stratum [online] Available from https://www.who.int/immunization/sage/meetings/2012/april/rvagerestriction_WHO_Mar28.pdf [Last accessed November, 2020].
15. World Health Organization. (2013). WHO Position paper on Rotavirus vaccine 2013. [online] Available from https://www.who.int/immunization/policy/position_papers/rotavirus/en/ [Last accessed November, 2020].

CHAPTER 19: Pneumococcal Conjugate Vaccines

Sanjay Srirampur

Q1. Describe the organism causing pneumococcal disease.

Ans. *S. pneumoniae* is a gram-positive, catalase negative, facultative anaerobic organism that grows as a single-coccus or as diplococci (identifiable because of their lanceolate shape) and also in chains of variable length. Polysaccharide capsule surrounding the cell wall is responsible for virulence, type specific identification and stimulation of protective antibody in the host.

Q2. What diseases are caused by *Pneumococcus*?

Ans. Spectrum of pneumococcal disease (PD) ranges from:
- Asymptomatic nasopharyngeal carriage
- Noninvasive diseases are due to contiguous spread and include otitis media, sinusitis, and pneumonia.
- *Invasive disease (hematogenous spread)*: Invasive pneumococcal disease, invasive pneumococcal disease (IPD) (septicemia), meningitis, pneumonia, others like soft tissue infections, osteomyelitis, and endocarditis.

Pneumococcal bacteremia in patients with sickle-cell disease, congenital asplenia, or postsplenectomy causes a rapidly progressive, fulminant course marked by abrupt onset, progressive purpura, disseminated intravascular coagulation and death in 24–48 hours.

Q3. What is a pneumococcal serotype? How many serotypes are there?

Ans. The capsular polysaccharide determines the serotype of the *Pneumococcus*. There are >90 serotypes. The composition and the quantity of the serotype determine the virulence. Pathogenic serotypes are limited. The serotype causing a specific disease depends on the age, geographical region, and site of infection and may also vary over a period of time.

Q4. Does *Pneumococcus* exist as a carrier in the nasopharynx? Is nasopharyngeal carriage (NPC) common in children?

Ans. *Pneumococcus* is often present as a carrier in the nasopharynx of children. In developed world, the carrier percentage is about 27%, whereas in the developing countries it may reach as high as 85%. Another characteristic is very early colonization in the developing countries.

Q5. What is the significance of nasopharyngeal carriage (NPC)?

Ans. It is significant for two reasons:
1. Pneumococcal disease will not occur without preceding nasopharyngeal colonization with the homologous strain.
2. Pneumococcal carriage is believed to be an important source of horizontal spread of this pathogen within the community.

Q6. What are the common serotypes which cause the disease?

Ans. More than 90 serotypes are recognized. Of these, the 10 most common serotypes isolated from 22 global alliance for vaccines and immunization (GAVI) eligible countries were (in order of frequency), 14, 5, 1, 6B, 19F, 23F, 6A, 7F, 2, and 19A. Serotypes 1 and 5 account for about 30% of IPD in the developing countries.

Q7. What is replacement phenomenon?

Ans. After the introduction of the seven valent pneumococcal vaccine, there was a reduction of disease by the vaccine serotypes and replacement of the disease by nonvaccine serotypes. This phenomenon is called as replacement phenomenon.

Among nonpneumococcal conjugate vaccine (PCV)-7 serotypes, 1 and 5 cause significant pneumococcal disease in India as well as in other developing countries. Serotypes 1, 5, and 14 together account for 28–43% of IPD across regions and for about 30% of IPD in 20 of the world's poorest countries. Serotype 3 can cause IPD which is associated with increased mortality. Serotype 19A which is prevalent worldwide causes disease in all age groups and is highly multidrug resistant. Serotype 19A is the most common replacement serotype currently prevalent. Inadequate coverage of serotypes by PCV7 led to the formulation of PCV10 that provides protection against 1, 5, and 7 and PCV13 which protects against 3, 6A, and 19A in addition to protection against PCV-10 serotypes.

Q8. Which serotypes are common in India? Are there any Indian studies?

Ans. There are two large studies IBIS (Invasive Bacterial Infection Surveillance) study and ASIP (Alliance for Surveillance of Invasive Pneumococcal disease in India) study. The other study is the "Pneumonet" study from Bangalore. There are some smaller studies from Delhi and Vellore (**Table 1**). The "Pneumonet" study is funded by M/s Pfizer and the ASIP is funded by M/s GSK. These are all hospital-based studies.

The common serotypes reported from these studies are 1, 3, 4, 5, 6A, 6B, 7, 12, 14, 19A, 19F, and 45. Serotype 1 and 5 accounted for almost 29% of cases.

SECTION 2: Individual Vaccines

Table 1: Serotype distribution in different studies.

IBIS 1999	6, 1, 19, 14, 4, 5, 45, 12, and 7
ANSORP study 2011	19F (43.5%), 23F (4.3%), 6B (8.7%), 1 (4.3%), 5 (13.0%), 7F (8.7%), 19A (13.0%), and 15 (4.3%)
Delhi study published in 2013	19 (26%), 6 (11%), 7 (10%), 1 (9%), 14 (7%), 9 (5%), 33 (4%), 17 (4%), 11 (2%), 3 (2%), 18 (1%), 23 (1%), 12 (1%), 32A (1%), 15B (1%), 22F (1%), 5 (1%), 29 (1%), nonvaccine type E (1%), F (1%), and H (7%)
Vellore study published in 2015	14, 19F, 5, 6A, and 6B
ASIP	14, 5, 1, 19F, and 6B

Q9. What is the burden of pneumococcal disease globally?

Ans. Globally 14.5 million episodes of IPD occur and >500,000 children die of IPD yearly. Case fatality rates for septicemia are 20% and for meningitis is 50%.

Q10. What is the burden of disease in India?

Ans. There is a lack of data on pneumococcal disease in the community. Most data are hospital based and are on meningitis. A Bengaluru based 2-year prospective study, found that in the first year of study, the incidence of IPD was 28.8 per 100,000 children <2 years. Of this, pneumonia contributed to ~55% and acute bacterial meningitis ~23.5%.

In 2010, 3.6 million episodes of severe pneumonia and 0.35 million deaths due to all-cause pneumonia occurred in under five children. Among these, 0.56 million severe episodes (16%) and 0.1 million deaths (30%) were attributed to pneumococcal etiology. Pneumococci were responsible for 27–39% of all acute bacterial meningitis in India.

Q11. What are the types of pneumococcal vaccines available?

Ans. At present, three types of pneumococcal vaccine are available in India.
1. Pneumococcal polysaccharide vaccine 23 valent (PPSV-23)
2. Pneumococcal conjugate vaccine 13 valent (PCV-13)
3. Pneumococcal conjugate vaccine 10 valent (PCV-10)

Q12. What is the composition of PPSV23? In whom is it used? What is the efficacy of PPSV23?

Ans.
- Pneumococcal polysaccharide vaccine 23 valent (PPSV23) is made up of the following serotypes 1, 2, 3, 4, 5, 6B, 7F, 8, 9N, 9V, 10A, 11A, 12f, 14, 15B, 17F, 18C, 19A, 19F, 20, 22F, 23F, and 30F. It is a T-cell independent vaccine. It should not be used in children <2 years. It should be given for a maximum of two doses. More than two doses result in immune

hyporesponsiveness. PPSV23 does not prevent NP carriage and does not provide any herd effect.

A single dose induces production of antibodies. Antibodies are of immunoglobulin G (IgG), immunoglobulin M (IgM), and immunoglobulin A (IgA) class. The IgG antibodies are of IgG2 class. The antibody production in the elderly is less.

A retrospective cohort analysis study based in the United States of America showed 57% [95% confidence interval (CI): 45–66%] overall protective effectiveness against invasive infections caused by serotypes included in PPSV23 in persons ≥6 years of age, 65–84% effectiveness among specific patient groups (e.g., persons with diabetes mellitus, coronary vascular disease, congestive heart failure, chronic pulmonary disease, and anatomic asplenia) and 75% (95% CI: 57–85%) effectiveness in immunocompetent persons aged ≥65 years of age.

PPSV23 is a clear and colorless solution. Each 0.5-mL dose of vaccine contains 25 µg of each polysaccharide type in isotonic saline solution containing 0.25% phenol as a preservative. The vial stoppers, syringe plunger stopper and syringe tip cap are latex-free. It is to be stored at +2°C to +8°C.

Q13. What is the advantage of conjugate vaccine over PPSV?

Ans. Pneumococcal conjugate vaccine is a T-cell dependent vaccine; hence, it is efficacious in a child of <2 years age. It is more immunogenic, boostable, provides herd effect, reduces NP carriage, and helps to contain antibiotic resistance.

Q14. What is the composition of pneumococcal conjugate vaccines currently available in India?

Ans. There are three pneumococcal conjugate vaccines being marketed in India. The compositions are:

PCV13: Prevenar13™: In infants and children from 6 weeks to 5 years of age, it is indicated for active immunization for the prevention of disease caused by *Streptococcus pneumoniae* serotypes 1, 3, 4, 5, 6A, 6B, 7F, 9V, 14, 18C, 19A, 19F, and 23F (including sepsis, meningitis, bacteremia, and pneumonia) and acute otitis media.

In the age groups 6–17 years of age and adults of 50 years and older age group, it is indicated for active immunization for the prevention of pneumonia and invasive disease caused by *Streptococcus pneumoniae* serotypes 1, 3, 4, 5, 6A, 6B, 7F, 9V, 14, 18C, 19A, 19F, and 23F.

Each 0.5-mL dose of the vaccine contains approximately 2.2 µg of each of *Streptococcus pneumoniae* serotypes 1, 3, 4, 5, 6A, 7F, 9V, 14, 18C, 19A, 19F, 23F saccharides, 4.4 µg of 6B saccharides, 34 µg CRM197 carrier protein, 100 µg polysorbate 80, 295 µg succinate buffer, and 125 µg aluminum as aluminum phosphate adjuvant. The tip cap and rubber plunger of the prefilled syringe are latex-free. The vaccine is to be stored at +2°C to +8°C.

PCV10: Synflorix™ is licensed for active immunization of infants and children from 6 weeks up to 5 years of age against disease caused by *Streptococcus pneumoniae* vaccine serotypes 1, 4, 5, 6B, 7F, 9V, 14, 18C, 19F, 23F, and crossreactive serotype 19A (including sepsis, meningitis, pneumonia, bacteremia and acute otitis media) and against acute otitis media caused by nontypeable *Haemophilus influenzae*.

Each 0.5-mL dose contains 1 µg of polysaccharide for serotypes 1, 5, 6B, 7F, 9V, 141, and 23F, and 3 µg of serotypes 4, 18C, and 19F. All serotypes are adsorbed on aluminum phosphate 0.5 mg. Serotypes 1, 5, 6B, 7F, 9V, 14, 23F, and 4 are conjugated to 13 µg of protein D (derived from nontypeable *Haemophilus influenzae*), serotype 23F is conjugated to 8 µg of tetanus toxoid carrier protein and serotype 4 is conjugated to 5 µg of diphtheria toxoid carrier protein. The vaccine is to be stored at +2°C to +8°C.

PCV10-Sii: Pneumosil™ is licensed for active immunization against invasive disease and pneumonia caused by *Streptococcus pneumoniae* serotypes 1, 5, 6A, 6B, 7F, 9V, 14, 19A, 19F and 23F in infants from 6 weeks of age group for 3 dose regimen (dosing schedule: 6, 10 and 14 weeks)as per the Drug Controller General India (DCGI) and for active immunization against invasive disease, pneumonia and acute otitis media caused by *Streptococcus pneumoniae* serotypes 1, 5, 6A, 6B, 7F, 9V, 14, 19A, 19F and 23F in infants and toddlers from 6 weeks up to 2 years of age, as per WHO and IAP.

Each 0.5 mL dose contains 2 µg of polysaccharide for serotypes 1, 5, 6A, 7F, 9V, 14, 19A, 19F, and 23F, and 4 µg for serotype 6B formulated with aluminum phosphate (0.125 mg) as an adjuvant and thiomersal 0.005%. The excipients include L-Histidine (1.55 mg), Succinic acid (1.18 mg), Sodium Chloride (4.5 mg), Polysorbate-20 90.05 mg and Water for Injection q. s. to 0.5 mL. The vaccine is to be stored at +20°C to +80°C.

Serotype composition of PCVs:

	SEROTYPES											
PCV10-GSK	1	xx	4	5	xx	6B	7F	9V	14	18C	xx	19F	23F
PCV 13	1	3	4	5	6A	6B	7F	9V	14	18C	19A	19F	23F
PCV10-Sii	1	xx	xx	5	6A	6B	7F	9V	14	xx	19A	19F	23F

Q15. What is the clinical development data about Pneumosil™?

Ans. In a phase 1/2 randomized, double-blinded, controlled trial in adults, toddlers, and infants in The Gambia, the infant postprimary seroresponse rates (IgG level > 0.35 mg/mL) were >89% for all serotypes except 6A (79%) in the SIIPL-PCV group. IgG geometric mean concentrations (GMCs) were >1 mg/mL for all serotypes in both SIIPL-PCV and PCV13 groups. The serotype-specific OPA GMTs following the primary series were comparable for the two vaccines for six (1, 5, 6B, 14, 19F, and 23F) of 10 serotypes, while the responses were lower following SIIPL-PCVTM for the remaining 4 serotypes. Post-booster GMCs were comparable between groups. Serum Institute of India Pvt. Ltd.-pneumococcal conjugate vaccine (SIIPL-PCV) was well-tolerated and had an acceptable safety profile.

A pivotal phase 3 infant safety, tolerability, lot-to-lot consistency, immunogenicity (including boostability), and concomitant expanded program on immunization (EPI) vaccine noninterference study in The Gambia, with Synflorix™ as the comparator vaccine, comparator vaccine. Both Synflorix™ and SIIPL-PCV elicited a significant booster immune response for all 10 serotypes except serotype 5, while the OPA GMTs showed a booster response for all 10 serotypes with persistence of antibodies for all serotypes till 1 year of follow up.

Q 16. What are the other conjugate vaccines under development?

Ans. An Indian company with the support of Department of Biotechnology is manufacturing a 15-valent vaccine. The additional serotypes other than PCV13 are 2 and 12F. Merck is manufacturing a 15-valent vaccine the additional serotypes other than PCV13 are 22F and 33F. The conjugate used in both these vaccines is CRM197.

Merck's 15-valent PCV which contains ST 22F and 33F, in addition to the STs in PCV13, has completed phase 2 studies in adults and infants. In the infant study, the percentage of subjects who achieved the WHO-accepted threshold of immune response (IgG ≥ 0.35 µg/mL) was noninferior to the percentage seen with PCV13 for the 13 serotypes shared between the two vaccines. For serotype 3, the percentage of subjects who achieved this threshold of immune response was higher for PCV15 (96.0% for lot 1; 94.1% for lot 2) compared with PCV13 (71.8%). For the two serotypes not included in PCV13, serotype 22F and serotype 33F, the percentage of subjects who achieved the defined threshold of immune response with PCV15 was above 98% (98.9% for lot 1 and 98.5% for lot 2) and above 87% (87.7% for lot 1 and 90.1% for lot 2), respectively. The adverse event (AE) profile for V114 including the number of serious AEs was found to be comparable to PCV13.

Pfizer's 20vPnC candidate includes the 13 serotypes contained in Prevnar 13 (1, 3, 4, 5, 6A, 6B, 7F, 9V, 14, 18C, 19A, 19F, and 23F) plus seven additional serotypes (8, 10A, 11A, 12F, 15BC, 22F, and 33F). The target group is adults >18 years for prevention of IPD. Enrollment has been completed in its phase 3 pivotal clinical trials evaluating 20vPnC for the prevention of invasive disease and pneumonia in adults 18 years and older.

Phase 2 trials in infants has been completed. PCV20 has received Breakthrough Therapy Designation by USFDA.

Q17. What is the correlate of protection for PCV?

Ans. Any new PCV has to meet the following criteria laid down by the World Health Organization (WHO):
- Immunoglobulin G (IgG) (for all common serotypes collectively and not individually) of ≥0.35 µg/mL measured by the WHO reference assay (or an alternative).

Both vaccines (PCV13 and PCV10) have comparable immunogenicity of serotype specific IgG > 0.35 µg/mL.

Although traditional antibody levels [enzyme-linked immunosorbent assay (ELISA) or WHO)] are useful as a surrogate marker of protection, they have limitations and a bioassay measuring the capacity of antibodies to opsonize pneumococci has been developed. This opsonophagocytosis assay (OPA) is a better reflection of protection by vaccine-induced antibodies. The lowest serum dilution routinely used in OPA assays is 1:8. Detection of opsonic antibodies at this dilution had been proposed to be predictive of protection against disease

Q18. What is the efficacy of pneumococcal conjugate vaccines?

Ans. The efficacy of pneumococcal conjugate vaccines is measured for:
- Invasive pneumococcal disease (IPD)
- Pneumonia
- Acute otitis media (AOM)

Invasive pneumococcal disease: IPD represents the most serious forms of disease caused by the *pneumococcus*. While the trials used different formulations of the vaccine administered in infants in either a 6-, 10-, and 14-weeks' schedule or a 2-, 4-, and 6-months schedule, the efficacy estimates were fairly consistent. In a systematic review and meta-analysis from seven studies, a pooled vaccine efficacy of 80% (95% CI: 58–90%, $P < 0.0001$) was observed against vaccine type invasive disease and 58% (95% CI: 29–75%, $P = 0.001$) against total invasive disease (irrespective of serotype).

Pneumonia: The pooled vaccine efficacy against radiologically defined pneumonia was 27%. Studies in South Africa have shown that there was a reduction in hospitalization of viral associated lower respiratory infection. This suggests that coinfection with *pneumococcus* increases the severity of the disease.

Acute otitis media: The PCVs were efficacious in preventing AOM caused by the serotypes of *pneumococcus* present in the vaccine, with very similar point estimates of efficacy, ranging from 56 to 57.6%. In two trials done with PCV7, there was a significant replacement phenomenon with increase in OM incidence with nonvaccine serotypes. It was also noted that the vaccines prevent serious and recurrent otitis media. A third trial with PCV10 showed a significant protection against AOM caused by nontypeable *Haemophilus influenzae* (NTHi) with observed efficacy of 35% (95% CI: 1.8–57.4); this protection was attributed to the immune response to protein D of NTHi, which was the protein carrier in this formulation of the vaccine. The Clinical Otitis Media and Pneumonia Study (COMPAS) in Latin America showed that PCV10 has a vaccine efficacy of 16.1% against otitis media. A study done in Israel with PCV13 showed that the incidence of AOM per 1,000 children decreased from 12.2 to 6.

Q19. What is the efficacy of PCVs on NP carriage?

Ans. Pneumococcal conjugate vaccine 10 valent (PCV10) in Finland showed a reduction by 23–38% with 2+1 schedule and by 19–56% with 3+1 schedule. COMPAS study showed a reduction by 25.5%. PCV13 in the United States of America showed efficiency of 51% in fully vaccinated children with vaccine serotypes.

Q20. What is the effectiveness (real world impact) of pneumococcal conjugate vaccines?

Ans. Many countries which have introduced the vaccine as a part of the immunization schedule have seen a significant reduction of the disease both in the vaccine-specific serotypes and others. Reduction of the disease has also been observed in the unvaccinated group (indirect effect).

After introduction of PCV13 in the United States, there was 90% decline in the six serotypes driven predominantly by 19A and 7F. Following introduction of PCV13 into the national immunization programs of Argentina, Uruguay, and United Kingdom, reductions in hospitalized chest X-ray confirmed pneumonia and empyema cases were noted. Similarly, following PCV13 introduction in Nicaragua—a low-middle income country, reduction in hospitalization and outpatient visits for pneumonia was found in children 1 year of age. However, at least one study failed to document any reduction in radiologically defined pneumonia. In one trial using PCV9, conducted in a high mortality setting in Gambia, reduction in overall mortality of 16% (95% CI: 3–28) was observed. Finland introduced PCV10 in its national immunization program in 2010. The vaccine efficacy was found to be 98% against vaccine serotypes. In a systematic review and meta-analysis of the impact of PCV10 and PCV 13 on hospitalizations for pneumonia, it was found that the incidence of clinical pneumonia and radiological pneumonia was reduced by 17% (95%CI: 11–22%) and 31% (95%CI: 26–35%), in those < 24 months of age and 9% (95%CI: 5–14%) and 24% (95%CI: 12–33%), in those between 24–59 months.

Q21. What is the duration of protection after pneumococcal conjugate vaccine?

Ans. Follow-up of subjects from the PCV9 trial in Gambia showed vaccine efficacy (VE) of 78%; (95% CI: 34–92%) against IPD up to 6.3 years. This was with a 3+0 schedule.

Q22. What is the effectiveness of incomplete series?

Ans.
- *One dose*: 48%
- *Two doses*: 87%
- *Three doses (2 + 1)*: 100%

Q23. Is pneumococcal vaccine safe?

Ans. The safety of PCV has been well studied and all formulations are considered to have an excellent safety profile. The main adverse events (AEs) observed are injection-site reactions, fever, irritability, decreased appetite, and increased and/or decreased sleep that were reported about 10% of the vaccines. Fever with temperature > 39°C was observed in 1/100 to <1/10 vaccines, vomiting and diarrhea in 1/1,000 to <1/100, and hypersensitivity reactions and nervous system disorders (including convulsions and hypotonic hyporesponsive episodes) were reported in 1/10,000 to <1/1,000 of the vaccines.

Q24. What is the serotype coverage of PCV13 versus PCV10?

Ans. A systematic review commissioned by the WHO found that both PCV13 and PCV10 covered >70% serotypes in all regions of the world. A recently published systematic review of seven studies showed that the weighted average difference in serotype coverage between the vaccines is 11% (**Fig. 1**).

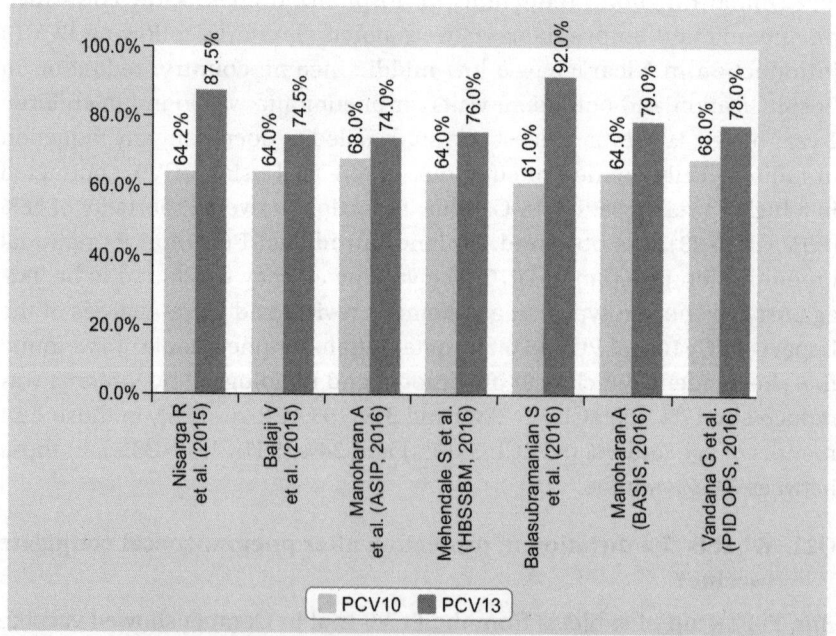

Fig. 1: A systematic review commissioned by the WHO: both PCV13 and PCV10 covered >70% serotypes in all regions of the world.

Q25. What is the dose and schedule of PCV13 and PCV10 as recommended by Advisory Committee on Immunizations and vaccine practices (ACVIP)?

Ans. The dose is 0.5 mL IM. Both the vaccines have been approved for use for children below the age of 5 years. As the age of incidence of pneumococcal disease above the age of 5 years is less, the routine use of this vaccine above 5 years is questionable (ACVIP 2018).

The ACVIP recommends the following schedule for PCV:
- *6 weeks to 6 months (PCV 10 and PCV 13)*: Three primary doses at 6–10–14 weeks (4 weeks interval), and a booster dose between 12 and 15 months of age. The booster can be administered 6 months after the third primary dose.
- *7–12 months (PCV10 and PCV13)*: Previously unvaccinated infants should receive two doses, at a minimum interval of 4 weeks between doses, followed by a booster dose in the second year of life.
- *12–24 months (PCV10 and PCV13)*: Two doses at least 8 weeks interval.
- *2–5 years*: PCV13: single dose
  PCV10: Two doses at least 8 weeks interval.
- *12 months to 5 years*: PCV 10—unvaccinated children should receive two doses with an interval of at least 8 weeks.

Q26. Are these vaccines interchangeable in the primary series?

Ans. Ideally, the vaccines are not interchangeable. In case of unavailability the schedule should be completed with the available vaccine. Restarting a series is not recommended even for the primary series.

Q27. Are the vaccines interchangeable for the booster dose?

Ans. In PCV13 primed infants, booster with PCV10 results in an inferior immunogenic response. In PCV10 primed infants, a robust response was seen for the 10 common serotypes and the extra serotype included in PCV13. However, interchangeability is not recommended.

Q28. Which are the high-risk groups for pneumococcal infections?

Ans. Very high risk: Immunocompromised conditions, anatomical or functional asplenia, sickle-cell disease (SCD), other hemoglobinopathies, cerebrospinal fluid (CSF) leaks or cochlear implants.

Moderate risk: Chronic heart disease (excluding hypertension), chronic lung disease (including asthma), chronic liver disease, alcoholism, or diabetes mellitus, and smokers or residents in nursing home or long-term care facilities.

Q29. How should we administer pneumococcal vaccines for high-risk individuals?

Ans. **Table 2** summarizes the recommendations in high-risk individuals.

Table 2: Administering pneumococcal vaccines for high-risk individuals.

Age	Previous doses of any pneumococcal vaccine	Recommendations
<23 months	Nil	Usual recommendations
24–71 months	Four doses of PCV13	One dose of PPSV23 at least 8 weeks after last dose of PCV13 One repeat dose of PPSV23 after 5 years
24–71 months	<3 doses of PCV13	Two doses of PCV13 at least 8 weeks apart Rest as above
24–71 months	One dose of PPSV23	Two doses of PCV13 at least 8 weeks apart and 8 weeks after last dose of PPSV23 One dose PPSV23 5 years after dose 1 of PPSV23 and 8 weeks after PCV13
6–18 years with medical conditions	Nil	One dose of PCV13 PPSV23 8 weeks later PPSV23 5 years after dose 1
	One dose of PCV13	One dose PPSV23 One dose PPSV23 5 years later *If HbSS:* 3 years later
	>1 dose of PPSV23	One dose PCV13 >8 weeks later One dose PPSV23 5 years later

(PCV: pneumococcal vaccines; PPSV: pneumococcal polysaccharide vaccine)

Notes:
a. Stand-alone PPSV23 should not be administered.
b. No more than two doses of PPSV23 are administered.
c. When elective splenectomy is planned than PCV/PPSV course should be completed 2 weeks before the scheduled surgery.
d. The ACVIP now includes preterm and very low birth weight (VLBW) babies also as a high-risk group. They have a ninefold risk of IPD when compared to normal babies. Pneumococcal vaccine should be administered to them on a priority basis.

Q30. Has Government of India (GOI) introduced pneumococcal conjugate vaccine in the National Immunization Program (NIP)?

Ans. Pneumococcal conjugate vaccine 13 valent (PCV13) has been introduced in the high-risk states of Himachal Pradesh, Bihar, Uttar Pradesh, Madhya Pradesh, and Rajasthan. This is being supported by global alliance for vaccines and immunization (GAVI) till 2021 after which the GOI will bear the cost of the program. In Haryana, the government has directly negotiated with GAVI and introduced it in the NIP.

Q31. What is the Government of India (GOI) schedule in the National Immunization Program (NIP)?

Ans. 2p+1 schedule. First two doses at 6 and 14 week and a booster at 9 months of age.

Q32. Why is it different from the Indian Academy of Pediatrics (IAP) schedule?

Ans. The NIP is aimed to make the vaccine available to maximum children with the greatest cost effectiveness and piggybacking to the existing schedule without the need for extra visits. A three-dose primary schedule results in significantly superior immunogenicity, at 1 month postvaccination, only for serotypes 6B and 23F and when measured at 1 year, this difference is not significant. Booster doses result in higher antibody levels. This will enhance the duration of protection, which may be more important for certain serotypes (e.g., serotype 1), which are more common in the second year of life.

Q33. What are the different shortened schedules? Are there any shortcomings?

Ans. The advantages of a shortened schedule are that it cuts down the costs and logistics moderately. The different shortened schedules are: 3p+0, 2p+1, and variant 2p+1 schedule.

3p+0: The shortcoming in those countries where serotype 1 is a significant cause, serotype 1 disease persists for a long time and disease may manifest in the second year of life. This schedule does not confer protection.

2p+1: The interval between the two primary doses is 8 weeks. This gives a better geometric mean titer (GMT) of antibodies. The shortcoming is that the protection during this window period is less for the serotypes 6B and 23F and may leave the child unprotected.

Variant 2p+1 schedule: In this schedule, the booster is brought forward in line with measles vaccine given at 9 months. This may address some of the shortcomings of the 3p+0 schedule.

Both PCV10 and PCV13 have been shown to be safe and effective and to have both direct (in vaccinated individuals) and indirect (in unvaccinated individuals living in communities with vaccinated children) effects against pneumococcal disease caused by the respective vaccine serotypes when used in a three-dose schedule (either 2p+1 or 3p+0) or in a four-dose schedule (3p+1). After the third dose of each schedule (post-booster for 2p+1 and post-primary for 3p+0), the 2p+1 schedule resulted in higher geometric mean concentrations (GMCs) but a similar percentage of responders as compared with a 3p+0 schedule for most serotypes, except for serotype 6B, for which the percentage of responders was higher with the 2p+1 schedule.

Q34. How will you compare PCV10 and PCV13?

Ans. Both PCV10 and PCV13 induce an antibody response to serotype 6A, which is included in PCV13 but not in PCV10, which contains 6B. Antibodies against 6A are cross protective against 6C, but antibodies against

6B are not cross protective against 6C which is responsible for a significant burden. PCV13 induces higher serotype 6A GMCs and a higher percentage of responders than PCV10. Both PCV10 and PCV13 induce an antibody response against serotype 19A, although PCV13 induces higher serotype 19A GMCs and a higher percentage of responders than PCV10.

Q35. What are WHO recommendations for PCV?

Ans. The World Health Organization (WHO) recommends the inclusion of pneumococcal conjugate vaccines (PCVs) in childhood immunization programs worldwide adding that it should be complementary to other measures, such as appropriate case management, promotion of exclusive breastfeeding for the first 6 months of life and reducing known risk factors such as indoor air pollution and tobacco smoke.

For administration of PCV to infants, WHO recommends a three-dose schedule administered either as 2p+1 or as 3p+0, starting as early as 6 weeks of age. In choosing between the 2p+1 and 3p+0 schedules, countries should consider programmatic factors including timeliness of vaccination and expected coverage. PCV13 may have an additional benefit in settings where disease attributable to serotype 19A or serotype 6C is significant.

The choice of product to be used in a country should be based on programmatic characteristics, vaccine supply, vaccine price, the local and regional prevalence of vaccine serotypes and antimicrobial resistance patterns. Once a PCV vaccination program has been initiated, product switching is not recommended unless there are substantial changes in the epidemiological or programmatic factors that determined the original choice of product, e.g., an increasing burden of serotype 19A.

Wherever possible, catch-up vaccination at the time of introduction of PCV should be used to accelerate its impact on disease in children aged 1–5 years, particularly in settings with a high disease burden and mortality.

Q36. What is the current Advisory Committee on Immunization Practices (ACIP)/The Centers for Disease Control and Prevention (CDC) recommendation for elderly adults?

Ans. All elderly adults over 65 years of age should receive one dose of PPSV23. A second dose is not recommended.

The administration of PCV13 in this age group, to those having risk factors, is recommended on "shared decision making". In this situation PCV13 is administered first followed by PPSV23 after 1 year.

If a PPSV23 dose has been received before 65 years of age, another dose of PPSV23 is recommended after the age of 65 years and 5 years after the previous PPSV23 dose.

Q37. Is this schedule relevant for India?

Ans. In India, coverage with PCV in infancy and toddler age is very low, so herd immunity is almost nonexistent. The previous schedule of one dose of PCV13 followed by PPSV23 after 6–12 months is probably more relevant.

Q38. What is the status of newer pneumococcal vaccines?

Ans. Currently available PCVs have restricted serotype coverage, are subject to serotype replacement with resultant increase of disease, and are expensive to manufacture.

Thus, there is a need to focus on potential targets for vaccines to overcome the drawbacks of the current type-specific capsular PS vaccines. Future vaccines to prevent IPD are focusing on noncapsular candidate antigens common to all serotypes, namely neuraminidase, autolysin, pneumolysin, pneumococcal surface protein A (PspA) and surface adhesion (PsaA).

The three component protein vaccine, being developed by Sanofi Pasteur, which comprises pneumococcal histidine triad protein D (PhtD), pneumococcal choline-binding protein A (PcpA), and pneumolysoid, has completed a phase 1 age de-escalation study in Bangladesh, demonstrating safety and immunogenicity. It is now in phase 2 trials.

An inactivated pneumococcal whole cell vaccine candidate is being developed by PATH in collaboration with Boston Children Hospital (BCH) which could provide broad protection and be inexpensive to produce and administer. This vaccine candidate is currently in a phase 1/2 age de-escalation clinical study in Kenya having completed a phase 1 study in healthy adults in the United States.

Pneumococcal vaccines that combine protein and conjugate vaccine technologies are being developed to provide protection against a broader range of pneumococcal disease than existing licensed vaccines. GSK is developing a bivalent protein vaccine comprising pneumococcal histidine triad protein D (PhtD) and pneumolysoid. This vaccine is in a phase 2 trial in "The Gambia".

SUGGESTED READING

1. Alicino C, Paganino C, Orsi A, Astengo M, Trucchi C, Icardi G, et al. The impact of 10-valent and 13-valent pneumococcal conjugate vaccines on hospitalization for pneumonia in children: A systematic review and meta-analysis. Vaccine. 2017;35(43):5776-85.
2. Anand Manoharan, et alfor the Alliance for Surveillance of Invasive Pneumococci (ASIP) Study Group. Invasive pneumococcal disease in children aged younger than 5 years in India: a surveillance study. Lancet Infect Dis 2017; 17: 305-12.
3. Balaji V, Jayraman R, Verghese VP, Baliga PR, Kurien T. Pneumococcal serotypes associated with invasive disease in under 5 children in Indian and implications for vaccine policy. Indian J Med Res. 2015;142:286-92.

4. Johnson HL, Deloria-Knoll M, Levine OS, Stoszek SK, Freimanis Hance L, Reithinger R, et al. Systematic evaluation of serotypes causing invasive pneumococcal disease in children under five: The pneumococcal global serotype project. PLOS Med. 2010;7(10):e1000348.
5. Masomian M, Ahmad Z, Gew LT, Poh CL. Development of next generation streptococcus pneumoniae vaccines conferring broad protection. Vaccines. 2020;8(1):132.
6. Molander et al. BMC Infectious Diseases 2013, 13:532.
7. Nisarga R, Premlatha R, Shivananada, Ravikumar KL, Shivappa U, Gopi A, et al. Hospital based surveillance of Pneumococcal disease and pneumonia in South Banagalore, India. Indian Pediatr. 2015;52:205-11.
8. Prospective multicentre hospital surveillance of Streptococcus pneumoniae disease in India. Invasive Bacterial Infection Surveillance (IBIS) Group, International Clinical Epidemiology Network (INCLEN). Lancet 1999; 353: 1216-21.
9. Shah AK. IAP Guide book on Immunizations 2018-2019, Advisory Committee on Immunizations and vaccine practices (ACVIP). New Delhi: Jaypee Brothers Medical Publishers (P) Ltd.; 2019. pp. 168-206.
10. Shariff M, Choudhary J, Zahoor S, Deb M. Characterization of Streptococcus pneumoniae isolates from India with special reference to their sequence types. J Infect Dev Ctries. 2013;7:101-9.
11. So Hyun Kim, Jae-Hoon Song, Doo Ryeon Chung, Visanu Thamlikitkul, Yonghong Yang, Hui Wang, Min Lu, et al. Changing Trends in Antimicrobial Resistance and Serotypes of Streptococcus pneumoniae Isolates in Asian Countries: an Asian Network for Surveillance of Resistant Pathogens (ANSORP) Study. Antimicrob. Agents Chemother. 2012, 56(3):1418.
12. Wahl B, O'Brien KL, Greenbaum A, Majumder A, Liu L, Chu Y, et al. Burden of Streptococcal Pneumonia and Hemophilus type b disease in children in the era of conjugate vaccines, global, regional and national estimates for 2000-2015. Lancet Glob Health. 2018;6(7):e744-e757.
13. World Health Organization. Pneumococcal Conjugate Vaccines in infants and children under 5 years of age, WHO Position Paper, Feb 2019. Weekly Epidemiol Record. 2019;8(94):85-104.

CHAPTER 20

Influenza Vaccines

Nitin Shah

Q1. What is influenza?

Ans. Influenza is a contagious respiratory tract infection caused by influenza virus A or B. Type C influenza virus does not lead to human infection. At present, type A influenza strains that are prevalent include pH1N1 and H3N2 and type B influenza strains that are prevalent include both Yamagata and Victoria strains.

Q2. Why do influenza outbreaks and pandemics occur?

Ans. Influenza viruses have two major surface antigens namely hemagglutinin (HA) and neuraminidase (NA) that are target for antibody formation and, thus, immune protection. Influenza viruses continually mutate when they replicate. There are two ways influenza virus mutates in to a new virus; antigenic drift or antigenic shift.

Antigenic drift: Minor changes in the HA or HA/NA antigens are known as antigenic drift. Such antigenic drift will lead to a new human influenza virus which will be still immunologically closer to the original virus and may still be recognized and cross protected by the existing antibodies to the original virus. However, it may escape recognition by the immune system when these minor changes accumulate enough over the time or there occurs a minor change in an important antigenic location. This, then, leads to an outbreak of influenza as is experienced every year. This is also the reason why influenza vaccine strains change every now and then.

Antigenic shift: When an abrupt and major change in HA or HA/NA antigens occurs a totally new influenza strain will emerge for which the community will have no existing immunity. This results in a major pandemic. One-way antigenic shift occurs is by reassortment between human and animal influenza viruses as happened in 2009 when a novel pH1N1 influenza virus strain emerged with genes from North American Swine, Eurasian Swine, humans and birds leading to the first pandemic of new millennium. Antigenic shift occurs only in influenza A virus and not type B influenza virus. Hence, pandemics are caused by only influenza A viruses. There have been four major pandemics in past 100 years including 1918-20 Spanish pandemic caused by H1N1 strain (estimated 33% of population infected resulting in 500 million cases, 20-100 million deaths, case fatality rate 2-3%), 1957-58 Asian pandemic caused by H2N2 strain (estimated 8-33% of population infected resulting in 250-1,000 million cases, 1-1.5 million deaths, case fatality rate < 0.2%), 1968-69 Hong Kong pandemic caused by H3N2 strain (estimated 7-28% of population infected resulting in 250-1,000 million cases, 0.75-1 million deaths, case fatality rate < 0.2%) and 2009 pandemic caused by pH1N1 (2009) strain (estimated 10-200 million cases, 0.1-0.4 million deaths, case fatality rate < 0.1%).

Q3. How does influenza present?

Ans. Influenza presents with fever which can be of high-grade and associated with chills, cough, sore throat, body ache, headache, fatigue, and in children often with diarrhea and vomiting.

In most cases influenza is mild and self-limiting. In some it can be severe and even fatal. Elderly subjects, pregnant women, children <5 years of age, those who have at risk conditions such as chronic respiratory, cardiac or metabolic diseases, and immune compromised hosts are at higher risk to develop severe influenza and even death.

Q4. What are the complications of influenza?

Ans. Influenza is often mistaken as common cough and cold caused by other respiratory viruses such as rhinovirus or adenovirus. However, influenza can be a serious disease with complications. It can lead to acute sinusitis or acute otitis media which then often gets secondarily infected with a bacterial cause such as nontypable *H. influenzae, Pneumococcus,* or *Moraxella*. Influenza can lead to serious complications such as pneumonia which often gets secondarily infected with bacteria like *Pneumococcus* or *Staphylococcus* and can lead to acute respiratory distress syndrome (ARDS) and death. Other complications include encephalitis, myocarditis, myositis, rhabdomyolysis, systemic inflammatory response (SIRS), multi-organ failure, and sepsis. It can lead to exacerbation of existing conditions such as asthma or heart failure.

Q5. What is the disease burden of influenza in children?

Ans. Typically, influenza infects subjects at two ends of life that is young children and the elderly. However, pH1N1 (2009) virus had predilection to infect adolescents and young adults who were otherwise healthy. Influenza incidence and mortality are higher in subjects who are immunocompromised or have a chronic illness such as pulmonary, cardiac, renal, or metabolic diseases.

During an outbreak approximately 10-30% of population gets affected. During pandemic approximately 30-50% of the population will get affected depending on the mutation as most of the population will be naïve and will have no immunity against the novel virus. Unfortunately, incidence of influenza episodes and acute respiratory tract infection (ARI) is two- to threefolds higher in children from developing countries as compared to children from developed countries. A recent meta-analysis has estimated that in children under the age of 5 years in 2008 there occurred 90 million cases of influenza, 20 million cases of ARI, 1-2 million cases of severe ARI and 28,000-111,500 deaths; most of these deaths occur in developing countries. Health utilization surveys conducted in Ballabhgarh (Haryana) and Vadu (Maharashtra) in 2010-12 showed that adjusted all-age influenza hospitalization incidence rates were 3.8-5.4 per 10,000 in Ballabhgarh and 20.3-51.6 per 10,000 in Vadu with significant burden in children. In children, outpatient visits increase by 6-15 per 100 outpatient visits during influenza season. Nearly 1-2% of children with influenza are hospitalized, 3% attend emergency care, 90% are prescribed antipyretics, 40% are prescribed antibiotics and 30% need a follow-up clinic visit.

Children are at the center of the outbreak as they transmit the infection among themselves to their family members and, in turn, to others in the community. Hence, vaccinating children with influenza vaccine can prevent influenza cases not only in children but also in the community.

During an influenza outbreak, generally hospitalization rates are 55 per 10^5 population with H1N1 strain, 99 per 10^5 with H3N2 strain, and 80 per 10^5 with type B strain.

Q6. What is the societal impact of influenza?

Ans. Influenza not only leads to medical disease in the affected child, it also leads to indirect societal impact in the form of school absenteeism for children and work absenteeism for the parents. Almost 75% of affected children remain absent in school from 1 or more days with average period of loss of schooling being 2-4 days. Similarly, nearly 65% of parents miss work with average days of lost work being 2-3 days. All these indirect societal costs add to the direct costs involved in managing children and adults with influenza.

Q7. Who are at risk to develop severe influenza?

Ans. Subjects at higher risk for developing severe influenza include children <5 years of age, pregnant women, elderly people >65 years of age, diabetics, obese patients with body mass index (BMI) > 40, patients younger than 19 years who are on chronic aspirin or salicylate containing medication, patients with sickle-cell disease, immunocompromised patients, and people with chronic systemic illnesses such as respiratory, cardiac, renal, neurological, hepatic, or metabolic diseases.

Children <2 years of age, pregnant women up to 2 weeks postpartum period, people living in healthcare facilities and elderly >65 years have higher chances of developing influenza in general.

Q8. What is the treatment of influenza?

Ans. Management of influenza includes general measures and antiviral therapy. General measures include hydration, antipyretics, nutrition, and personal hygiene to prevent further spread such as gloves, masks, gowns, and hand hygiene. Specific treatment includes giving antiviral agents such as "oseltamivir" or "zanamivir". Oseltamivir should be given to severe and progressive cases of influenza based on the national guideline and should be started as soon as possible preferably within 48 hours of onset of symptoms. Prior testing for influenza or waiting for its result is not required as negative result does not exclude influenza. Dose is based on the age and weight of the child. Dose for the 0–1-year-old is 3 mg/kg/dose twice a day and for >1-year-old it is based on weight bands. For <15 kg weight, it is 30 mg twice a day, for 15–23 kg 45 mg twice a day, for 24–40 kg 60 mg twice a day, and for >40 kg it is same as adult dose which is 75 mg twice a day. It should be given for 5 days, however, can be continued for a maximum of 10 days in a sick child with progressive disease. Zanamivir or peramivir is the drug of choice for all those with oseltamivir resistance and should be given by intravenous (IV) route. However, zanamivir is not easily available in India. In a patient at risk for severe influenza who is in contact with a case of influenza can be given oseltamivir prophylaxis using same amount per dose as treatment but given once a day for 10 days.

Q9. How can we prevent influenza?

Ans. Prevention of influenza includes general measures, chemoprophylaxis, and influenza vaccination.

General measures include avoiding contact with sick people, personal habits such as cough etiquette, use of face mask, hand hygiene, avoiding touching nose, mouth and eyes when sick, and keeping away from school and work when sick. Similarly, at school and at workplaces one must take general precautions to prevent spread of influenza including keeping schools or workplaces closed during peak of outbreaks. One must also ensure availability of hand sanitizers at such places and clean up periodically places and items used by people at such places such as door knobs, toilet knobs, etc.

Chemoprophylaxis is already discussed above and influenza vaccines are discussed in subsequent questions.

Q10. Which are the types of influenza vaccine?

Ans. Basically, there are two types of influenza vaccines: injectable inactivated influenza vaccines (IIV) and cold-adapted live-attenuated intranasal vaccines (LAIV). Each of them can be trivalent or quadrivalent. IIV can be split virion or subunit vaccines. Theoretically, split virion vaccines are more immunogenic but also more reactogenic. Practically, there is not much difference in efficacy between these two types of vaccines at least in children and one can use any on them in clinical practice.

CHAPTER 20: Influenza Vaccines

Q11. What is the composition of influenza vaccines?

Ans. Influenza vaccines consist of three strains (trivalent, pH1N1, H3N2, and one of the two B types either Yamagata or Victoria strains) or four strains (quadrivalent, pH1N1, H3N2, and both Yamagata and Victoria type B strains) of influenza viruses. The composition of vaccines changes from time to time as the influenza viruses constantly mutate leading to antigenic drifts as discussed before. Influenza vaccines also contain gelatine as stabilizer, antibiotics, aluminum salts, formaldehyde, thiomersal (or thimerosal), and egg proteins as most influenza vaccines are grown in chick embryos. This is also the reason influenza vaccine is contraindicated in subjects with severe egg allergy.

Q12. What are the Northern and the Southern influenza vaccines and which one should we use in India?

Ans. Influenza vaccines come in market twice in a year that is the northern vaccines and the southern vaccines. Making influenza vaccines is a race against the time. World Health Organization (WHO) collects nasopharyngeal swab samples from patients suspected to have influenza-like illness periodically from various parts of the world throughout the year and collates the data from time to time. Based on the data, it meets twice a year and recommends representative strains that will best match the circulating strains in last 6 months all over the world to be included in the NH and the SH vaccines. Each year in the months of February to March, it meets and provides strains for the northern vaccines which come in market in the month of September of that year for use before the subsequent winter season as influenza season peaks in winter in the northern zone countries. It also meets in the months of August and September each year to suggest strains to be included in southern vaccines that then come out in market in March the next year to be used before the monsoon as influenza peaks during monsoon in the southern zone countries. So, one should use appropriate vaccine based on whether the peak of influenza is in winter (use northern vaccine) or monsoon (use southern vaccine). *Influenza peaks are in monsoon months and hence behaves like a southern zone country and, hence, we should use southern vaccine in the months of April to August to cover the monsoon peak, except in Jammu and Kashmir where the influenza peaks during winter and, hence, we should use northern vaccine there. In the northern parts of India, there is an equal peak during winter as during monsoon and, hence, one can use either of the vaccines.*

Q13. In case a subject comes during the winter period should one give the northern vaccine or wait till next southern vaccine becomes available?

Ans. One should use influenza vaccine before the peak of influenza season for better protection, which in India would mean using the southern vaccine in the months of April to August before monsoon season. However, if the person comes for the first time say in the month of November after monsoon peak is over one should give any available IIV at the first contact without waiting for the next season SH vaccine and then try to convert to southern vaccine at the earliest possibility for the subsequent years. None should be denied the vaccine irrespective of the time of the year.

Q14. Why is type B influenza so important in clinical practice to include both type B strains in the current quadrivalent vaccines?

Ans. Type B influenza is more common in children and elderly subjects staying in nursing home settings. It is as infective as type A influenza. It does not lead to antigenic shift so does not lead to pandemics; however, it leads to frequent antigenic drifts that occur slowly leading to outbreaks every 2–4 years. Hospitalization rates following type B influenza is almost as common as H3N2 and much higher than that with pH1N1 influenza. Similarly, mortality due to type B influenza is next to that by H3N2 influenza and more than that with pH1N1 influenza. Type B influenza contributes nearly 34% of childhood influenza deaths. Type B contributes to 20–30% of all influenza cases all over the world. A group of researchers from Asian countries on influenza (GARI) showed that it was as high as 50% of in a study done from various Asian countries. Same study showed that in India type B contributed 37.8% of all influenza cases.

Q15. Why are both the types B influenza strains included in recent quadrivalent influenza vaccines?

Ans. Since 1985 two lineages of influenza virus are circulating namely Yamagata and Victoria strains. Natural and vaccine induced protection against type B strains is homotypic with minimum cross protection. Since 2013, the World Health Organization (WHO) has been recommending to use both Victoria and Yamagata strains of influenza B making it a quadrivalent vaccine. This is because it is difficult to predict which of the type B strain will circulate in next season. In studies done in various parts of the world it has been shown that 46–58% of the time there is a mismatch between circulating type B strain and type B vaccine strain in a trivalent vaccine. Besides this many times both the types of B virus cocirculate during a season making efficacy of the vaccine suboptimal if you use a trivalent vaccine. So, failure to predict accurately the circulating type B strain and cocirculation of both type B strains along with minimum cross protection make it logical to include both type B strains in the vaccine making it a quadrivalent influenza vaccine.

Q16. How much more protection quadrivalent influenza vaccines (QIV) will offer as compared to trivalent influenza vaccines (TIV)?

Ans. This would depend on the circulating influenza virus during the season and, hence, would differ from season to season. However, on an average

4-5% more overall influenza 11% more of type B influenza will be prevented by QIV as compared to TIV. Modeling studies have predicted that there will be 17-28% more type B influenza prevented by QIV as compared to TIV.

Q17. What about the dose, schedule, and route of administration of inactivated influenza vaccines?

Ans. Dose of inactivated influenza virus vaccines (IIV) is 0.25 mL for 6-36 months old subjects and 0.5 mL for >36 months old subjects. However, as discussed below, recently 0.5 mL dose is found to be as safe but more immunogenic than 0.25 mL even for 6-36 months old subjects and, hence, is preferred dose even at that age. For children 6 months to 9 years of age, two doses are recommended for the first time (unprimed children) and subsequently one dose every year. For those >9 years, only one dose is recommended for the first year and thereafter every year. IIV is given intramuscularly in anterolateral aspect of the thigh in infants or deltoid region in older children.

Q18. How do you store IIV and what is the expiry period?

Ans. Inactivated influenza virus vaccine (IIV) is stored in refrigerator at 2-8°C. It should not be frozen, and if by mistake frozen should be discarded. As discussed before, IIV is manufactured and brought to the market twice a year that is southern vaccine in February and northern vaccine in September. Hence, one should use the latest vaccine that is available even though technically expiry of IIV is 1 year. Even Indian Academy of Pediatrics (IAP) recommends using the latest available vaccine.

Q19. What are the side effects of IIV?

Ans. In general, IIVs are safe vaccines. Local side effects include pain, swelling and redness which are seen in 10-30% of subjects and are usually mild and resolve in 1-2 days with or without oral paracetamol. Systemic side effects include fever, loss of appetite, irritability, drowsiness, and crying which are seen in 10-40% of subjects and are again mild and self-resolving.

Q20. Can influenza vaccine lead to Guillain-Barré syndrome (GBS)?

Ans. Guillain-Barré syndrome is a rare autoimmune disorder and no additional cases over and above the background rates have been reported with IIV except with use of a special swine influenza vaccine in 1976 when there was some extra risk to the tune of one additional case per 100,000 doses used. At other times, GBS rates fluctuate from time to time and if at all there is extra risk it is rare and is usually 1-2 additional cases per million doses used. However, one should also keep in mind that person developing GBS is more likely to get it following influenza disease than with influenza vaccine.

Q21. What are the contraindications for IIV?

Ans. An anaphylactic allergic reaction to egg or other components of influenza vaccine is an absolute contraindication to use of any influenza vaccines in future. People who are moderately sick due to any reason should wait for influenza vaccination till they recover. Guillain-Barré syndrome (GBS) within 6 weeks following past influenza vaccine is a precaution to its further use and if such a subject is not at risk of severe influenza should generally not receive further influenza vaccine.

Q22. What is the efficacy of IIV?

Ans. Various studies have looked at efficacy or effectiveness of IIV in different setups. The efficacy will vary according to endpoint used in the study such as efficacy against acute respiratory infections (ARI), influenza-like illness (ILI), or more specific endpoint-like culture or polymerase chain reaction (PCR) proven influenza or PCR-proven matched strain influenza. Other endpoints used include efficacy or effectiveness against acute otitis media, antibiotic prescription, excess hospitalization during influenza season, excess outdoor visits during influenza season, school absenteeism, work absenteeism, etc.

One study in the United States of America looked at vaccine efficacy of TIV in a case-controlled trial in children 6–50 months old over eight influenza seasons from 1999–2000 season to 2006–2007 season comparing PCR proven cases with PCR negative controls for their vaccination status. The results showed that vaccine efficacy was 86% (95% CI: 29–97) with full vaccination and 73% (95% CI: 3–93) for partial vaccination. Another study in China looked at vaccine efficacy against other endpoints and found that there was 84.8% reduction in influenza such as illness, 41% reduction in upper respiratory infections, and 35% reduction in common cold like illness. One study from Finland showed that IIV reduced acute otitis media with influenza by 83% ($p < 0.001$) and all cause AOM by 36%. ($p < 0.02$). It is believed that 24–85% of exacerbations of asthma occur due to influenza infection although impact of IIV on asthma exacerbation has always been a debatable issue with studies showing results which are favorable or otherwise. Lastly, IIV can help to reduce spread of infections to household contacts leading to indirect benefits. One study compared incidence of influenza-like illness (ILI) with fever, school absenteeism, parents work absenteeism, physician's visits, and antibiotic prescriptions in household contacts of IIV vaccinated children compared to household contacts of unvaccinated children. Results showed that there was almost 80% reduction in all the above parameters in the household contacts of IIV vaccinated children compared to those in contact with unvaccinated children.

Q23. Can we use 0.5 mL instead of 0.25 mL of IIV even in 6–36-month-old children? Why?

Ans. It has been standard practice to use 0.25 mL per dose of IIV for 6–36-month-old children and 0.5 mL per dose for older subjects. The main reason was the fear of toxicity with 0.5 mL in young children which was so evident with the old whole cell vaccine. However, recent studies have compared 0.5 mL with 0.25 mL in children 6 months to 3 years. It was found that geometric mean titers (GMT) were almost 1.5 times higher with 0.5 mL meaning better protection and no significant difference in the adverse effects in the two groups. Influvac Tetra˙ 0.5 mL is recently approved for use in 6-36-month-old children in India. Fluquadri˙ has submitted dossier to the Drugs Controller General of India (DCGI), India for approval of 0.5 mL for 6-36 months. Fluquadri® 0.5 mL is already licensed for use in 6-36 months old in countries such as the United States of America, the United Kingdom, Australia, Canada, and others. Same vaccine available as Vaxigrip Tetra® has approval for 0.5 mL for 6-36 months old in more than 50 countries. Hopefully, over the years 0.5 mL will replace 0.25 mL for 6-36 months old all over the world. While 0.25 mL vaccine is still available for 6-36 months old, based on better immunogenicity and similar reactogenicity of 0.5 mL compared to 0.25 mL, the 0.5 mL dose may become a universal dose from the age of 6 months. The Advisory Committee on Immunization Practices (ACIP), USA, and the World Health Organization (WHO) recommend using 0.25 mL or 0.5 mL for 6-36-month-old children, the Green book, UK, Canadian Immunization Guide, and National Influenza Specialist Group (NSIG), New Zealand recommend only 0.5 mL for 6-36-month-old children.

Q24. What is the efficacy of quadrivalent influenza vaccines (QIV) in 6-36-month-old children?

Ans. Recently two placebo controlled randomized studies have looked at the efficacy of 0.5 mL of QIV in 2,721 6-36-month-old children. Results showed that efficacy against vaccine similar strain severe influenza was 72% (95% CI: 44-87) and vaccine similar strain any severity influenza was 69% (95% CI: 52-81). Efficacy against any strain severe influenza was 57% (95% CI: 37-71) and any strain any severity influenza was 52% (95% CI: 40-62). Efficacy against acute otitis media (AOM) was 68.7%, acute lower respiratory infections (ALRI) 78.2%, healthcare visits 59.2%, parents' absenteeism 70.2%, and antibiotic use 60.9%.

Another phase III observer blind nonflu vaccine placebo controlled randomized multicentric study was conducted in 13 countries over five influenza seasons between 2010 and 2013 in children who were 6-36 months old. Results showed that efficacy against matched strain moderate to severe polymerase chain reaction (PCR) confirmed influenza was 63% (95% CI: 51-72) and matched strain any severity PCR conformed influenza was 50% (95% CI: 42-57). Efficacy against any strain moderate to severe culture confirmed influenza was 64% (95% CI: 53-72) and any strain any severity culture confirmed influenza was 51% (95% CI: 44-58). Efficacy against general practitioner (GP) visits was 47%, emergency room (ER) visits was 79%, and antibiotic use was 50%.

Q25. What about live-attenuated influenza vaccines (LAIV)? How do they work?

Ans. Live-attenuated influenza vaccines (LAIV) have been developed that are cold adapted which limits its replication in cool temperature found in nasopharynx when given intranasally without replicating in lower respiratory tract making them safe to use. Two manufactures make LAIV, Flumist made by AstraZeneca (since 2003 and is cell culture based) available in the United States of America and a Russian origin vaccine (since 1954 and is egg culture based) available in Russia for decades and then made in India too by Serum Institute of India.

Live-attenuated influenza vaccine is a 6:2 reassortant vaccine where candidate live wild virulent vaccine virus of interest is reassorted in embryonated chicken eggs (or cell culture for the United States vaccine) with master donor nonvirulent virus (Indian vaccine master donor virus is A/Leningrad/134/17/57 (H2N2) and B/USSR/60/69 and US vaccine master donor is A/Ann Arbor/6/60 (H2N2) and B/Ann Arbor/1/66). The resultant reassortant vaccine virus now expresses two antigens of the candidate vaccine virus namely hemagglutinin and neuraminidase that trigger protective antibody and six genes of the donor virus that code for internal viral proteins to confer nonvirulent properties (ca, ts, and att, phenotypic characteristics; allows reassortant viruses to replicate efficiently in embryonated chicken eggs).

The resultant vaccine virus has some important properties. It is cold adapted (Ca) that allows efficient viral replication at 25°C in cooler regions of the upper respiratory tract. It is temperature sensitive that restricts replication at higher temperatures above 39°C in the warmer lower respiratory tract making it safe for use. It is attenuated so it does not cause classical influenza-like illness. It is genetically stable and, hence, does not mutate or revert into wild form.

Q26. What is the dose, route of administration, and storage of LAIV?

Ans. Indian live-attenuated influenza vaccine (LAIV) pack contains a glass vial containing freeze dried cake of vaccine, plastic twist-to-open ampule containing sterile water as diluent, a needle to withdraw diluent, a 1 mL plastic syringe with luer-lock for administering reconstituted vaccine, a dose divider device that allows the dose to be distributed equally while injecting in each nostril and a nasal spray device. The vaccine is reconstituted and is withdrawn back in the syringe, the dose divider is fixed on the plunger of the syringe, spray device is attached to the syringe, and vaccine is delivered in each nostril. It is a bit cumbersome procedure at the end and needs patience. The vaccine is stored at 2–8°C in refrigerator. Under no circumstances, LAIV should be injected.

Dose is 0.25 mL per nostril (total of 0.5 mL) for Indian LAIV and 0.1 mL per nostril (total 0.2 mL) for the US LAIV. Only one dose is recommended for the Indian vaccine at any age whereas two doses are recommended for the first time for children 2–9 years for the US LAIV.

Q27. What are the side effects of live-attenuated influenza vaccine (LAIV)?

Ans. Side effects of LAIV include local side effects such as nasal discomfort, nasal stuffiness, sneezing, loss of smell, red eyes, lacrimation and facial swelling; and systemic side effects that include fever, headache, chills, fatigue, sore throat, cough, myalgia, arthralgia, irritability, wheezing, and loss of appetite. These are seen in around 5% of vaccinees, are mild and self-limiting in most, and resolve with or without paracetamol. One study done in Bangladesh in 24–59-month-old children found no statistical difference in side effects between LAIV and placebo. Another study looked at wheezing following LAIV or placebo given to children with medical history of treatment or hospitalization for asthma in past and found no statistical difference in incidence of wheezing between vaccinees (7.7%) and placebo (19.7%).

Q28. What is the efficacy of live-attenuated influenza vaccine (LAIV)?

Ans. One placebo-controlled randomized efficacy study was done in Bangladesh in 24–59-month-old children who were given one dose. Results showed that LAIV efficacy against laboratory confirmed influenza was 57.5% against vaccine matched strains and 41% against any strains in first year and efficacy persisted at 27% against vaccine matched strain and 20.5% against any strain in second year. One case controlled study was done in five tertiary care hospitals in Pune, India in 2011-12 using monovalent pH1N1 LAIV in subjects > 2 years (age range 2 years to 79 years for cases and 2 years to 87 years for the controls) old presenting with influenza like illness to look for efficacy against laboratory proven influenza (essentially pH1N1 strain as that was the only circulating strain in 2010 following the pandemic that started in 2009 in India with Pune being the epicenter of spread that time). Results showed that adjusted efficacy of monovalent (pH1N1) LAIV was 76% (95% CI: 42.1–89.7).

Meta-analysis of studies using the US LAIV when compared to IIV in children have shown that efficacy against vaccine matched strains has been 85% (77–91) with LAIV compared to 43% (14–63) with IIV and against unmatched strains has been 60% (20–81) with LAIV compared to 47% (–63 to 83) and regardless of matching has been 80% (70–87) with LAIV compared to 48% (31–61). Hence, in children LAIV seemed to score over IIV. In between, the United States Centers for Disease Control and Prevention (US-CDC) and some other world agencies had recommended against using LAIV due to poor effectiveness; however, now this adverse recommendation has been removed by CDC and it recommends using either LAIV or TIV as appropriate without any preference of one over the other.

Q29. What are the contraindications of live-attenuated influenza vaccine (LAIV)?

Ans. An anaphylactic allergic reaction to egg or other components of influenza vaccine is an absolute contraindication to use of any influenza vaccines including the Indian LAIV. People who are moderately sick due to any reason should wait for any influenza vaccination till they recover. Guillain-Barré syndrome (GBS) within 6 weeks following past influenza vaccine is a precaution to its further use and if such a subject is not at risk of severe influenza should generally not receive further influenza vaccine. In addition, LAIV is not licensed below 2 years and above 50 years of age. LAIV is contraindicated during pregnancy, in immunocompromised host, contacts of immunocompromised host, children between 2 and 5 years with asthma, subjects on aspirin therapy (due to fear of Reye syndrome), and receipt of antiviral influenza medication within previous 48 hours. Asthma in >5 years of age and conditions that might predispose to complications of influenza such as chronic cardiorespiratory or metabolic diseases, etc. is taken as precaution to use of LAIV. Antiviral drugs should not be administered for up to 2 weeks following LAIV and if given by mistake, vaccine should be repeated.

Q30. What are the recommendations by Indian Academy of Pediatrics (IAP) on use of influenza vaccine?

Ans. Indian Academy of Pediatrics has published, in 2018, revised recommendations on immunization schedule and updates on vaccines for 0-18-year-old children. 2018 recommendations took cognizance of high disease burden of influenza in children especially below the age of 5 years which leads to high hospitalization rates as well as mortality in this age group. Influenza burden and mortality are higher in children from developing countries as compared to those in developed countries. It also recognized that both strains of type B influenza are reported from India round the year and they often co-circulate. There is round the year influenza activity in India with major monsoon peak in most of the parts of the country giving it the southern hemisphere type of seasonality (suggesting the use of southern hemisphere vaccine) and an equal winter peak in the northern part of the country giving it the northern hemisphere type of seasonality (suggesting use of either of the northern or southern vaccine).

2018 IAP guidelines recommend routine use of influenza vaccines in children from 6 to 60 months and recommend to continue to use influenza vaccines at all ages in all those children who are at high risk to develop severe influenza such as immunocompromised host, children with chronic systemic or metabolic diseases such as chronic cardiac illness, chronic respiratory illness, diabetes, chronic renal disease, obesity, sickle-cell disease, splenectomized children, cochlear implant recipients, etc. It also says to use quadrivalent/trivalent inactivated influenza vaccine (implying not to use

LAIV at present). The latest available vaccine should be used (implying to start vaccination at the first contact with the patient without waiting for the peak season). Vaccination should start at least 2-4 weeks before influenza season giving two doses for children below 9 years of age for the first year followed by one dose annually.

Q31. A 3-year-old child comes for flu vaccine, he had taken only one dose last year. How many doses should this child receive this year?

Ans. Any child, who has received less than two doses in the past, should receive two doses again in this season.

Q32. A 2-year-old child has received two doses in 2017, none after that. He comes in 2020 for the flu shot. How many doses should the child receive?

Ans. Any child who has received two or more doses in the past (these doses need not be in the same season), should receive only one dose again in this season.

Q33. A child has received two doses of TIV this year. Father learns that a better vaccine, quadrivalent influenza vaccine (QIV) is available and comes to you for an additional dose. Will you administer a dose of QIV now, third dose in same season?

Ans. There is no recommendation for more than one or two doses (depending on age and number of doses taken in past) in a season. So, this child preferably should not be administered the third dose in this season.

Q34. An unimmunized child has just recovered from swine flu. Does he need a flu shot and when?

Ans. Yes, he needs a flu vaccine to protect him from the other strains in the vaccine. He can receive the vaccine after clinical recovery. live-attenuated influenza vaccines (LAIV) should be administered 48 hours after stopping antiviral medications.

Q35. What precautions are to be taken while administering the flu vaccine to a child with suspected egg allergy?

Ans. If the child can eat lightly cooked egg (e.g., scrambled egg) without reaction, administer influenza vaccine as per usual protocol. After eating eggs or egg-containing foods, the child experiences mild reactions such as hives, administer IIV and one may observe the child for 30 minutes. But, if the child has severe egg allergy such as cardiovascular changes (e.g., hypotension), respiratory distress (e.g., wheezing), gastrointestinal symptoms (e.g., nausea or vomiting), reaction requiring epinephrine or reaction requiring emergency medical attention, IIV should be administered by a physician with experience in the recognition and management of severe allergic conditions in a setting with facilities for resuscitation and further care. Observe for reaction for at least 30 minutes after vaccination. Lastly, there is influenza vaccine like "Flublok" that is grown on other cell culture lines and not eggs and can be considered for a person with egg allergy, though this vaccine is not available in India at present.

SUGGESTED READING

1. Balasubramanian S, Shah A, Pemde HK, Chatterjee P, Shivananda S, Guduru VK, et al. Indian Academy of Pediatrics (IAP) Advisory Committee on Vaccines and Immunization Practices (ACVIP) Recommended Immunization Schedule (2018-19) and Update on Immunization for Children Aged 0 Through 18 Years. Indian Pediatr. 2018;55:1066-74.
2. Brooks WA, Zaman K, Lewis KDC, Ortiz JR, Goswami D, Feser J, et al. Efficacy of a Russian-backbone live attenuated influenza vaccine among young children in Bangladesh: a randomised, double-blind, placebo-controlled trial. Lancet Glob Health. 2016;4:e946-54.
3. Claeys C, Zaman K, Dbaibo G, Li P, Izu A, Kosalaraksa P, et al. Prevention of vaccine-matched and mismatched influenza in children aged 6–35 months: a multinational randomised trial across five influenza seasons. Lancet. 2018;2(5):338-49.
4. DiazGranados CA, Denis M, Plotkin S. Seasonal influenza vaccine efficacy and its determinants in children and non-elderly adults: a systematic review with meta-analyses of controlled trials. Vaccine. 2012;31(1):49-57.
5. Grohskopf LA, Alyanak E, Broder KR, Walter EB, Fry AM, Jernigan DB. Prevention and Control of Seasonal Influenza with Vaccines: Recommendations of the Advisory Committee on Immunization Practices—United States, 2019–20 Influenza Season. MMWR. 2019;69(3):1-21.
6. Heikkinen T, Ruuskanen O, Waris M, Ziegler T, Arola M, Halonen P. Influenza Vaccination in the Prevention of Acute Otitis Media in Children. Am J Dis Child. 1991;145(4):445-8.
7. Hirve S, Krishnan A, Dawood FS, Lele P, Saha S, Rai S, et al. Incidence of influenza-associated hospitalization in rural communities in western and northern India, 2010-2012: A multi-site population-based study. J Infect. 2015;70:160-70.
8. Hurwitz ES, Haber M, Chang A, Shope T, Teo S, Ginsberg M, et al. Effectiveness of influenza vaccination of day care children in reducing influenza-related morbidity among household contacts. JAMA. 2000;284(13):1677-82.
9. Jianping H, Xin F, Changshun L, Bo Z, Linxiu G, Wei X, et al. Assessment of effectiveness of Vaxigrip. Vaccine. 1999;17(Suppl 1):S57-8.
10. Joshi AY, Iyer VN, St Sauver JL, Jacobson RL, Boyce TG. Effectiveness of inactivated influenza vaccine in children less than 5 years of age over multiple influenza seasons: a case-control study. Vaccine. 2009;27:4457-61.
11. Kramarz P, Destefano F, Gargiullo PM, Chen RT, Lieu TA, Davis RL, et al. Does influenza vaccination prevent asthma exacerbations in children? J Pediatr. 2001;138(3):306-10.
12. Kulkarni PS, Agarkhedkar S, Lalwani S, Bavdekar AR, Jog S, Raut SK, et al. Effectiveness of an Indian-made attenuated influenza A (H1N1)pdm2009 vaccine : a case control study. Hum Vaccin Immunother. 2014;10(3):566-71.
13. Montomoli E, Torelli A, Manini I, Gianchecchi E. Immunogenicity and Safety of the New Inactivated Quadrivalent Influenza Vaccine Vaxigrip Tetra: Preliminary Results in Children ≥6 Months and Older Adults. Vaccines (Basel). 2018;6(1):14.
14. Nair H, Brooks WA, Katz M, Roca A, Berkley JA, Madhi SA, et al. Global burden of respiratory infections due to seasonal influenza in young children: A systematic review and meta-analysis. Lancet. 2011;378:1917-30.

15. Ortiz JR, Goswami D, Lewis KDC, Sharmeen AT, Ahmed M, Rahman M, et al. Safety of Russian-backbone seasonal trivalent, live-attenuated influenza vaccine in a phase II randomized placebo-controlled clinical trial among children in urban Bangladesh. Vaccine. 2015;33(29):3415-21.
16. Reichert TA, Sugaya N, Fedson DS, Glezen WP, Simonsen L, Tashiro M. The Japanese experience with vaccinating schoolchildren against influenza. N Engl J Med. 2001;344(12):889-96.
17. Saha S, Chadha M, Shu Y, GARI. Influenza and other Respiratory Viruses. Influenza Other Respir Viruses. 2016;10(3):176-84.
18. Simonsen L, Fukuda K, Schonberger LB, Cox NJ. The impact of influenza epidemics on hospitalizations. J Infect Dis. 2000;181:831-7.
19. The Advisory Committee on Immunization Practices (ACIP), Centers for Disease Control and Prevention. (2020). Immunization update 2019. [online] Available from https://www.pharmacytoday.org/article/S1042-0991(19)30653-X/pdf; https://www.cdc.gov/vaccines/acip/meetings/downloads/slides-2018-10/Influenza-03-Mercer-508.pdf [Last accessed November, 2020].
20. World Health Organization. WHO recommendations on the composition of influenza virus vaccines. [online] Available from https://www.who.int/influenza/vaccines/virus/recommendations/en/ [Last accessed November, 2020].

CHAPTER 21

Measles, Mumps and Rubella Vaccines MR/MMR/MMRV Vaccines

Rohit Agrawal

Q1. What is the importance of measles elimination and rubella control?

Ans. Measles is a highly infectious disease and in pre-vaccination era >90% of the individuals were infected by the age of 10 years globally.

Measles elimination is very important since it contributes significantly in achieving millennium development goal 4 (MDG4).

One of the three indicators for monitoring achievement of MDG4 is the proportion of 1 year old children immunized against measles.

While measles is now rare in many developed countries, it still prevails as a common illness in many developing countries including India.

According to the World Health Organization (WHO) estimates, in 2001 alone >23 million DALY (Disability Adjusted Life Years) were lost due to measles.

Measles can be readily prevented by vaccination.

After reaching worldwide coverage of one dose of measles vaccine to 82% in 2007, the estimated number of deaths from measles dropped from 750,000 to 197,000.

While India has made significant progress in child survival, measles still remains a leading cause of death and disability among young children.

The estimated 50,000–100,000 children die of measles annually making it a leading cause of child mortality.

The measles and rubella initiative is a global partnership aimed at ensuring no child dies of measles or is born with congenital rubella syndrome (CRS).

Since 2001 the initiative delivered >1 billion doses of measles vaccines to help to raise and maintain measles vaccination coverage to 85% globally and thereby reduce global measles death by 74%.

These efforts have contributed significantly in reducing child mortality as per MDG4.

In many developing countries including India, measles continues to be a serious public health problem.

After the introduction of measles vaccination in universal immunization program (UIP) since 1985, measles deaths have been reduced from 106,000 in

2005 to 65,000 in 2010 and 29,336 in 2012, but still India contributes to almost 47% of global measles deaths.

India reported 74 measles outbreaks in 2012 and 61 outbreaks in 2013.

With these high number of measles deaths, high birth cohort, and relatively poor vaccine coverage, India possess a challenge. In a nutshell, measles disease burden is still huge particularly in developing countries.

Q2. What are the modalities for measles prevention and elimination?

Ans. Apart from effective vaccination and sustained vaccination coverage of >95% in the community (herd immunity), a multiprong strategy including improved routine coverage with two doses through routine public immunization system, periodic supplemental immunization activities, careful surveillance, outbreak preparedness, research and development, addressing the issues of vaccine hesitancy and building public confidence in immunization are the preventive modalities.

Q3. What is the contribution of vaccination in elimination of measles and rubella?

Ans. Vaccination is the only strategy; however, to control measles our country needs sustained vaccination coverage of >95%.

However, unfortunately, a recent vaccination survey in India showed overall vaccine coverage of 71% of measles containing Vaccine (MCV) at 9–12 months.

Considering 85% vaccine efficacy for vaccination at 9 months, the actual protection was conferred to only 60% of annual birth cohorts and 40% cohorts remained susceptible (including unimmunized and 15% of vaccine failure to seroconvert)

Another challenge for India is a considerable difference in vaccination coverage in different states. Whereas states such as Kerala, Goa, Sikkim, and Punjab have achieved almost 90% of coverage, the states such as Uttar Pradesh, Bihar, Madhya Pradesh, and Rajasthan have achieved a coverage of only 70%, the least being from Uttar Pradesh and Bihar.

Hence, if a country like India succeeds in sustaining >95% coverage universally, with two doses of measles-rubella (MR), measles and rubella can certainly be controlled.

Q4. What is the composition of measles-rubella/measles, mumps, and rubella (MR/MMR) vaccines?

Ans. Measles vaccine is derived from live-attenuated strains of Edmonton-Zagreb measles virus (Tresivac^{TM}) or Shwartz strain (Priorix^{TM}).

Rubella vaccine is derived from live-attenuated strains of Wistar RA-27/3 rubella virus in both vaccines.

Mumps vaccine is derived from different formulations having different strains of the virus which include Leningrad-Zagreb (Tresivac^{TM}),

Leningrad-3, Urabe-AM9, Jeryl-Lynn and RIT-4385 strengths, derived from Jeryl Lynn strain (Priorix™).

All the three vaccine strains are grown and propagated on human diploid cell cultures/chick embryo.

Measles, mumps, and rubella vaccines are available in lyophilized forms and should be frozen for long-term storage. In clinical practice, the vaccine may be stored at 2–8°C, should be protected from light, and the reconstituted vaccine should be used within 4–6 hours.

It is available as single-dose vial and needs to be administered subcutaneously or intramuscularly; the dose is 0.5 mL. The vaccine should be diluted with the diluent provided with the vaccine.

Each 0.5 mL dose of Tresivac™ contains not <1,000 median cell culture infective doses ($CCID_{50}$) of live measles virus and 1000 $CCID_{50}$ of rubella virus and 5000 $CCID_{50}$ of the mumps virus.

It is the World Health Organization (WHO) prequalified vaccine and shelf life is 24 months at 2–8°C.

Each 0.5 mL dose of Priorix™ contains not <10^3 median cell culture infective doses ($CCID_{50}$) of live measles virus and 10^3 $CCID_{50}$ of rubella virus and 10^3 $CCID_{50}$ of the mumps virus.

Measles containing vaccine vials, especially multidose, can get contaminated with the puncture of cap and multiple uses leading to bacterial growth in the vial as it does not contain preservatives.

Staphylococcus is the most common organism which can cause severe toxic shock in the recipient through its exo-toxins-toxic shock syndrome (TSS).

Stringent injection safety norms and protocols need to be adhered to prevent TSS.

Q5. What is the adverse events profile of measles, mumps, and rubella (MMR) vaccines?

Ans. Measles, mumps, and rubella vaccine is quite safe and effective. Minor adverse events following immunization (AEFIs) are not very common and usually mild. The common events encountered within 24 hours are mild pain, tenderness at the injection site, and mild fever can occur in 5–15% of vaccinees between 7 and 12 days postvaccination period and is self-limiting.

Rash may occur in approximately 2% of the recipients, starting between 7 and 10 days postvaccination and may last for 2–3 days. A mild measles like illness may appear between 7 and 12 days postvaccination in 2–5% of the vaccinees. Thrombocytopenic purpura is very rare, approximately at a frequency rate of 1:30,000 vaccinees. There is mild depletion of CMI for a transient period. Serious AEFIs like encephalitis is very rare and being reported at a frequency rate of one case/million doses, although the causal link is not totally established.

Febrile seizures are known to occur rarely in toddlers (with second dose), particularly when given concomitantly or in combination with varicella vaccine especially in naïve children who did not receive the first dose.

Transient parotitis may occur in <1% vaccinees. Mild aseptic meningitis can very rarely occur 2–3 weeks postvaccination. The virus is nontransferable from the vaccinees to the contacts.

Measles component can very rarely cause an anaphylactic reaction. A mild anaphylactic reaction may also occur due to neomycin component in the vaccine. The rubella component may commonly cause arthralgia and arthritis to the tune of 10–25% in adolescents and young adult females lasting for few days to 2 weeks. However, they are found to be rare in young children. Low-grade fever, rash, lymphadenopathy, myalgia, and paresthesia are being reported not commonly in clinical practice. The vaccine may very rarely cause allergic reactions such as urticaria and pruritus within 24 hours of vaccination.

Q6. What are the contraindications for measles, mumps, and rubella (MMR) vaccines?

Ans. Being a live vaccine, and due to its influence on both, humoral and cell-mediated immunity, MCV is contraindicated in severely immunocompromised subjects and during pregnancy.

Should the benefits of vaccination overweigh the contraindications it can be given as early as 6 months, e.g., in the human immunodeficiency virus (HIV) child wherein the CD4 counts are well preserved in early stages of life with a note of suboptimal response.

The vaccine is contraindicated in those with history of severe allergic reactions to the constituents of the vaccine like neomycin.

Measles, mumps, and rubella vaccine is an absolute contraindication in pregnant women; however, if given inadvertently in pregnancy, termination of pregnancy is not indicated. Pregnancy may be planned after an interval of at least 3-month postvaccination.

Malnutrition, low-grade fever, mild upper respiratory tract infections (URTI), diarrhea, and other minor illnesses are not contraindications, on the contrary, vaccination should be ensured in a malnourished child.

Q7. What is the efficacy and immunogenicity of measles, mumps, and rubella (MMR) vaccines?

Ans. There are no robust and accurate efficacy data of measles or rubella vaccination globally. However, a drastic reduction in the deaths due to measles and congenital rubella syndrome (CRS) cases in industrialized nations with high vaccination coverage has shown a very high impact and effectiveness of the vaccine. Few vaccine efficacy-studies from India have reported varying degree of efficacies ranging from 60 to 80% when initiated at the age of 9 months with an effectiveness under field conditions around 85%.

SECTION 2: Individual Vaccines

Immunogenicity: Multiple studies have demonstrated immunogenicity around 80–85% at the age of 9 months while 95% and more at the age of 12–15 months. Seroconversion rates are found to be around 60% if administered at the age of 6 months, most probably due to interference by the pre-existing maternal antibodies, along with primary vaccine failure for measles vaccine to the tune of 20%. At 9 months of age, primary vaccine failure is reported to be around 15%. While antibody titers wane over the years measles specific cellular immunity persists and may provide a very long duration of protection. Secondary vaccine failures are very rare. Paradoxically, superior seroconversion rates are seen at 6 months as compared to 9 months in HIV infected infants due to progressive decline in the immune status. The immunogenicity with mumps component with one dose is 78%, while with two doses is almost 88–90%. The exact disease burden of mumps is less specified and mainly sporadic outbreaks have been reported. Rubella component of the MMR vaccine gives more robust and long-term immunity with a single dose. Seroconversion rates of rubella component with single dose is 95% and >95% with two doses. It is essential to achieve >80% coverage of immunization against rubella in young children or else indiscriminate use of rubella vaccine as monovalent or as MR/MMR may prove to be counter protective as it may shift the rubella epidemiology to the right with more cases occurring in young adults leading to increase in cases of CRS. This has been proved by direct evidences from Greece and Latin American countries.

Q8. Association of autism, inflammatory bowel disease (IBD), Guillain-Barré syndrome (GBS), encephalitis with measles vaccinations. Are they myths or facts?

Ans. Earlier a temporal relationship of MMR vaccine was corelated with autism, IBD, GBS, encephalitis. As a result, many countries in the west ceased MCV in their national program and consequently suffered many measles outbreaks.

However, there is no conclusive evidence to establish a causal relationship between MMR vaccine and these conditions. Hence, associations of MMR vaccine with autism/IBD/GBS/subacute sclerosing panencephalitis (SSPE) are myths and not facts.

Q9. What are the national and Indian Academy of Pediatrics (IAP) recommendations for routine and catch-up immunization for measles, mumps, and rubella (MMR)?

Ans.

Recommendations IAP (Individual Use)

At least two or three doses of measles containing vaccines are recommended as: First dose as MMR at the completion of 9 months, second dose as MMR at 15–18 months and third dose as MMR at 5 years of age.

Despite of three doses of MCV, 5–8% vaccinnees may still remain susceptible.

Administration of the vaccine within 2 days of exposure may protect or modify the severity of the clinical disease.

The vaccine should be given irrespective of prior history of any exanthematous illness which may more often be confused with measles.

Measles, mumps, and rubella vaccine at 9 months is not the best as it has almost 15–20% primary vaccine failure due to maternal antibodies.

It is best when given at 12 months, however, a significant proportion of measles cases in India occur below the age of 12 months, hence, in order to balance best between early protection and high seroconversion, completed 9 months is a compromised but the most appropriate age for MMR vaccinations.

- First dose MCV-1 as MR/MMR at 9 months
- Second dose MCV-2 as MMR ideally delivered between the age of 15 and 18 months
- Third dose MCV-3 as MMR between 4 and 6 years of age

Public Health Perspective

Apart from two doses of MR vaccines, Ministry of Health and Family Welfare, Government of India (MoHFW-GOI) who is a committed signatory to the global measles and rubella strategic plan has launched one of the world's largest MR vaccination campaigns to eliminate measles and control rubella in the country from the year 2020.

The phased MR campaign is just being concluded and has vaccinated 410 million children in the age group 9 months to 14 years.

A follow-up MR campaign is a periodical event guided by country specific surveillance data, routine immunization (RI) coverage, existence of pockets of unprotected children and vaccine efficacy. The target age group for immunization in these follow-up campaigns will include all children above age 9 months who are born after the previous MR vaccination campaign.

Catch-up Vaccination

All the school-aged children above 5 years of age, if not vaccinated earlier should at least be vaccinated with MMR vaccine with minimal interval of 4 weeks between the two doses.

Only one dose should be given, if previously vaccinated with MMR.

Q10. What about postexposure prophylaxis?

Ans. Measles, mumps, and rubella vaccine, if administered within 72 hours of initial measles exposure or immunoglobulins IG if administered within 6 days of exposure, may provide some protection or modify the clinical course of the disease. If MMR vaccine is not administered within 72 hours of exposure as postexposure prophylaxis (PEP), MMR should still be offered at any interval following exposure to the disease in order to offer protection from future exposures. People who are at risk for severe illness and complication from measles such as infants younger than 12 months of age, pregnant women without evidence of measles immunity and people with severely compromised immune system should receive IV IgG.

Q11. Initially in universal immunization program (UIP), the recommendation was for one dose of measles, then it was changed to two doses, then from standalone measles to MR. Why so?

Ans. Switch from one dose of measles vaccine to two doses of MR needs following consideration.

As per World Health Organization recommendations, achieving and maintaining measles vaccination coverage of 80% or greater is a must. As per WHO, all countries that are providing two doses of measles vaccine through routine immunization (RI)/supplemental immunization activity (SIA) or both have done exceedingly well in sustaining coverage of >80%.

One dose measle was included in 1985 in UIP, but the chances of dropouts, poor coverage, vaccine failures, waning immunity, and vaccine efficacy of 85%, >40% cohort remained unimmunized. Hence, two doses of measles containing vaccine (MCV) one at 9 months standalone measles and second as MR at 15 months was initiated.

Though exact rubella disease burden estimates are not known and difficult to assess but since India has committed to the elimination of measles and control of rubella by the year 2020, rubella vaccine will be introduced in national immunization program (NIP), as MR vaccine replacing both doses of MCV at 9 months and 16–24 months.

Though one dose of rubella vaccine probably induces a long duration protection, more than one dose could render lifelong immunity.

Q12. Why is there a deviation between Indian Academy of Pediatrics (IAP) and government recommendations, e.g., MR in government and MMR in IAP?

Ans. Indian Academy of Pediatrics now recommends MMR vaccine in place of measles/MR at 9 months and 16–24 months. Government of India (GOI) does not recognize the burden of mumps in public health in view of less morbidity-mortality with lack of substantial disease burden data. Hence, GOI recommends MR in NIP in place of MMR.

However, IAP considers mumps morbidity as significant as much as rubella. There are cluster of complications of mumps such as aseptic meningitis, encephalitis, pancreatitis, orchitis, transverse myelitis, polyradiculitis, etc. with lifelong repercussions or disabilities.

Mumps can also cause fetal aqueduct stenosis leading to congenital hydrocephalus in fetus when afflicts the pregnant woman.

Though epidemiology of mumps is not clear in India it is estimated that outbreaks do occur every 5–10 years.

Globally, most countries use MMR vaccine instead of monovalent or MR and thereby the burden of mumps has reduced substantially in developed countries following use of MMR vaccine.

In MMR vaccine, the protective immune response to each of the component remains unchanged, noninterfering and noninferior.

Q13. Why measles containing vaccine (MCV) after 9 months and not earlier?

Ans. Ideally, MMR vaccine should be immunologically given at 12 months for the advantage of higher seroconversion rates at this age with fewer cases of primary vaccine failure.

In countries with low rates of transmission, the World Health Organization recommends first dose at 12 months. In developing countries like India where the ongoing process of transmission is high and significant proportion of measles occurs below 12 months of age to achieve the best balance between the early protection and high seroconversion, completed 9 months of age is being recommended as the appropriate age for measles vaccination in India.

The 9-month schedule is an epidemiological compulsion and has almost 20% primary vaccine failure due to maternal antibodies. Thus, at least two to three MCV doses are required for protection and despite this 5–8% population may remain susceptible.

The vaccine cannot be given at 6 months of age for the reason of poor immune response and seroconversion due to circulating maternal antibodies. However, in case of an outbreak the vaccine can be given to infants as young as 6 months old.

The studies have shown seroconversion rates are around 60% at the age of 6 months, 85% at the age of 9 months, and >95% at the age of 12–16 months.

Q14. If there is an outbreak, can we vaccinate children younger than 9 months?

Ans. Measles, mumps, and rubella can be given to children as young as 6 months of age who are at high risk of exposure such as during a community outbreak. However, doses given *before* 9 months of age should be considered as invalid and cannot be counted towards the three-dose series for MMR.

Q15. What are measles and rubella (MR) vaccination campaigns and their role?

Ans. According to the global measles and rubella strategic plan 2012, all the six WHO regions have committed to measles elimination and rubella control.

Government of India is a signatory in this mission of measles elimination and rubella control by 2020; however, with two dose routine immunization it was a challenging task to cover almost all children with uncertain vaccine records. Based on the huge success of polio vaccination campaign in eliminating polio from the country, MR campaign was designed as one dose campaign irrespective of previous vaccination or disease status in the age group between 9 months and 15 years.

Immediately after the completion of campaign, MR vaccine will be introduced in two-dose schedules at 9–12 months and 16–24 months instead of standalone measles vaccine.

The MR dose received during the campaign will not be counted and will be an extra dose on an above two doses of MR.

An additional dose, does not harm and in fact, is beneficial for a miniscule group of children who do not seroconvert even after 2/3 doses.

Government of India has just initiated the phase MR campaign and completed with vaccinating 31 crores of children between 9 months and 15 years.

A follow-up MR campaign will be required as a periodic event every 3–5 years guided by country-specific surveillance data.

The periodicity will depend on RI coverage, existence of pockets of unprotected children, and vaccine efficacy.

This follow-up campaign will target only those children, born after the last campaign aged above 9 months, to achieve and sustain high level of population immunity.

Q16. Why so much hype about rubella control?

Ans. Rubella also known as German measles is basically a mild exanthematous viral illness with fever and milder complications. It was first understood as a significant health problem when a pandemic of rubella [congenital rubella syndrome (CRS)] occurred in 1964–65. Rubella, if contracted in the first trimester of pregnancy, can lead to CRS with disastrous consequences in the fetus/newborn as stillbirth, mental retardation (MR), congenital heart diseases (CHD), cataracts, blindness, deafness, etc.

Developed countries have drastically reduced the burden of CRS by universal immunization against rubella. There is no evidence of true burden of rubella in India; however, GOI estimates that there are around 30,000 cases annually. WHO estimates that around 100,000 cases of CRS occur annually in developing countries alone. Data of 2008 estimates suggest the highest CRS burden is in southeast Asia to the tune of approximate 48% and India is a major contributor. In 2012 and 2013, India reported 28 and 48 rubella outbreaks, respectively.

In view of this, all the regions of the World Health Organization have made declarations for elimination of measles and rubella control, India is a signatory to this declaration made at SEARO Summit at Kathmandu in 2013.

Q17. Why are two or more doses of rubella vaccine recommended, when one dose can confer long duration immunity (nearly lifelong)?

Ans. Undoubtedly, single dose of rubella vaccine renders long duration immunity probably lifelong in 95% of vaccinees. However, a small cohort of subjects remains seronegative and with suboptimal vaccine coverage of about 71% a substantial pool remains susceptible to acquire the infection in late childhood or adolescence. To control rubella, it is essential to have >80% coverage. Indiscriminate use of rubella vaccine as mono or as a constituent of MR/MMR through private-public sector may shift the rubella epidemiology to right, thereby more rubella cases occurring in young adults leading to paradoxical increase in CRS cases.

In a multicentric study across the country conducted at Amritsar, Jammu, and Maharashtra showed rubella susceptibility in young female adults between the age groups of 11 and 18 years to the tune of 36%, 32%, and 23%. It has also been observed that around 40–45% of women in child bearing age are susceptible to rubella. Hence, it is prudent to administer a second dose of rubella which will give a lifelong immunity.

Q18. What is measles, mumps, rubella, and varicella (MMRV) vaccine?

Ans. Measles, mumps, rubella, and varicella is a fixed dose combination of MMR and varicella vaccine which was available in India since last 7–8 years under the name Priorix tetra™ by GSK but presently unavailable.

The advantage is that it reduces one additional prick to the recipient. Multiple studies in the western world have shown increased risk of febrile seizures with MMRV as compared to MMR + V given concomitantly.

Review of MMRV safety indicated that the risk of febrile seizures for children 12–23 months receiving MMRV vaccine was 7–9 per 10,000 children, compared to 3–4 per 10,000 for the children receiving separate MMR and varicella vaccines. This risk peaked 5–12 days after vaccination. The relative risk of febrile seizures after vaccination with MMRV compared to MMR+V was 1.96 (95% CI: 1.43–2.73) for children 12–23 months.

However, the incidence of febrile seizures was much less in the cases that were already primed with measles vaccine at 9 months.

The clinical studies have also demonstrated increased reactogenicity when administered concomitantly with conjugated quadrivalent measles containing vaccine.

However, no increased reactogenicity of MMRV vaccine with hepatitis A and/or diphtheria, tetanus, and pertussis (DTaP)/inactivated poliovirus (IPV)/*Haemophilus influenzae* type b (Hib) were demonstrated. High cost of the vaccine is a constraint in our country.

Measles, mumps, and rubella vaccine is an appropriate cost-effective strategy even with three doses, in view of high diseases burden and complications of mumps and measles and number of cases of congenital rubella syndrome (CRS).

It is the only modality for the commitment of measles elimination and rubella control by 2020.

SUGGESTED READING

1. Balasubramanian S, Shah A, Pemde HK, Chatterjee P, Shivananda S, Guduru VK, et al. Indian Academy of Pediatrics (IAP) Advisory Committee on Vaccines and Immunization Practices (ACVIP) Recommended Immunization Schedule (2018-19) and Update on Immunization for Children Aged 0 Through 18 Years. 2018;55:1066-74.
2. Centers for Disease Control and Prevention. (2013). Status_Report_Measles_Rubella 21Oct2013_FINAL.pdf. [online] Available from: http://www.who.int/biologicals/areas/vaccines/mmr/mumps/e. [Last accessed November, 2020].
3. Ministry of Health and Welfare, Govt. of India. (2017). National operational guideline for introduction of Measles-Rubella vaccine, 2017. [online] Available from: http://origin.searo.who.int/india/topics/measles/measles_rubella_vaccine_guidelines.pdf [Last accessed November, 2020].
4. UNICEF. (2009). UNICEF Coverage Evaluation survey, 2009 National Fact Sheet. [online] Available from: http://www.unicef.org/india/National_Fact_Sheet_CES_2009.pdf. [Last accessed November, 2020].
5. World Health Organization. (2011). Rubella vaccines, Summary of WHO position paper published in WER July 2011. [online] Available from: http://www.who.int/immunization/position_papers/PP_rubella_July_2011_summary.pdf [Last accessed November, 2020].
6. World Health Organization. (2012). Immunization, Vaccines and Biologicals: The Measles and Rubella Initiative Welcomes World Health Assembly Commitment to Measles and Rubella Elimination Goals. [online] Available from: https://www.who.int/immunization/newsroom/measles_rubella_wha_elimination_goals_statement_may12/en/ [Last accessed November, 2020].
7. World Health Organization. (2013). SAGE Working Group on Measles and Rubella (17 October 2013): Status Report on Progress Towards Measles and Rubella Elimination. [online] Available from: http://www.who.int/immunization/sage/meetings/2013/november/ [Last accessed November, 2020].
8. World Health Organization. Global Measles and Rubella Strategic Plan: 2012-2020. Geneva: World Health Organization Press; 2012. pp. 10-21.
9. World Health Organization: Regional Office for South-East Asia (WHO: SEARO). (2013). Measles Elimination and Rubella Control 2013. [online] Available from: http://www.searo.who.int/mediacentre/events/governance/rc/66/9.pdf. [Last accessed November, 2020].

CHAPTER 22

Typhoid Vaccines

Vijay Yewale

Q1. How prevalent is "typhoid fever"?

Ans. Typhoid is a public health problem in low and middle income countries (LMIC). An estimated 17.8 million cases occur each year in LMIC of Asia. Among the *population-based studies* the incidence is 377 per 100,000 person years and 105 per 100,000 person years for typhoid and paratyphoid, respectively. In 2016, India had 6.6 million typhoid cases (499 cases/100,000 population) and 66,439 typhoid deaths, more than half were in children below 15 years of age. As per the systematic review and meta-analysis of literature between 1990 and 2015, about 10% of fever in *hospitalized patients* is culture-confirmed typhoid fever and paratyphoid is approximately 1/10th of typhoid fever. Children aged 2–4 years having the highest incidence. The incidence varies from region to region and the disease incidence is the highest among children aged 2–4 years.

Q2. What are the preventive measures for typhoid fever?

Ans. Sanitation, hygiene, and safe drinking water, which are the primary preventive measures for food and water-borne pathogens, show slower results, require significant behavioral changes, and require significant investment for infrastructure development. On the other hand, vaccination yields quicker results, is affordable, cost-effective, and does not require significant behavioral changes. Most policymakers agree that routine public health use of typhoid vaccines should be integrated with other control strategies.

Q3. What are the different types of typhoid vaccines?

Ans. There are different generations of vaccines developed so far:
- Whole-cell inactivated typhoid-paratyphoid vaccine (TAB)
- Live-attenuated Ty21 oral vaccine
- Vi-antigen polysaccharide vaccine (ViPS)
- Typhoid conjugate vaccine (TCV)

Q4. What is the whole-cell inactivated typhoid/paratyphoid vaccine TAB?

Ans. Typhoid, paratyphoid A, and paratyphoid B (TAB) vaccine was the first heat inactivated phenol preserved vaccine against typhoid and paratyphoid.

It had efficacy of 51–88% in children and young adults lasting up to 7 years.

One-third of the vaccinees developed fever and local pain and headache was seen in 10% of the vaccines. It was withdrawn from the public health program for the high reactogenicity and is no longer available.

Q5. Which is the oral typhoid vaccine?

Ans. Live-attenuated Ty21 vaccine is the oral vaccine in which several genes of the Ty2 strain have been attenuated by chemically induced mutagenesis. It lacks the Vi antigen. It contains 2 to 6×10^9 CFU of Ty21a (attenuated Ty2 strain of *S. typhi*).

It is available in a liquid form for use in children above 2 years and enteric-coated capsules administered orally as three doses on alternate days to children above the age of 6 years. Revaccination is recommended after 3–7 years. This vaccine cannot be administered to the immunocompromised and those on antibiotics.

This vaccine is not available in India.

Q6. How efficacious is the live-attenuated Ty21 vaccine?

Ans. It induces adequate cell-mediated immune response in addition to antibodies to O, H, and other surface antigens. However, it does not induce Vi antibodies as it lacks Vi antigen. The human challenge trials demonstrated 87–96% efficacy. In the Santiago, Chile trial demonstrated progressively increasing efficacy with age of the subject. The overall efficacy was 67% over 3 years, reducing to 62% efficacy over 7 years.

Q7. What are the characteristics of the typhoid Vi polysaccharide vaccine?

Ans. Contents: 25 micrograms of the purified Vi capsular polysaccharide from the *Ty2 S. typhi* strain in 0.5 mL in a fully liquid formulation.

It has to be stored between +2°C and 8°C. It is stable for 6 months at 37°C and for 2 years at 22°C.

The route of administration is intramuscular or subcutaneous.

It is recommended above 2 years of age and has to be repeated every 3 years.

The cumulative efficacy at 3 years against culture confirmed typhoid fever is reported as 55%.

Anti-Vi antibodies and 1 µg/mL are proposed as the serologic correlate of protection.

Effectiveness: Cluster randomized trial at Kolkata slums demonstrated effectiveness of 61% at 2 years follow-up; it was 80% in children below 5 years with herd effect of 44% in unvaccinated children in the vaccinated cluster. The effectiveness has not been uniform. In Pakistan field trial, it demonstrated effectiveness of 38% with no herd effect.

Q8. What are the different typhoid conjugate vaccines?

Ans. There are different typhoid conjugate vaccines made from the polysaccharide derived either from *S. typhi* or *Citrobacter freundii* conjugated with a carrier protein which is either *Pseudomonas aeruginosa* ExoProtein A (rEPA), tetanus toxoid (TT), diphtheria toxoid (DT) or cross-reactive material (CRM 197), a nontoxic mutant of diphtheria toxin.

Q9. Which conjugate vaccine is WHO prequalified?

Ans. Typhoid-conjugate vaccine made by conjugation of the 25 µg of Vi polysaccharide of *S. typhi* Ty2 conjugated with TT.

Typhoid Conjugate Vaccine (S. Ty2 + TT)

Contents: 25 µg Vi polysaccharide antigen linked to tetanus toxoid protein (also referred to as Vi-TT conjugate vaccine).

Preparation: Fully liquid, 0.5 mL administered IM, 6 month onward up to 45 years.

Storage: +2°C to +8°C

Route of administration: Intramuscular

Schedule: The World Health Organization (WHO) and The Indian Academy of Pediatrics (IAP) recommend single dose of TCV beginning at 6 months of age. The need for a booster dose is unclear at this point in time.

The best practicable schedule for TCV would be to give it with measles containing vaccine (MCV) at 9 months. It also allows flexibility of adopting either one- or two-dose schedules, in case there is a need-based change in future, wherein the second dose can be given at the time of the second dose of MCV at 16–18 months.

Immunogenicity

Prelicensure phase III trial consisted of two cohorts: *Cohort 1*: >6 months to 2 years (n = 327); open label was given 1 dose of the Vi-TT and *Cohort 2*: 2 years to 45 years (n = 654); double-blind randomized Vi-TT was given to 340 and typhoid polysaccharide was given to 314 subjects. Immunogenicity was demonstrated by measuring the IgG Vi antibody geometric mean titer (GMT). The cohort was followed up till 5 years. On day 720, a subcohort of 174 was given a booster of Vi-TT or tetravalent polysaccharide vaccine (TPSV) and followed up till 5 years.

Significant seroconversion and GMTs were demonstrated at day 42 in both the cohorts. The GMTs were higher in Vi-TT recipient compared to the polysaccharide vaccine recipient in the randomized controlled trial (RCT).

Vi-tetanus toxoid elicited significantly higher GMTs than unconjugated ViPS at 6 weeks after the first dose and 6 weeks after the second dose at day 720.

At 3 and 5 years, subjects in RCT who received a single dose demonstrated persistence of antibodies and the levels were higher as compared to the unconjugated ViPS recipient.

In cohort 1, infants aged 6–11 months and children aged 12–23 months, a single dose of Vi-TT elicited high titers of IgG anti-Vi antibody [1937.4 (95% CI: 1785.0–2102.9, N = 307)] that persisted up to 5 years in approximately 84% of children **(Table 1)**.

The avidity of the IgG Vi-antibody was higher with TCV compared to the ViPS and the avidity index demonstrated a booster response.

As shown in the **Table 1**, high titers of anti-Vi IgG were seen in all cohorts till 5 years, even in the unboosted cohort. This is the basis of the WHO and the IAP recommendation of a single dose at all ages above 6 months of age.

Serologic Correlate of Protection

There is no established serologic correlate of protection for typhoid disease or vaccines hence the immunogenicity of typhoid vaccine cannot be equated with the efficacy of the vaccine. Based on the efficacy data of the experimental Vi conjugate vaccine [Vi-rEPA, a conjugate of the capsular polysaccharide of *Salmonella typhi*, Vi, bound to nontoxic recombinant *Pseudomonas aeruginosa* exotoxin A (rEPA)]. It is estimated that a level of 3.52 enzyme-linked immunosorbent assay (ELISA) unit/mL offers adequate protection.

Table 1: geometric mean titers (GMTs) and seroconversion rate (SCR) in nonboosted and boosted cohorts open label trial (OLT): 6–23 months. Randomized controlled trial (RCT): 2–45 years.

Time point	TCV-OLT: GMTs		TCV-RCT: GMTs		TCV-OLT: SCR (%)		TCV-RCT: SCR (%)	
	Boosted	Non-boosted	Boosted	Non-boosted	Boosted	Non-boosted	Boosted	Non-boosted
Day 0	9.56	9.56	10.4	10.4	7.17	7.17	10.24	10.24
Day 42	1,937.4	1,937.4	1,292.5	1,292.5	98.05	98.05	97.29	97.29
Day 540	58.7	58.7	92.8	92.8	62.3	62.3	78.3	78.3
Day 720	48.3	48.3	81.7	81.7	59.55	59.55	74.07	74.07
Day 762	1,721.9	XXXXX	1,685.3	XXXXX	98.39	XXXXX	85.76	XXXXX
Day 1,095	307.69	114.5	276.34	64.42	90.54	78.05	71.43	76.56
Day 1,825	132.29	80.16	190.67	51.78	83.75	76.6	75.75	74.07

Source: From Background paper on typhoid vaccines for SAGE meeting (October 2017).

Efficacy

In the absence of established serologic correlates of protection, it was important to have efficacy data on the Vi-TT.

Vi-tetanus toxoid had efficacy of 87.1% (95% CI: 47.2, 96.9%) compared to 52.3% (95% CI: -4.2, 78.2%) with the comparator ViPS vaccine at 1 month after vaccination in a human challenge study in a population of immunologically naïve 112 adult volunteers between 18 and 60 years of age.

The seroefficacy was estimated as 85% (95% CI: 80–88%). This seroefficacy was derived from reanalysis of data from a proportion of subjects enrolled in the Vi-TT phase III immunogenicity trial with presumed clinical or subclinical infection.

Field Effectiveness

Large and double-blind randomized trials of between 20,000 and 42,000 children are ongoing in Nepal, Bangladesh, and Malawi to assess the vaccine's effectiveness when administered to children in endemic settings. In addition, the population impact of vaccine introduction is being assessed in Navi Mumbai.

Results of the Nepal Efficacy Study

Efficacy of 81.6% (58.8–91.8) was demonstrated in the Nepal study of 20,000 subjects given TCV and meningococcal serogroup A (MenA) in 1:1 distribution. This study is done using single dose of TCV.

The immunogenicity calculated in the subgroup showed seroconversion of 99% in the TCV group and 2% in the MenA vaccine group.

Q10. Is a second (booster) dose of the TCV needed?

Ans. The World Health Organization Strategic Advisory Group of Experts (WHO-SAGE) does not recommend a second dose especially in the endemic setting where there is an opportunity of natural boosting especially for children above the age of 2 years.

This is based on the persistence of GMTs with high avidity at the end of 5 years in the single-dose recipient subgroup.

Q11. What is the data about PedaTyph™?

Ans. In a small efficacy trial of the above TCV available in India (5 µg ViPS conjugated with TT), single-dose recipient (n = 140) had no breakthrough disease till 2.5 years follow-up.

The Pedatyph™ study has important limitations regarding information about the studies done including an apparent nonrigorous study design. No clarifications or additional data has been supplied by the manufacturer. Hence, the WHO has not prequalified or recommended this vaccine.

Q12. Is there a need for a second dose for children vaccinated before 1 year of age?

Ans. Young children below 2 years may not provide a robust long-lasting immune response due to lack of certain key "immunological edifices" needed for providing a long-lasting immunity owing to the immaturity of the immune system. The opportunity for natural boosting will also be less in the young below 2 years of age. However, the available data does not support the need for a second dose.

Q13. Which are the other TCVs available in India?

Ans.
1. 25 µg of ViPS conjugated with TT, by Zydus. This vaccine was licensed based on noninferiority with the comparator WHO qualified 25 µg TCV + TT vaccine.
2. 25 µg of ViPS derived from *Citrobacter freundii* conjugated with CRM197

    This vaccine, manufactured by an Indian company, Biological Evans, has demonstrated high immunogenicity and good safety in the age groups 6 months to 45 years of age, which was noninferior to licensed comparator TCV and is licensed by the Drugs Controller General of India (DCGI) in February 2020. The WHO approval is pending.

Q14. Do you need to give the typhoid vaccine after the child has had a culture proven typhoid? If yes, how many days after recovery?

Ans. Immunity after typhoid disease is neither complete nor long lasting. We need to give a typhoid injection after complete recovery from the illness.

Q15. Which are the other TCVs in development?

Ans.
1. A Vi-rEPA vaccine, manufactured by Lanzhou Institute of Biological Products Co. Ltd., PR China, has gained national licensure.
2. Other Vi-polysaccharides conjugated to DT are in various phases of clinical development.

Q16. Is 5 microgram of ViPS immunogenic and adequate in the Vi-TT?

Ans. The anti-Vi IgG antibody response is dose dependent. 12.5 µg of the experimental rEPA vaccine elicited the presumed protective cut off of 3.53 ELISA units/mL (4.3 µg/mL).

However, levels of 2 µg/mL of anti-Vi IgG antibody levels were found to be effective in the efficacy trial in Vietnam of the rEPA. If this is taken as the level required for protection, perhaps 5 µg may also produce the desired adequate immune response.

Q17. Is there any progress in development of paratyphoid vaccine?

Ans. Bharat Biotech is in the process of developing a quadrivalent vaccine which will include typhoid, paratyphoid A and B, along with nontyphoid salmonella (NTS).

Q18. Can TCV be administered simultaneously with measles containing vaccines (MCV)?

Ans. Studies have shown that coadministration of TCV and MCV do neither result in any significant decrease in anti-Vi IgG nor in the levels of anti-measles IgG titers. Similar results have also been observed with the other antigens in measles, mumps, and rubella (MMR) vaccine.

Hence, TCV and MCV can be given on the same day.

Q19. What are the IAP ACVIP recommendations on typhoid vaccines?

Ans. For the primary schedule, a single dose of TCV 25 µg is recommended from the age of 6 months onward routinely.

Typhoid conjugate vaccine and measles-containing vaccine can be administered simultaneously when it is offered at the age of 9 months or beyond.

For a child who has received only typhoid polysaccharide vaccine, a single dose of TCV is recommended at least 4 weeks following the receipt of polysaccharide vaccine.

Routine booster for TCV at 2 years is not recommended as of now.

Q20. Can TCV be given to adults?

Ans. The TCV-TT vaccine is licensed and can be given till 45 years of age.

■ SUGGESTED READING

1. Advisory Committee on Vaccines and Immunization Practices, Indian Academy of Pediatrics. (2020). IAP Guidebook on Immunization 2018-19. [online] Available from https://iapindia.org/pdf/124587-IAP-GUIDE-BOOK-ON-IMMUNIZATION-18-19.pdf [Last accessed October, 2020].
2. John J, Van Aart CJ, Grassly NC. The Burden of Typhoid and Paratyphoid in India: Systematic Review and Meta-analysis. PLoS Negl Trop Dis. 2016;10(4):e0004616.
3. Vashishtha VM, Kalra A. The need and the issues related to new-generation typhoid conjugate vaccines in India. Indian J Med Res. 2020;151(1):22-34.
4. World Health Organization. Typhoid vaccines: WHO position paper, March 2018—Recommendations. Vaccine. 2019;37(2):214-6.

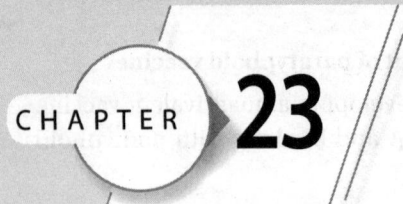

CHAPTER 23: Hepatitis A Vaccines

Jaydeep Choudhury

Q1. What is the epidemiology of hepatitis A infection in India?

Ans. According to the estimation of the World Health Organization (WHO), there are >100 million cases of hepatitis A annually, resulting in an estimated 15,000–30,000 deaths per year. The disease burden is related to the economic development of a country.[1] India was categorized as a high endemic country for hepatitis A. Due to transition of some areas in cities and in higher socioeconomic strata to intermediate endemicity, India is considered as a mixed endemic country. As the endemicity shifts toward intermediate category due to improvement in sanitation and hygiene, the dwelling population is at a greater risk of disease.[2,3] In this stage of endemicity, a certain population of children remains susceptible and the risk of hepatitis A transmission continues due to prevailing poor sanitation and contaminated water supply.

Hepatitis A seroprevalence study in Pune revealed a fall in seroprevalence from 85% to 50% in 6–10-year-old children and 92% to 45% in 11–15-year-old children from 1992 to 1998.[4] A cross-sectional multicentric seroprevalence study in children 1–16 years showed that seroprevalence in children 6–11 years was 10.3% in Kochi, 40.2% in Kolkata, 63.2% in Jaipur, 71.4% in Patna, and 91.6% in Indore.[5]

Several sporadic outbreaks of hepatitis A have been noted in various parts of India, in Kerala (1980), Pune (2004), Kottayam (2005), and Shimla (2005) in various age groups.

Hepatitis A infections in older age groups are the result of a natural epidemiological shift of age of infection due to improvements in hygiene, sanitation, and availability of clean drinking water.

Hepatitis A virus infection remains the most common cause of viral hepatitis in children in developing countries. Acute viral hepatitis A and E are waterborne and are the major cause of contamination of drinking water.

There is no chronic infection or carrier state with hepatitis A infections.

Q2. What is the infective period of a case of hepatitis A infection?

Ans. Generally 2 weeks prior to the development of symptoms to 1 week after.

CHAPTER 23: Hepatitis A Vaccines

Q3. Can hepatitis A infection recur in a previously infected individual?

Ans. Infection with hepatitis A provides life-long protection by anti-HAV antibody. An immunocompetent person does not suffer from reinfection.

Q4. When was the first hepatitis A vaccine developed?

Ans. The first inactivated vaccine was licensed in 1995.[1] It was produced by GSK (Havrix®).

Q5. What are the different vaccines against hepatitis A?

Ans. Both inactivated and live-attenuated hepatitis A vaccines are available. The inactivated vaccine is derived from HM 175/GBM strains grown on MRC-5 human diploid cell lines.[3] The live-attenuated vaccine is derived from H2 strain of hepatitis A virus after serial passage in human diploid cell line.[6]

Q6. What are the currently available inactivated hepatitis A vaccines?

Ans.
- *Havrix® 720*: Each 0.5 mL pediatric dose of vaccine contains 720 EL.U. of viral antigen, adsorbed onto 0.25 mg of aluminum as aluminum hydroxide.
- *Havrix® 1,440*: Each 1 mL adult dose of vaccine contains 1,440 EL.U. of viral antigen, adsorbed on 0.5 mg of aluminum as aluminum hydroxide.
- Havrix® is preservative free.
- It should be stored at 2–8°C. Havrix 1440, presently, is not available in India.
- Anterolateral thigh or over deltoid muscles are the preferred sites for administration.
- Avaxim® (Sanofi) is marketed in two formulations, 80 U and 160 U.
- The 80 U formulation is recommended from 12 months to 15 years of age. It contains 80 U in 0.5 mL dose with 0.15 mg of aluminum hydroxide per dose.
- The 160 U formulation is recommended >15 years of age. It contains 80 U in 0.5 mL dose with 0.3 mg of aluminum hydroxide per dose.

Q7. What is the schedule of inactivated hepatitis A vaccine?

Ans. Minimum age of administration of inactivated hepatitis A vaccine is 12 months of age. Two doses should be given 6–18 months apart.

Q8. If more than 18 months has elapsed after the first dose then should the course be restarted?

Ans. No. The second dose has to be given. Only two doses of the vaccine are indicated irrespective of the time gap.

Q9. What will happen if the inactivated hepatitis A vaccine is accidentally frozen?

Ans. The vaccine has to be discarded. The adjuvants precipitate. It will cause increased reactogenicity and decreased efficacy.

Q10. What is the currently available live-attenuated hepatitis A vaccine?

Ans. Live-attenuated hepatitis A vaccines are manufactured in China and available in other countries including India. The vaccines are derived from H2 strain or *Lactobacillus acidophilus* (LA)-1 strain of hepatitis A virus. The H2 strain was developed from hepatitis A virus grown from feces of a 12-year-old child suffering from hepatitis A. It was subsequently propagated in human diploid cells. Initial field efficacy trials were done using live-attenuated hepatitis A vaccine in China in 1–9 years age group seronegative children where 68,546 subjects received the single test dose against 66,794 controls. In another study in China 191,571 seronegative 1–9-year-old children received a single dose against 168,441 controls. The results showed a combined efficacy of 100% (95% CI: 92.2–100%).[7] Several global studies (Zhuang et al. 2001, Zhuang et al. 2005, and Zhuang et al. 2010) have proved effectiveness of live vaccines by demonstrating high rates of seroprotection ranging from 80 to 81%.[8-10] The dose is 0.5 mL subcutaneous single dose age 12 months onward.[11]

Live-attenuated hepatitis A vaccine is well-studied in Indian subjects. There are published evidences on long-term follow-up in Indian subjects with live-attenuated vaccine. 10-year follow-up study from India showed long-term immunity after single dose.[11] In the long-term follow-up study[11] 98.1% subjects showed seroprotective titer of IgG antibodies (>20 mIU/mL). The GMT of anti-HAV antibodies among seroprotected children was 100.5 mIU/mL. No significant safety concern was reported in the study. Other studies from India have also reported immunogenicity and safety of live-attenuated hepatitis A vaccine.[12,13]

Q11. What is the catch-up schedule for hepatitis A vaccine?

Ans. Two doses, at least 6 months apart of inactivated hepatitis A vaccine or a single dose of live vaccine. For inactivated vaccine, pediatric formulation is recommended till 18 years of age and adult formulation thereafter.

Q12. What is the safety profile of the available hepatitis A vaccines?

Ans. The inactivated hepatitis A vaccine is generally safe. Mild and transient injection site reactions such as pain, tenderness, and redness may occur particularly in older children. Rare systemic effects are headache, fever, fatigue, diarrhea, and vomiting.

Live hepatitis A vaccines are also well-tolerated. Local reactions such as pain, redness, swelling, and pruritus are rare features. Systemic features are also rare.

Q13. What are the correlates of protection following hepatitis A vaccination?

Ans. The anti-hepatitis A virus concentrations are measured in comparison with the World Health Organization (WHO) reference immunoglobulin reagent. Antibody levels 10–33 IU/mL have been proposed as the threshold for protective level.[1] But, the absolute lower limit of antibody needed to prevent infection has not been determined. Generally, a level of 20 IU/mL is considered as protective.

Q14. What is the efficacy and effectiveness of the available hepatitis A vaccines?

Ans. Both inactivated and live-attenuated hepatitis A vaccines are safe and effective in providing protection in children as well as adults.[14] No vaccine (inactivated or live) is licensed for children <1 year of age. Scientific evidence on long-term immunogenicity is available for both types of hepatitis A vaccines. In a large study of approximately 40,000 children in the age group 1–16 years, the efficacy of inactivated vaccine HM175 strain, used to prepare Havrix® (GSK), was 94% (CI: 79–99%) after two doses administered 1 month apart. There are many studies which have demonstrated the effectiveness of inactivated hepatitis A vaccines in preventing and controlling hepatitis A in endemic communities.[1]

In India, a 5-year follow-up study showed a single dose of live hepatitis A vaccine provides long-term immunogenicity. Another follow-up study demonstrated 10-year protection.[11,12]

Single dose of live-attenuated vaccine offers advantages over inactivated hepatitis A vaccine in terms of better compliance and convenience. Live and killed vaccines differ in stimulation of the immune system. Live-attenuated vaccines provide both cellular and humoral immunity and hence result in robust immune responses and long-lasting immunity. Inactivated vaccines produce weaker immune response because it acts predominantly by activating humoral response and very less due to cellular immunity. Chances of waning of immune protection achieved with single dose in two dose schedules of killed vaccine are more than live vaccine. Live vaccines due to presence of memory cells can provide long-term immunity even if antibody titers are not up to the WHO recommended level of 20 IU. A long-term follow-up study showed antibody persistence and immunological memory even after 17 years of single dose live vaccine administration.[15]

Q15. What is the duration of protection after vaccination?

Ans. The exact duration of protection after hepatitis A vaccination is not known. Studies have shown persistence of antibody for at least 17 years after vaccination with live-attenuated hepatitis A vaccine.[15]

The average incubation period for hepatitis A is 4 weeks. The anamnestic response after the second dose of inactivated vaccine is rapid and robust. Hence, the vaccine recipients who have seroconverted will be protected by anamnestic response even if their antibody level has fallen below the protective level. A two-dose schedule is expected to confer lifelong protection.

Q16. Is there any role of hepatitis A vaccine for postexposure prophylaxis?

Ans. Hepatitis A vaccine may be given for postexposure prophylaxis to the household contacts of a hepatitis A case, those with immune-deficiency and chronic liver disease. It should be given as early as possible and preferably within 14 days.[3] Hepatitis A vaccine for postexposure prophylaxis is recommended for healthy persons 12 months to 40 years of age.[1,6] Serum immunoglobulin is useful for postexposure prophylaxis below 1 year and above 40 years of age. Availability and cost are the challenges for use of serum immunoglobulins.

Live or killed vaccine can be an option for postexposure prophylaxis against hepatitis A. Immunogenicity of the vaccine may be decreased in people with old age.

Q17. What is the role of hepatitis A vaccine in hepatitis B carriers?

Ans. There are evidences from some countries that hepatitis A infection is more severe in hepatitis B carriers with increased case fatality. The ACVIP recommends Hepatitis A vaccine to all Hepatitis B and Hepatitis C carriers.

Q18. What is the role of hepatitis A vaccine in chronic liver disease (CLD)?

Ans. Patients with chronic liver disease (CLD) are at increased risk of complications when they are infected with hepatitis A. Hence, patients suffering from CLD should receive hepatitis A vaccine.

Q19. Is there any indication for prevaccination serology testing for adolescent who come for hepatitis A vaccination?

Ans. Generally, it is not required. It is more costeffective to vaccinate than do prevaccination serology. Hepatitis A vaccination in those already immune is not associated with any adverse effects.

Q20. Is there any role for a single-dose schedule for inactivated hepatitis A vaccines?

Ans. Protective anti-hepatitis A vaccine (HAV) antibody levels after a single dose of inactivated HAV can persist for almost 11 years and increase or reappear after booster vaccination.

In 7.5-year Observational Pilot Study in Nicaraguan children who received a single dose of inactivated hepatitis A vaccine, an estimated protective effectiveness of 98.3% (95% confidence interval: 87.9–99.8) was observed. Boosting elicited an average 29.7-fold increase of anti-HAV levels.

In 2005, a single-dose vaccine schedule in 12-month-old children was implemented all across Argentina. The incidence of hepatitis by HAV decreased to <1 case every 100,000 inhabitants per year (6–12 cases of hepatitis every 100,000 inhabitants per year between 2000 and 2005) and no liver transplants associated with HAV had been reported since 2007.

It must be emphasized that this single dose schedule is for public health and not for individual use.[3]

REFERENCES

1. Averhoff FM, Khudyakov Y, Nelson NP. Hepatitis A vaccines. In: Plotkin SA, Orenstein WA, Offit PA, Edwards KM (Eds). Plotkin's Vaccines, 7th edition. Philadelphia: Elsevier Inc.; 2018. pp. 319-41.
2. Mathur P, Arora NK. Epidemiological transition of hepatitis A in India: issues for vaccination in developing countries. Indian J Med Res. 2008;128(6):699-704.
3. Advisory Committee on Vaccination and Immunization Practices (ACVIP), Balasubramanian S, Shastri DS, Shah AK, Pemde HK, Chatterjee P, et al. IAP Guidebook on Immunization 2018–2019, 3rd edition. New Delhi: Jaypee Brothers Medical Publishers (P) Ltd.; 2020. pp. 265-77.
4. Arankalle VA, Chadha MS, Chitambar SD, Walimbe AM, Chobe LP, Gandhe SS. Changing epidemiology of hepatitis A and hepatitis E in urban and rural India (1982–98). J Viral Hepatitis. 2001;8:293-303.
5. Mall ML, Rai RR, Philip M, Naik G, Parekh P, Bhawnani SC, et al. Seroepidemiology of hepatitis A infection in India: changing pattern. Indian J Gastroenterol. 2001;20:132-5.
6. Thacker N, Shah NK. Immunization in Clinical Practice, 2nd edition. New Delhi: Jaypee Brothers Medical Publishers (P) Ltd.; 2016. pp. 153-62.
7. Xu Z, Xuanyi W, Rongchen L, Zongda M, Yanting L. Preliminary results of a randomized and controlled trial of live, attenuated hepatitis A vaccine. Chinese Med Sci J. 1999;14:8-10.
8. Zhuang F, Jiang Q, Gong Y. Epidemiological effects of live-attenuated hepatitis A vaccine (H(2)-strain): results of A 10-year observation. Zhonghua Liu Xing Bing Xue Za Zhi. 2001;22:188-90.
9. Zhuang FC, Qian W, Mao ZA, Gong YP, Jiang Q, Jiang LM, et al. Persistent efficacy of live-attenuated hepatitis A vaccine (H2-strain) after a mass vaccination program. Chin Med J (Engl). 2005;118:1851-6.
10. Zhuang FC, Mao ZA, Jiang LM, Wu J, Chen YQ, Jiang Q, et al. Long-term immunogenicity and effectiveness of live-attenuated hepatitis A vaccine (H2-strain)-a study on the result of 15 years' follow-up. Zhonghua Liu Xing Bing Xue Za Zhi. 2010;31:1332-5.
11. Bhave S, Sapru A, Bavdekar A, Kapatkar V, Mane A. Long-term immunogenicity of single dose of live-attenuated hepatitis A vaccine in Indian children. Indian Pediatr. 2015;52:687-90.
12. Faridi MM, Shah N, Ghosh TK, Sankaranarayanan VS, Arankalle V, Aggarwal A, et al. Immunogenicity and safety of live and attenuated hepatitis A vaccine: a multicentric study. Indian Pediatr. 2009;46:29-34.
13. Mitra M, Shah N, Faridi MMA, Ghosh A, Sankaranarayanan VS, Aggarwal A, et al. Long term follow-up study to evaluate immunogenicity and safety of a single dose of live-attenuated hepatitis a vaccine in children. Hum Vaccin Immunother. 2015;11:1147-52.
14. WHO position paper on hepatitis A vaccines—June 2012. Wkly Epidemiol Rec. 2012;87(28/29):261-76.
15. Chen Y, Zhou CL, Zhang XJ, Hao ZY, Zhang YH, Wang SM, et al. Immune memory at 17-years of follow-up of a single dose of live attenuated hepatitis A vaccine. Vaccine. 2018;36:114-21.

CHAPTER 24

Varicella Vaccines

Tanu Singhal

Q1. What is the epidemiology of varicella in India relevant to vaccination?

Ans. Varicella is caused by the very highly contagious varicella-zoster virus (VZV), which has a worldwide distribution. Varicella spreads through inhalation of droplet nuclei and less commonly through contact with contaminated surfaces/lesions of the infected. It is highly communicable with secondary attack rates of >90% in the susceptible in household exposure and 15% in community exposure. The disease is usually benign in most children but can be severe in neonates, pregnant women, adults, and the immunocompromised. Absenteeism from schools and work places is another societal consequence.

The epidemiology of varicella largely depends on the climate and vaccination status of the population. Before the advent of immunization, the annual incidence was equal to the birth cohort. In temperate climates, most people were infected in early childhood and disease in adolescents and adults was rare. However, in tropical countries the age of natural infection is shifted upward. The exact reason is not known but may be due to reduced longevity of the virus in the vesicular fluid and surfaces due to higher temperatures and humidity.

Varicella is a common childhood illness in India. One study published from Kerala in 1978 reported the incidence as 74/100,000 population in 1973, 197.5/100,000 population in 1974, and 224.9/100,000 in 1975. Venkitaraman reported the incidence in medical staff and students between 1977 and 1982 as 720/100,000 population (0.72%), with the highest incidence in young adults aged 17–24 years. As a comparison, the incidence reported from the United States in the prevaccine era was 1,600 cases/100,000 inhabitants. Data from Asia Pacific about varicella rates in the absence of a universal vaccination program ranges from 100/100,000 in China (2007) to 2,530/100,000 in Taiwan (2000). There is no recent data available from India about incidence of varicella in the community. There is scanty data on mortality, complications, and hospitalizations in India. One study from Kolkata reported a mortality rate of 6% in 300 hospitalized cases of varicella.

A cross-sectional multicentric study on seroprevalence of varicella was performed in four major cities of India: Kolkata (formerly Calcutta) (outpatients), Mumbai (outpatients), Lucknow (walk-in patients to a diagnostic laboratory, orphanage, and factory workers), and Bengaluru (outpatients and walk-in patients to a diagnostic laboratory). A total of 1,609 volunteers from birth to 40 years of age were included in the study. The overall seroprevalence of anti-VZV antibodies was 68%. The age-related seroprevalence rate of anti-VZV antibodies was 29% in the age group of 1–5 years, 51% in 5–10 years, 72% in 11–15 years, 80% in 16–20 years, 88% in 21–30 years and 91% in 31–40 years. In another study done before the vaccine was available in India (1995–96), seroprevalence was 96.6% in the urban population versus 69.9% in the rural population. In a study in 5,000 nurses at the tertiary care hospital in Mumbai between 2014 and 2017, 28% were seronegative. Most of these nurses were from Kerala and in the age group of 21–30 years.

To summarize, there is limited recent data on the incidence and consequences of the disease in India. Seroprevalence data, however, indicates that a significant proportion of adolescents and adults are susceptible to the virus.

Q2. What is the risk of herpes zoster after natural varicella?

Ans. Varicella remains latent in the dorsal root ganglion to reactivate later in life. These reactivations may be subclinical or clinical as herpes zoster. The incidence of herpes zoster rises with advancing age. The lifetime risk of reactivation of herpes zoster is around 30%. Around 15% of all cases of herpes zoster present in children.

Q3. When was varicella vaccine first available in India? What is the uptake?

Ans. In India, varicella vaccine is available for immunization in the private sector since 1999. There are two studies reporting the uptake of the vaccine in the private sector; one reports this as 2.8% in children below 5 years in Chandigarh in 2004–2005 (doses not mentioned). Paradoxically, in another study interviewing educated mothers in the top socioeconomic sections of the society, coverage rates of 96.6% were reported and cost and access to the vaccine were not considered as barriers to vaccine uptake.

Q4. Which are the varicella vaccines available?

Ans. Monovalent varicella vaccines available in India currently are as under:
- *Variped (MSD)*: 1350 PFU/0.5 mL dose
- *Varilrix (GSK)*: $10^{3.3}$ PFU/dose
- *Biovac-V (Mf. China, Mkt-Wockhardt)*: 2,500 PFU
- *Varivax (Mf. China, Mkt-VHB Life Sciences)*: At least 2,000 PFU
- *Nexipox (Mf. China, Mkt-NovoMedi Sciences)*: 2,000 PFU
- *Zuvicella (Mkt Zuventus healthcare)*: At least 2,000 PFU

- Other varicella containing vaccines include the MMRV vaccine (Measles, Mumps, Rubella with Varicella) and the Herpes Zoster vaccines.

Q5. What is the composition of the varicella vaccine?

Ans. All current vaccines are derived from the vOka strain. The Oka strain undergoes 11 passages in human embryonic lung cells, 12 passages in guinea pig embryo cells and 1 passage in WI 38 cells. This is common to all available varicella vaccines. Individual manufacturers subject this bulk substrate to further passages before producing the final vaccine product. *It needs to be emphasized that the number of passages has no relationship to the efficacy of the vaccine.* The World Health Organization (WHO) has not offered any guidelines regarding the choice of stabilizer.

Q6. How should the varicella vaccine be stored?

Ans. The vaccine is available in a lyophilized form and should be stored between 2 and 8°C in the refrigerator and has a shelf-life of approximately 2 years when stored appropriately. The diluent should be stored at 2-8°C or at room temperature; it should not be frozen. The vaccine should be reconstituted using the diluent provided and used preferably within 30 minutes of reconstitution.

Q7. What is the method for administration of varicella vaccine?

Ans. It is to be administered subcutaneously. It can be co-administered safely with all other vaccines. If given with measles, mumps, and rubella (MMR), then it should be administered either on the same day or 4 weeks apart. It can be given at any time interval with other killed or live vaccines. Salicylates should be avoided within 6 weeks of the vaccine owing to the risk of Reye's syndrome. The vaccine should not be given within 9–12 months of administration of intravenous immunoglobulin (IVIG).

Q8. What if varicella vaccine is administered intramuscularly?

Ans. Inadvertent intramuscularly (IM) administration has not been found to be associated with decreased seroconversion. Hence, it need not be repeated.

Q9. What is the immunogenicity of the vaccine?

Ans. The glycoprotein enzyme-linked immunosorbent assay (gp-ELISA) was the first test used to assess the immunogenicity of the vaccine. A gp-ELISA cut-off of 5 units/mL was seen to correlate better with protection against clinical disease as compared to seroconversion and this level was achieved in 86% of children following a single dose. Subsequent studies used fluorescent antibody to membrane antigen (FAMA) titers of >1:4 after 16 weeks of vaccination as a correlate of protection. FAMA antibody titers correlate better with protection against varicella as compared to ELISA and indirect fluorescent antibody (IFA) assays. It is postulated that the initial burst of antibodies that is measured by ELISA/IFA is inadequate to instill a T-cell memory response. By FAMA, a lower percentage of children (76%) achieve the protective cutoff following receipt of single dose of the vaccine as compared to the ELISA studies. Follow-up studies indicate persistence of antibodies for 7–10 years and even 20 years following vaccination. Since immunity to varicella is also cell-mediated, T-lymphocyte proliferation responses have been studied and found to be present in 87–90% of children for up to 5 years postvaccination.

The immunogenicity improves with a second dose of the vaccine in all respects, after one dose of varicella vaccine, 85-89% of children achieve protective antibody levels, and after two doses, >99% achieve this level.

The immunogenicity is similar whether the second dose is given 3 months or 4–6 years after the first dose **(Table 1)**.

The immunogenicity of the vaccine is lower in adolescents and adults and studies have demonstrated seroconversion rates of 72–94% following a single dose of the vaccine and 94-99% after two doses of the vaccine administered 4–8 weeks apart. Some studies indicate that 25–31% of adults lose their detectable antibodies by FAMA at multiple intervals (1–11 years) following vaccination.

Q10. What is the effectiveness of the varicella vaccine?

Ans. The pooled one-dose vaccine effectiveness (VE) was 81% (95% CI: 78–84%) against all varicella and 98% (95% CI: 97–99%) against moderate/severe varicella with no significant association between VE and vaccine type or study design ($P > 0.1$). For one dose, median VE for prevention of severe disease was 100% (mean = 99.4%).

Table 1: Immune response among children aged 12 months–12 years at 6 weeks postvaccination, by vaccine type and vaccination schedule—United States, 1988–2002 (MSD vaccine).

Immune response	6 weeks after dose 1		6 weeks after dose 2 (after 3 months)		6 weeks after dose 2 (at 4–5 years)	
	Varicella	MMRV	Varicella	MMRV	Varicella	MMRV
VZV IgG gp-ELISA > 5 units/mL	85.7	91.2	99.6	99.2	99.4	98.9
GMT VZV IgG gp-ELISA units/mL	12.5	13	142.6	588	212.4	317
Mean SI	28.6		36.9		58.6	

(GMT: geometric mean titers; gp-ELISA: glycoprotein enzyme-linked immunosorbent assay; IgG: immunoglobulin G; MMRV: measles-mumps-rubella and varicella; VZV: varicella zoster virus)

Vaccine effectiveness for prevention of polymerase chain reaction (PCR)-confirmed varicella was 98% after two doses, compared with 86% for one dose ($P < 0.001$).

Q11. What is breakthrough varicella (BV)?

Ans. Varicella which occurs in children vaccinated >6 weeks after vaccination is called breakthrough varicella. It is generally milder and may present with just short-lasting maculopapular rashes and may not progress to the vesicular stage. BV has lesser fever, lesser number of lesions and a shorter duration of illness. However, it is infective, can result in transmission to susceptible contacts, and rarely result in severe complications and death.

Q12. Which are the risk factors for breakthrough varicella (BV)?

Ans.
- Vaccination below 12 months of age
- Not observing 28 days interval with MMR
- Immunocompromised child

Q13. Why is breakthrough varicella milder compared to varicella occurring in unimmunized persons?

Ans. In some individuals, one dose of the vaccine results in a suboptimal immune response resulting in the generation of an insufficient number of virus specific memory T-cells. While priming has occurred, the immunological response has been less than optimum resulting in suboptimal immunity and the resulting modified disease.

Q14. What is the effect of varicella vaccine on breakthrough varicella?

Ans. The risk of breakthrough varicella following one dose of the vaccine varies from 15 to 20%. Increased risk of primary vaccine failure is seen with lower age at first vaccine (12 months), lower titer vaccine, time since use of other live vaccines (within 4 weeks), receipt of oral or inhaled corticosteroids, and history of eczema or asthma.

In a 14-year prospective cohort study of the long-term effectiveness of varicella vaccine, it was noted that the highest incidence of breakthrough varicella was in the 1st year postvaccination (26.6/1,000 PY), but remained high in the first 6 years after vaccination (17.4/1,000 PY in the 6th year).

This tends to suggest that most of the vaccine failure is primary and not secondary. However, where the natural wild virus circulates, periodic boosting of immunity may lead to reduction in secondary vaccine failures.

Q15. What is the impact of varicella vaccination on herpes zoster?

Ans. The interplay between varicella vaccination and herpes zoster is complex. While both the vOka and wild virus establish latency, the capability of the vOka to reactivate is lesser than that of the wild virus. Studies also indicate lower incidence of herpes zoster in both immunocompromised and immunocompetent individuals vaccinated previously as against those who had natural varicella infection.

In immunocompromised children with leukemia, vaccination reduced the incidence of herpes zoster by 67%.

In the 14-year prospective cohort study of the long-term effectiveness of varicella vaccine, a 40% reduction in incidence of herpes zoster was noted.

But at a population level, matters are different. Universal vaccination is likely to reduce circulation of wild varicella virus and reduced exogenous boosting of older individuals with increased tendency for shingles.

Following the introduction of universal varicella vaccination in the United States of America, herpes zoster incidence has continued to increase in a generally steady manner among the younger adult age strata (i.e., aged 35 through 50–55 years), without any clear accelerations or decelerations during the study interval (1996–2016). However, among the older age strata (i.e., aged ≥50–55 years), a deceleration has been noted since 2006.

Q16. What are the adverse effects of varicella vaccination?

Ans. The vaccine is generally well tolerated and the side effects reported are mild and transient. Approximately, 6% of recipients develop vaccine-associated rash either generalized or localized or both, 1 month after vaccination. This is similar to varicella rash but less extensive. Other adverse events associated with varicella vaccine include fever (10–14%), and injection-site reactions (in up to 20%). The overall incidence of adverse effects following vaccination is 2–4/10,000 doses.

Case-control studies did not find any significantly increased risk of exacerbation or induction of diseases such as systemic lupus erythematosus, Guillain-Barré syndrome, multiple sclerosis, neuritis, thrombocytopenia, or vasculitis. One of the most comprehensive systematic studies reports 30 neurological adverse effect cases out of 16,683 adverse events reported. In none of these, however, was the vaccine strain found in the cerebrospinal fluid of subjects. Extensive rashes with pneumonia or neurologic symptoms have been reported in immunocompromised children who have been inadvertently administered the vaccine but these cases are but a handful. The excellent safety of the varicella vaccine is attributed to the fact that it is highly attenuated and does not revert to virulence and remains susceptible to the usual antiviral drugs. One study on use of two doses of varicella vaccine in children with acute lymphoblastic leukemia, given the vaccine after the intense chemotherapy was over, showed rash appearing in almost 40% of children with the first dose but not with the second dose.

Q17. What are the contraindications to varicella vaccination?

Ans.
- History of hypersensitivity to one or more components of the vaccine (including neomycin and gelatin) and previous varicella vaccine.

- Immunodeficiency:
    - Any cell-mediated or combined immunodeficiency. It may be given in severe B-cell immunodeficiency such as agammaglobulinemia but is unlikely to be effective. Here, the monthly intravenous immunoglobulin therapy provides some passive protection. It can, however, be given in less severe B-cell immunodeficiencies such as immunoglobulin A (IgA) and immunoglobulin G (IgG) subclass deficiency and also in complement and phagocyte immunodeficiency.
    - Human immunodeficiency virus (HIV) infected children/adults with a CD4 count of ≤15% or clinical symptoms of HIV disease.
    - Persons receiving high-dose systemic immunosuppressive therapy, including persons on oral steroids ≥2 mg/kg of body weight (if <10 kg weight) or a total of ≥20 mg/day of prednisone or equivalent for persons who weigh ≥10 kg, when administered for ≥2 weeks. It may be given 1 month after cessation of steroid therapy.
    - Patients with cancer on chemotherapy and following solid organ transplant/hematopoietic stem cell transplant (HSCT). For cancer survivors varicella vaccine may be given 3–6 months after cessation of all chemotherapy. It may be given 24 months after HSCT if the patient is not on immunosuppressive drugs, does not have graft versus host disease, and the antivaricella IgG is negative.
    - Persons who have a family history of congenital or hereditary immunodeficiency in first-degree relatives (e.g., parents and siblings) unless the immune competence of the potential vaccine recipient has been clinically substantiated or verified by a laboratory.
    - The vaccine can be given safely to family contacts of immunodeficient hosts including those with HSCT. However, if the vaccinee develops a vaccine-induced rash then contact with the immunodeficient patient should be avoided.
- Pregnant women or women planning to become pregnant. Pregnancy should be avoided for a minimum 1 month and preferably 3 months following the vaccine. Registry data, however, indicates no increased risk of congenital birth defects following accidental vaccination in pregnancy or in women who become pregnant within a month after vaccination. Hence, medical termination of pregnancy (MTP) is not indicated in this setting.
- The safety of varicella vaccination in breastfeeding mothers has not been adequately studied.
- The efficacy and adverse event profile has not been studied in infants below the age of 9–12 months. However, there is need for studies of varicella vaccination in infants born to seronegative mothers and especially if there are due for solid organ transplants (liver transplant in infants with metabolic liver disease or extrahepatic biliary atresia).

Q18. What are the ACVIP recommendations for the use of varicella vaccines?

Ans. Advisory Committee on Vaccines and Immunization Practices (ACVIP) 2018 recommends offering the vaccine to all healthy children with no prior history of varicella with special emphasis in all children belonging to certain high-risk groups as enumerated below:
- Children with humoral immunodeficiencies
- Children with HIV infection but with CD4 counts 15% and above the age-related cutoff
- Leukemia but in remission and off chemotherapy for at least 3–6 months
- Children on long-term salicylates. Salicylates should be avoided for at least 6 weeks after vaccination.
- Children likely to be on long-term steroid therapy. The vaccine may be given at any time if the children are on low-dose steroids/alternate day steroids but only 4 weeks after stopping steroids if the patients have received high-dose steroids (>2 mg/kg) for 14 days or more.
- In household contacts of immunocompromised children
- Adolescents who have not had varicella in past and are known to be varicella IgG negative, especially if they are leaving home for studies in a residential school/college.
- Children with chronic lung/heart disease
- Seronegative adolescents and adults if they are inmates of or working in the institutional setup, e.g., school teachers, daycare center workers, military personnel, and healthcare professionals.

Q19. What is the IAP schedule for vaccine administration?

Ans. The Indian Academy of Pediatrics (IAP) recommends administration of the first dose at 15–18 months and the second dose is recommended preferably 3 months after the first dose or at 4–6 years.

For catch-up vaccination in children aged 12 months to 12 years, two doses should be given 12 weeks apart; the minimum interval should be 4 weeks. For catch-up vaccination in children 13 years and above, two doses should be given 4–12 weeks apart. Here, the interval between the two doses can be short to ensure early protection.

Q20. What is the optimum timing for the second dose?

Ans. The timing of the second dose has been debated. Vaccine failure following varicella is more due to primary rather than secondary vaccine failure. Most cases of breakthrough varicella occur early after vaccination. Hence, shifting the second dose to the 2nd year of life should reduce the risk of breakthrough varicella further without compromising the safety and efficacy of the vaccine A modeling study estimates that shortening the interval between two doses could reduce twofold the cumulative number of cases of breakthrough varicella. The second dose should be administered 12 weeks after the first dose; the minimum acceptable interval is 4 weeks.

Q21. What is the protocol for administration of varicella vaccine in children with acute lymphatic leukemia (ALL), with no evidence of immunity?

Ans. Since varicella is a devastating illness in the immunocompromised especially acute lymphatic leukemia (ALL), exclusive recommendations exist for administration in ALL.

In children between 12 months and 17 years of age with a negative history of varicella in whom leukemia is in remission for at least 12 months, the peripheral blood lymphocyte count ≥ 700 cells/mm^3 and the platelet count is ≥100,000/mm^3, two doses of varicella vaccine may be administered. Maintenance chemotherapy should be withheld for 7 days before and after at least the first dose.

Q22. If a child had a very mild chickenpox, will it provide adequate immunity? Is vaccine necessary?

Ans. Any varicella illness, whether mild or severe will confer immunity and hence vaccination is not necessary following the illness. However, if the diagnosis is in doubt, it is preferable to administer the vaccine, as vaccine administered to an immune child will not result in any increased adverse effects.

Q23. Can varicella vaccine be administered to a 10-month-old infant for postexposure prophylaxis?

Ans. No. Varicella vaccine is not licensed for use below the age of 1 year. Even if inadvertently administered before 1 year of age, it should be counted as an invalid dose.

Q24. Is postvaccination serology necessary following varicella vaccination?

Ans. Postvaccination serological testing is not recommended for anyone, including the high-risk groups.

Q25. How useful is varicella vaccination in postexposure prophylaxis?

Ans. Among children, protective efficacy was reported as ≥90% when vaccination occurred within 3 days of exposure.

Protective efficacy in preventing any type of disease was 62.3% [confidence interval (CI) 95%: 47.8–74.9)] and 79.4% (CI 95%: 66.4–88.9) in preventing moderate and severe disease, up to 5 days after exposure.

Vaccination still recommended for those with no other evidence of immunity even after 5 days of exposure because it will help provide protection against future exposures. Thus, vaccination >5 days postexposure is recommended to help protect against subsequent exposures and limit VZV transmission during an outbreak.

Q26. What is the public health impact with varicella vaccination?

Ans. There are basically three approaches for varicella vaccination: universal vaccination with one or two doses, selective immunization of high-risk individuals, and finally immunization of patients who can pay for the vaccine. The WHO recommends that countries can consider introducing the varicella vaccine in the public program if they consider varicella a significant health problem and are able to maintain sustained coverage rates of >80%.

Universal vaccination has been implemented in some high-income countries including USA (two doses at 12 months and 4–6 years), Germany (two doses in the second year), Greece, Latvia, and some provinces of Italy and Spain. In the Asia Pacific, universal vaccination is practiced in Australia (two doses), New Zealand (two doses), Japan (two doses), South Korea (one dose), Taiwan (one dose), and Hong Kong (two doses). In the USA, in the prevaccination era there were about 4 million cases (about 1,600 cases per 100,000 inhabitants), 11,000–13,000 cases of hospitalization and 100–150 deaths per year in the early 1990s. With the introduction of vaccination in 1995, the number of cases decreased by 79% in the 2000–2010 period compared to the prevaccination era and, since the introduction of a second vaccine dose, by 93% in 2012. In the same year, hospital admissions and deaths from varicella decreased by 90%. No impact on the incidence of herpes zoster in adults was noted. Closer home, in Asia Pacific, rise in incidence of varicella following implementation of the universal vaccination program in Australia, South Korea, and Taiwan probably due to better reporting rather than true increase.

In some countries including areas of Spain and Italy, varicella vaccination has been recommended for high-risk patients.

In the rest of the countries including India, varicella vaccine is administered outside the national immunization program to children and patients who can afford the vaccine. Since only a small proportion of the population undergoes vaccination, it is not possible to study the public health impact of the program. At the author's institute since implementation of a varicella vaccination program for seronegative nurses in 2014, a significant decline in incidence of varicella in nurses was observed.

■ SUGGESTED READING

1. Balasubramanian S, Shah A, Pemde HK, Chatterjee P, Shivananda S, Guduru VK, et al. Indian Academy of Pediatrics (IAP) Advisory Committee on Vaccines and Immunization Practices (ACVIP) Recommended Immunization Schedule (2018-19) and Update on Immunization for Children Aged 0 Through 18 Years. Indian Pediatr. 2018;55(12):1066-74
2. Bonanni P, Gershon A, Gershon M, Kulcsár A, Papaevangelou V, Rentier B, et al. Primary versus secondary failure after varicella vaccination: implications for interval between 2 doses. Pediatr Infect Dis J. 2013;32(7):e305-13.
3. Chartrand SA. Varicella vaccine. Pediatr Clin North Am. 2000;47:373-95.

4. Freer G, Pistello M. Varicella-zoster virus infection: natural history, clinical manifestations, immunity and current and future vaccination strategies. N Microbiol. 2018;41(2):95-105.
5. Goh AEN, Choi EH, Chokephaibulkit K, Choudhury J, Kuter B, Lee PI, et al. Burden of varicella in the Asia-Pacific region: a systematic literature review. Expert Rev Vaccines. 2019;18(5):475-93.
6. Harpaz R. Do varicella vaccination programs change the epidemiology of herpes zoster? A comprehensive review, with focus on the United States. Expert Rev Vaccines. 2019;18(8):793-811.
7. Lachiewicz AM, Srinivas ML. Varicella-zoster virus post-exposure management and prophylaxis: A review. Prev Med Rep. 2019;16:101016.
8. Lokeshwar MR, Agrawal A, Subbarao SD, Chakraborty MS, Ram Prasad AV, Weil J, et al. Age related seroprevalence of antibodies to varicella in India. Indian Pediatr. 2000;37(7):714-9.
9. Marin M, Güris D, Chaves SS, Schmid S, Seward JF; Advisory Committee on Immunization Practices, et al. Prevention of varicella: Recommendations of Advisory Committee on Immunization Practices (ACIP). MMWR Recomm Rep. 2007;56(RR-4):1-40.
10. Marin M, Marti M, Kambhampati A, Jeram SM, Seward JF. Global Varicella Vaccine Effectiveness: A Meta-analysis. Pediatrics. 2016;137(3):e20153741.
11. Shah S, Singhal T, Naik R, Thakkar P. High prevalence of varicella seronegativity in nurses at a tertiary care private hospital in Mumbai, India. Indian J Med Microbiol. 2018;36(2):294-5.
12. Takahashi M, Otsuka T, Okuno Y. Live vaccine used to prevent the spread of varicella in children in hospital. Lancet. 1974;ii:1288-90.
13. Yin M, Xu X, Liang Y, Ni J. Effectiveness, immunogenicity and safety of one vs. two-dose varicella vaccination: a meta-analysis. Expert Rev Vaccines. 2018;17(4):351-62.

CHAPTER 25: Human Papillomavirus (HPV) Vaccines

Sanjay Marathe

Q1. What is human papillomavirus (HPV)?

Ans. Human papillomaviruses are nonenveloped, double-stranded deoxyribonucleic acid (DNA) viruses from the family of Papillomaviridae. The HPV genome is enclosed in a capsid shell comprising major (L1) and minor (L2) structural proteins. More than 100 HPV genotypes are known. Of these, at least 13 oncogenic types may cause cervical cancer or are associated with other anogenital and oropharyngeal cancers. Worldwide, HPV types 16 and 18 cause about 70% of all cases of invasive cervical cancer with type 16 having the greatest oncogenic potential.

Q2. What are the diseases caused by HPV?

Ans. About 80% of the population gets infected with HPV. HPV infection is an essential factor in cervical carcinogenesis and cervical carcinoma is the second most common cause of cancer among women worldwide. Other malignancies in both men and women such as esophageal, oropharyngeal, penile, vulvar, vaginal cancer, and anal cancer have been causally associated with this virus.

The low-risk HPV types 6 and 11 are responsible for about 90% of anogenital warts and almost all recurrent respiratory papillomatosis. About 1% of sexually active adults in the US have visible genital warts at any point in time. Cancer is the most serious possible complication from HPV infection. As per 2018 HPV center data, cervical cancer was estimated to cause over 569,847 new cases and 311,365 deaths each year of which 96,922 cases and 60,078 deaths occur in India alone. Approximately 90% of the squamous cell carcinomas which are positive for HPV DNA are related to HPV types 16, 18, 45, 31, 33, 52, and 58.

Q3. What are the symptoms of HPV infection?

Ans. About 80% of unvaccinated adults will have an HPV infection at some point in their life. In most people, it causes no symptoms so is therefore unavoidably shared mainly through sexual activity (or close skin-to-skin contact) with someone who is infected. The interval between infection with HPV and the appearance of genital warts or a cervical smear abnormality can vary from months to many years.

Q4. How is HPV infection contracted?

Ans. Human papillomavirus is usually acquired by direct skin-to-skin contact during intimate sexual activity with someone who is infected. The virus can be transmitted by penetrative as well as nonpenetrative sexual contact (genital-genital, oral-genital, anal-genital, and oral-anal).

Human papillomavirus can infect areas that are not covered by a condom, so condoms may not fully protect against HPV.

Sex partners tend to share HPV, even when both partners do not show signs of HPV. HPV can lie dormant for many years so there is no way to know from which partner it was transmitted or since how long.

Having HPV does not mean that a person or the partner is having sex outside the marital relationship.

Q5. What are the risk factors for HPV infections?

Ans. The various factors are: (1) multiple sexual partners, (2) multiple pregnancies, (3) early sexual debut, (4) immune suppression [including human immunodeficiency virus (HIV) infection], (5) previous sexually transmitted infection, (6) history of sexual abuse, (7) inconsistent condom use, (8) uncircumcised male partner, and (9) tobacco or marijuana use.

Q6. How does HPV infection progress to disease?

Ans. The progression to cervical cancer begins with normal epithelial cells becoming infected with HPV. Cervical cancer develops at the transformation zone that corresponds to that area where the columnar epithelium is being replaced by squamous epithelium. During this process, glandular columnar cells changing into squamous cells are more prone for being infected with HPV. Within months or years, persistent infections can cause the development of premalignant glandular or SILs, and then to cancer. However, 70–90% of HPV infections are asymptomatic, most infections clear spontaneously in 1–2 years, and most cervical lesions never progress to cancer. Mild lesions are common in the cervix, especially for women in their 20s and 30s. However, precancerous conditions, while not yet cancer, cause changes to cells that result in a higher probability of developing cancer, especially with persistent untreated infection with high-risk HPV types. The time from infection to cancer usually takes 10–20 years or longer, but it can take less time than that. Premalignant lesions are histologically classified as cervical intraepithelial neoplasia (CIN) using the CIN classification system; or cytologically classified as squamous intraepithelial lesions (SILs), using the Bethesda system.

Q7. How long after an HPV infection does it take for cancer to develop in the body?

Ans. While most people who are infected with HPV do not develop cancer, persistent infection with a high-risk HPV type that is undetected or inadequately treated can progress to invasive carcinoma. When this happens, the time from infection to disease will usually take 10-20 years or longer, but it can sometimes take less time than that. Immunocompromised individuals, including those with HIV, are more likely to have persistent HPV infection and faster progression to cancer.

Q8. What is the magnitude of the cervical cancer problem in India?

Ans. India alone accounts for one-quarter of the worldwide burden of cervical cancers. Cervical cancer is the second most common cancer of women after breast cancer. In India, cervical cancer contributes to approximately 6-29% of all cancers in women. It is the one of the leading causes of cancer mortality, accounting for 17% of all cancer deaths among women aged between 30 and 69 years. In 2018, in India, there were 96,922 cases of cervical cancer and 60,078 deaths due to it. The prevalence of 16/18 in women with normal cytology was 5%, in low-grade cervical lesions it was 28.2%, in high-grade cervical lesions it was 62.8%, and 83.2% in cervical cancer.

Q9. If most women develop natural infection then does natural infection not provide immunity?

Ans. Genital HPV infection is followed by seroconversion and type-specific antibody to L1 protein after 6-18 months after infection. The antibody concentrations after natural infections are very low. The lack of a viremia because of poor access to vascular and lymphatic channels may explain the poor antibody response. Only 20-25% of women remain antibody positive over 10 years. These low levels of antibodies are not protective against future infections.

Q10. If there is poor access to vascular channels then how will vaccine help in local lesions?

Ans. Vaccines induce very high levels of specific antibodies. Antibody concentrations in cervical secretion are however very low, 10-1,000 times less than those in the serum and likely to be undetectable in many subjects 18-24 months postvaccination. Microabrasion of the genital epithelium results in epithelial denudation and favors HPV binding to this exposed basement membrane by the L1 receptor. Then the keratinocytes migrate along basement membrane to reepithelialize the small wound. Rapid serous exudation occurs in the wound which contains high levels of specific antibodies in the vaccinated. This leads to virus neutralization and provides an opportunity to encounter with circulating B memory cells which initiates a memory response. High levels of L1 antibodies prevent infection by blocking association with basement membrane heparan sulfate proteoglycans (HSPGs) and low levels of L1 virus-like particle (VLP) antibodies prevent infection by blocking transfer from basement membrane HSPGs to the keratinocyte surface receptors.

Q11. What is the immune response to the HPV vaccine?

Ans. After natural infection, only 70–80% of women develop serum antibodies to HPV and the degree of protection is low. After vaccination, however, the serological response is much stronger (1–4 logs higher) than that of natural infection. The mechanism of protection is likely mediated by polyclonal neutralizing antibodies against the L1 surface protein, which have better affinity and avidity. One likely reason that this immune response to vaccination is so much higher than natural infection is the route of immunization. Natural infection is entirely intraepithelial, so antigens have little access to the lymphatics and draining lymph nodes where immune responses start. But the HPV vaccine, like most VLP vaccines, is administered intramuscularly and this greatly enhances immunogenicity. Intramuscular deltoid injection gives immediate access to lymph nodes, rapidly activating helper T cell and B cell responses. Additionally, VLPs are inherently highly immunogenic due to the repeating L1 capsomer pattern that triggers the innate immune sensors and leads to strong adaptive immunity. Long-term HPV-specific antibody persistence is a result of long-lived plasma cells in the bone marrow, which regularly produce immunoglobulin G (IgG) antibodies. Immune responses are highest in 9–11-year-old girls prior to sexual debut, and high coverage in girls (>80%) provides herd protection for boys. Even with lower antibody titers the HPV vaccine continues to provide protection, and there is no evidence that the vaccine response wanes over time.

Q12. What is HPV vaccine?

Ans. The current HPV vaccines are based on VLPs that are formed by HPV surface components and resemble the viral surface. VLPs lack viral DNA and hence are not infectious. VLPs, being highly immunogenic, induce high levels of antibody production by the body. Addition of adjuvants renders the vaccines more immunogenic.

Q13. What are the vaccines to prevent HPV infection?

Ans. Three HPV vaccines are now being marketed in many countries throughout the world—a bivalent, a quadrivalent, and a nonavalent vaccine. All the three vaccines are produced by recombinant technology and contain VLPs of the dominant L1 capsid protein.
- Gardasil®, made by Merck Sharp & Dohme (MSD or Merck) is a quadrivalent vaccine [4-valent HPV (4vHPV)]. It contains L1 VLPs of types 16, 18, 6, and 11 with aluminum as adjuvant.
- Cervarix®, made by GlaxoSmithKline (GSK) is a bivalent vaccine (2vHPV). It contains L1 VLPs of types 16 and 18 adjuvanted with adjuvant system 04 (AS04).
- Gardasil 9®, made by MSD and licensed in 2014, is a nonavalent vaccine (9vHPV), containing types 6, 11, 16, 18, 31, 33, 45, 52, and 58. Not yet

available in India as of May 2020. There are five additional oncogenic types that will increase the coverage for oncogenic HPV-related disease from 70 to 90%.

All three vaccines are very effective in preventing infection with the most common HPV types responsible for cervical cancer and most other HPV-related types of cancer, as long as the recommended number of doses is taken. The quadrivalent and nonavalent vaccines also prevent external genital lesions like benign genital warts.

Q14. What is the efficacy data with bivalent HPV (bHPV) and quadrivalent HPV (qHPV) in controlled trials?

Ans. Pivotal field efficacy trials and subsequent extensions of these trials were conducted with both vaccines, PATRICIA trial for bHPV and Future I and II trials for qHPV. The efficacy data is shown below.

The VE against CIN2+ was 92.9 (79.9-98.3) for bHPV in the according to protocol (ATP) analysis and 98.1% (88.4-100) in the ATP-E analysis, in which probable causality to HPV type was assigned in lesions infected with multiple oncogenic types. Against qHPV, in the per protocol (PP) analysis, the vaccine efficacy (VE) was 98.2 (93.3-99.8).

In the total vaccine cohort/intention to treat (TVC/ITT) cohort, the VE against CIN2+ was 52.8 (37.5-64.7) for bHPV and 51.5 (40.6-60.6) for qHPV.

In the TVC-naïve cohort, VE against CIN2+ was 98.4 (90.4-100) for bHPV and 100 (91.9-100) for qHPV.

Against CIN3, the VE with bHPV was 80.0 (0.3-98.1) in the ATP cohort, 33.6 (1.1-56.9) in the TVC cohort and 100 (64.7-100) in the TVC-naïve cohort. Corresponding VE for qHPV was 96.8 (88.1-99.6) in the PP cohort, 45.1 (29.8-57.3) in the ITT cohort and 100 (90.5-100) in the TVC-naïve cohort.

For qHPV, the VE in the HPV-naïve cohort, against genital warts was 96.4 (91.4-98.8), against VIN1/VaIN1 was 95.2 (70.0-99.9) and against VIN2/VaIN2 95.4 (71.5-99.9).

In the ITT cohort, VE against genital warts was 79.5 (73.0-84.6), against VIN1/VaIN1 76.0 (54.2-88.3) and against VIN2/VaIN2 78.5 (55.2-90.8).

- *According to protocol*: Received three vaccinations, seronegative/DNA-negative to respective HPV types at day 1; DNA-negative to respective HPV types at month 6; normal or low-grade Pap test at day 1; case counting began 1 day after vaccine dose 3.
- *Per protocol*: Received three vaccinations, seronegative/DNA-negative to vaccine HPV types; remained DNA-negative through 1 month post dose 3; case counting started 1 month after dose 3.
- *Total vaccinated cohort and ITT*: Received at least one vaccination, regardless of baseline HPV-related infection or disease; case counting began after day 1.

- *Total vaccinated cohort-naïve and HPV-naïve*: Received at least one dose; polymerase chain reaction (PCR) negative at entry for HPVs 16, 18, 31, 33, 35, 39 45, 51, 52, 56, 58, and 59 (and 66 and 68 for TVC-naïve); seronegative for vaccine types and Pap cytology normal at day 1; case counting after day 1.
- *According to protocol-E*: Analysis in which probable causality to HPV type was assigned in lesions infected with multiple oncogenic types (ATP-E cohort).

In the FUTURE trial, 99–100% efficacy was seen against vaccine type related genital warts.

Q15. What impact has the HPV vaccine had so far?

Ans. Human papillomavirus vaccination is having a clear impact in reducing the spread of HPV. The immediate signs of this are reductions in the number of women with cervical lesions and a dramatic drop in the number of men and women suffering from genital warts. Rapid reductions up to 90% in HPV infections and genital warts in teenage girls and young women were demonstrated in Australia, Belgium, Germany, Sweden, United Kingdom, United States, and New Zealand. Subsequently, as vaccinated cohorts began cervical screening, reductions in cervical abnormalities became apparent. For example, in Australia and Denmark where HPV vaccine was introduced early and programs achieved high coverage, studies showed reductions of 80% for high-grade cervical abnormalities, which are likely to lead to cancer if left untreated.

Q16. What are Advisory Committee on Vaccine and Immunization Practices (ACVIP) recommendations on HPV schedule?

Ans. The ACVIP and WHO recommendations are as follows:
- *Girls 9 through 14 years*: Two doses of either of the two HPV to be administered at an interval of 6 months, 0–6 months.
- *Girls 15 years and older*: Three doses recommended in the schedule 0–1–6 months for the bHPV and 0–2–6 months for the qHPV.
- *In immunocompromised*: Three doses recommended in the schedule 0–1–6 months for the bHPV and 0–2–6 months for the qHPV.

For the three-dose schedule, the minimum acceptable interval between dose one and two is 4 weeks and the minimum acceptable interval between dose two and three is 12 weeks. For two-dose schedule, the minimum acceptable interval between doses is 5 months. The third dose in both vaccines is given 6 months after the first dose and minimum 12 weeks gap from second dose. The upper limit of the last dose is not specified but best given at 6–12 months from the first dose. The vaccine can be administered at the same visit as other needed vaccines.

Q17. Is there evidence of effectiveness of two-dose schedule in children below 15 years age and will two-dose schedule work as well as the three-dose schedule?

Ans. The WHO's Strategic Advisory Group of Experts (SAGE) working group on HPV has recommended revision of vaccination schedule for preadolescent and adolescent girls from three doses to two in its April 2014 meeting. The committee has reviewed the background material and various trials conducted in this regard. Review of the data from four randomized, two nonrandomized and observational studies on two- versus three-dose schedule, concluded that two doses of HPV vaccine in girls 9–14 years of age are noninferior in terms of immunogenicity when compared to three doses in girls 9–14 years or 15–24 years of age. A two-dose vaccine schedule is likely to be as efficacious as three doses, even though long-term outcome and clinical efficacy data are not yet available. Study done in India by Dr Sankarnarayanan in 2015 also had similar observations.

Q18. Is the vaccine useful in older sexually active women?

Ans. People who are sexually active may benefit from vaccination. People who have not been infected with any vaccine HPV type, would receive the maximum benefit of vaccination. Those who have been infected with one of the two oncogenic HPV types in the vaccine, would get protection from the other vaccine type they have not acquired. Natural infection with HPV infection may elicit a poor systemic immune response and reinfections with the same serotype may occur. In the FUTURE 3 study, qHPV vaccine demonstrated high efficacy, immunogenicity, and acceptable safety in women aged 24–45 years, regardless of previous exposure to HPV vaccine type. However, the vaccine will not have any effect on existing Pap test abnormalities, HPV infection, or genital warts.

Q19. Why is it recommended to wait 6 months between the two doses?

Ans. Memory B cell responses are activated after the first dose of the vaccine and take at least 4–6 months to mature into high-affinity B cells. The second dose reactivates these high-affinity B cells and kick starts their differentiation into antibody-secreting plasma cells. Thus the 6-month gap allows the body to develop long-term immunity, whereas with shorter dose gaps between doses, affinity maturation may not occur, and protection duration may be shorter.

Q20. Can the HPV vaccines be used interchangeably with one another?

Ans. There is limited evidence concerning the safety and efficacy of the HPV vaccines when used interchangeably with one another. These three vaccines are comparable in terms of immunogenicity for the common HPV types and prevention of vaccine type related cervical cancers, but the three vaccines contain different components and indications. As such, every effort should be made to use the same vaccine for every dose. If the vaccine used for previous doses is unavailable or unknown, it is acceptable to use any of the HPV vaccines to complete the scheduled doses.

Q21. How long is the vaccine effective? Do we need booster doses?

Ans. As the vaccine was first introduced in 2006, the full duration of protection is not yet known. Data of quadrivalent HPV vaccine FUTURE II trials with qHPV showed undiminished protection in participants up to 14 years. bHPV follow-up studies in a subset of participants over 9.4 years shows no evidence of waning immunity. It is postulated that at present there is no need for boosters.

Q22. How much cross-protection is offered by HPV vaccine for nonvaccine serotypes?

Ans. In regard to cervical cancer prevention, the two HPV vaccines provide high protection against HPV 16 and HPV 18, the types which are associated with 71% of cervical cancer cases globally (82% in India). HPV vaccines also provide some cross-protection against HPV types not included in the vaccines. HPV 16 is phylogenetically related to HPV types 31, 33, 52, and 58 (A9 species); and HPV 18 is related to HPV 45 (A7 species). Based on evidence from clinical trials and post-introduction impact evaluations, the bHPV and qHPV vaccines provide some level of cross-protection against high-risk HPV types other than 16 and 18, in particular for types 31, 33, and 45. However, cross-protection has not been seen to be long lasting.

Q23. What is the data with nonavalent HPV (nHPV) vaccine?

Ans. A phase 2–3 multicentric double-blind qHPV controlled trial in 16–26-year-old women using three doses of 9vHPV for its immunogenicity, safety, and efficacy against persistent infection or disease caused by 9 vaccine HPV types. 14,215 healthy women enrolled with no more than four sexual partners and no history of positive Pap smear or abnormal cervical biopsy in past. Primary endpoints calculated as PP analysis (seronegative on day 1 and PCR negative for vaccine types from day 1 to 7 months) were efficacy against additional five vaccine type high grade cervical, vaginal, and vulvar lesions and noninferior immune response with lower bound 95% confidence interval (CI) geometric mean antibody titer (GMT) ratio of >0.67 for HPV types 6, 11, 16, and 18 comparing nHPV with qHPV. The GMT ratio for the common serotypes was 0.8–1.2 passing the noninferior criteria. Efficacy for additional serotypes against high grade cervical, vulvar or vaginal lesions was 96.7% (95% CI 80.9–99.8).

Q24. Why should we vaccinate at such an early age when the child is not even sexually active?

Ans. First, immune responses are superior in 9–14-year-old girls, compared to young women. Second, girls between 9 and 14 years are assumed to be sexually naïve and are considered ideal for administration of a prophylactic vaccine. Third, in this age group only two doses are required and help in reducing the total cost. Fourth, in this age group, it can be clubbed with the adolescent immunization schedule. Moreover, high coverage in girls (>80%) provides herd protection for boys also.

Q25. What is "gender-neutral vaccination (GNV)"?

Ans. Gender-neutral vaccination is universal vaccination with the HPV vaccine irrespective of sex. The primary goal of HPV vaccination is to prevent cervical cancer. Investing in high coverage among girls of the recommended age (9–14 years) is considered by WHO to be the most effective use of resources to achieve this goal. However, HPV vaccination has benefits for men as well as it protects against penile, anal and oral cancer, diseases which have a strong relation to HPV infection and diseases whose incidence have increased remarkably in the past decade. HPV vaccination of boys alongside girls would reduce transmission, increase herd immunity, and effectively prevent HPV-associated diseases. Limiting HPV vaccination to girls will not lead to eradication. However, it is believed that vaccinating males provides only small additional benefit and is not cost-effective, especially if female programs obtain >75% coverage. If countries have the resources, they may choose to offer the vaccine to boys as well.

Q26. How should the vaccine be stored?

Ans. Human papillomavirus vaccines should be stored at 2–8°C, not frozen, and administered as soon as possible after being removed from the refrigerator. However, for the bivalent vaccine, stability has been demonstrated when stored outside the refrigerator for up to 3 days at temperatures between 8 and 25°C, or for up to 1 day at temperatures between 25 and 37°C. For the quadrivalent vaccine, stability studies demonstrate that the vaccine is stable for 3 days when stored at temperatures from 8 to 42°C.

Q27. Should individuals be screened before getting vaccinated?

Ans. Girls/women do not need to get an HPV test or Pap test to find out if they should get the vaccine. This is because even if they have infection with one strain the vaccine will protect against others. Moreover, natural infection provides limited immunity.

Q28. If we do regular screening, do we still need the vaccine?

Ans. Screening is testing of all asymptomatic women at risk of cervical cancer, with the aim to detect precancerous changes, which, if not treated, may lead to cancer. Women who are found to have abnormalities on screening need follow-up, diagnosis, and possibly treatment, in order to prevent the development of cancer or to treat cancer at an early stage. Screening is only effective if there is a well-organized system for follow-up and treatment and the population is motivated. In developed countries, screening led to a significant reduction in the incidence of cervical cancer, but could not eliminate it. In developing countries, the uptake of screening programs is dismal. Hence, there is need for vaccination in tandem with screening.

Q29. Do women still need to get a Pap test if they have been vaccinated against HPV?

Ans. Yes, women should continue regular cervical cancer screening for three reasons. First, the vaccine does not provide protection against all types of HPV that cause cervical cancer. Second, women may not receive the full benefits of the vaccine if they were infected with HPV before receiving the vaccine. Third, if a woman does not complete the series, she may not be completely protected.

It is imperative that we would need both vaccination as well as efficient screening schemes and rapid intervention like "screen and treat" protocol.

Q30. Can the vaccine be administered to a 18 years young man proceeding going to US for further education?.

Ans. Human papillomavirus vaccines are approved for boys in over 24 countries across the globe. However, it is not approved by the Drugs Controller General of India (DCGI) in India, for boys. So, as of date in India it will be an off-label use. For boys only 4HPV (or 9HPV when it becomes available) is to be used not 2HPV. Nonavalent vaccine will be licensed for both girls and boys.

Q31. If an adolescent 13 years old had a fainting attack on first dose can I still give the second dose after six months?

Ans. Yes, the second dose has to be given but with precautions. The child should not be vaccinated standing or sitting. Should be made to lie down and then give the vaccine. Observe the child for 15 minutes after vaccination.

Q32. Can HPV vaccine cause HPV?

Ans. Human papillomavirus vaccines are inactivated (no live organism) so they cannot cause disease-like symptoms or HPV disease.

Q33. Is revaccination with 9vHPV advised for people who have previously received a series of 2vHPV or 4vHPV?

Ans. Centers for Disease Control and Prevention (CDC) has not recommended routine revaccination with 9vHPV for persons who have completed a series of another HPV vaccine though there is data that a revaccination series with 9vHPV is safe.

Q34. A 12-year-old was started on a three-dose series at another facility. She has received the first two doses, 2 months apart. As she is less than 15 years, is her HPV vaccine series complete or does she need a third dose?

Ans. Adolescents aged 9 years through 14 years who received two doses of HPV vaccine separated by less than 5 months should receive a third dose 6–12 months after dose one and at least 12 weeks after dose two.

Q35. What should be done if a young female becomes pregnant after initiating the vaccination series?

Ans. The remaining dose(s) should be delayed until after the pregnancy is completed.

Q36. Should termination of pregnancy be advised if HPV vaccine was given inadvertently during pregnancy?

Ans. Termination of pregnancy is not indicated if vaccination was carried out inadvertently during pregnancy.

Q37. Can we give HPV vaccine to a lactating mother?

Ans. Breastfeeding is not a contraindication for HPV vaccination. Available evidence does not indicate an increased risk of adverse events linked to the vaccine in either the mothers or their babies after administration of HPV vaccine to lactating females.

Q38. How many doses will be required by a child who has received one dose when she was 14 years and 8 months old and now she is 15 years and 3 months old?

Ans. Only one more dose is needed to complete her schedule. Any girl primed before 15 years of age and even if older than 15 years at the time of second dose, a two-dose schedule is applicable.

Q39. A child received one dose of 4vHPV at 11 years of age. She forgot the second dose and now comes at 14 years of age. Should I restart the schedule?

Ans. The second dose should be given ideally after 6–12 months of the first dose but there is no upper age limit and it is never required to restart the schedule.

Q40. If someone is infected with one type of HPV and their immune system clears it, are they immune to other types of HPV too?

Ans. Immunity to one type of HPV does not offer protection against the other types. The protection is type-specific only, that too not absolute.

Q41. What does it mean when people say HPV infection "cleared"? Is the infection gone or is it dormant? Can it still be spread to someone else?

Ans. Human papillomavirus can cause persistent infections. This means that when a person is infected, the virus is reproducing in the cells that line the infected area. It does not live silently inside of cells like herpes viruses. This means that when the immune system "clears" the infection, it is no longer present, and therefore it cannot be spread to someone else.

Q42. Can someone be infected with more than one type of HPV?

Ans. Yes, you can be infected with more than one type of HPV at a time.

Q43. If a series was started with 4vHPV or 2vHPV, can it be completed with 9vHPV?

Ans. Yes, 9vHPV may be used to continue and complete a series started with a different HPV vaccine product.

Q44. Are additional 9vHPV doses recommended for a person who started a series with 4vHPV or 2vHPV and completed the series with one or two doses of 9vHPV?

Ans. There is no recommendation for additional 9vHPV doses for persons who started the series with 4vHPV or 2vHPV and completed the series with 9vHPV.

Q45. If a series was started with 4vHPV or 2vHPV and will be completed with 9vHPV, what are the intervals for the remaining doses in a three-dose or two-dose series?

Ans. If the first dose of any HPV vaccine was given before the 15th birthday, vaccination should be completed according to a two-dose schedule by giving the second dose 6–12 months from the first dose.

If the first dose of any HPV vaccine was given on or after the 15th birthday, vaccination should be completed according to a three-dose schedule. The second dose is recommended 1–2 months after the first dose, and the third dose is recommended 6 months after the first dose, (0, 1–2, and 6) month schedule.

If a vaccination schedule is interrupted, vaccine doses do not need to be repeated. Number of recommended doses is based on age at administration of the first dose.

Q46. What are the side effects of HPV vaccines?

Ans. Quadrivalent vaccine: Local reactions reported were pain at the injection site in 83% of vaccines (mainly mild and moderate intensity) and swelling and erythema in 25%. Systemic adverse effects such as fever reported in 4% of vaccines.

Bivalent vaccine: Local side effects with bivalent vaccines reported were pain (mild and moderate intensity) in 90% and swelling and erythema in 40%. Systemic side effects such as fever were seen in 12%.

Both the vaccines have very good safety record. They are all minor adverse effects and no serious vaccine-related adverse events have been reported either in trials or postmarketing surveillance studies. CDC states that syncope (fainting) can occur among adolescents following vaccination. To decrease the risk of falls and other injuries that might follow syncope, Advisory Committee on Immunization Practices (ACIP) recommends that clinicians consider observing patients for 15 minutes after vaccination and in apprehensive patients give the vaccine lying down.

Q47. Do HPV vaccines promote earlier sexual activity?

Ans. There is no evidence that being vaccinated against HPV encourages earlier sexual activity. A study published in October 2018 in the Canadian Medical Association Journal showed that since the implementation of the school-based HPV vaccination program, sexual risk behaviors reported by adolescent girls have either reduced or stayed the same. These findings contribute evidence against any association between HPV vaccination and risky sexual behavior.

Q48. Is there any evidence available to support a link between HPV vaccination and postural orthostatic tachycardia syndrome (POTS)?

Ans. There is no evidence to suggest a link between POTS and HPV vaccination. POTS is a condition that causes lightheadedness or fainting and a rapid increase in heartbeat upon standing. The cause is unknown, but doctors think POTS may be associated with a number of medical conditions including: a recent viral illness, prolonged physical inactivity, chronic fatigue syndrome, and nervous system problems. About 80 million doses of HPV vaccine were administered in the United States in the period from June 2006 through September 2015. CDC monitoring in this period through the Vaccine Adverse Event Reporting System (VAERS) did not detect any increase in incidence of POTS following HPV vaccination.

Q49. Is the vaccine safe for people who are immune compromised and/or infected with HIV?

Ans. The vaccine can be used safely in individuals who are immune compromised (whether by disease or by medication) and/or individuals who are HIV-infected, and they should receive three doses even if age is less than 15 years at the time of first dose. However, there is limited data on the immunogenicity of the vaccine in immune compromised and/or HIV infected patient.

Q50. Is there any indication that the HPV vaccine may affect fertility?

Ans. No. HPV vaccination does not affect fertility. Clinical trials before the first HPV vaccine was licensed in 2006 and safety monitoring and studies since its introduction have confirmed that the vaccine does not cause any reproductive problems in women. In fact, the HPV vaccine helps to protect fertility by preventing precancerous cervical lesions and cervical cancer.

Q51. Has HPV vaccination been linked to Guillain–Barré syndrome or any other syndrome or disease?

Ans. The Global Advisory Committee on Vaccine Safety (GACVS) collected large population-level country data on the following safety concerns: Bell's palsy, complex regional pain syndrome (CRPS), POTS, premature ovarian insufficiency, primary ovarian failure, and venous thromboembolism. They found no evidence of causal association between the HPV vaccine and any of these conditions.

Q52. What are the contraindications for HPV vaccine?

Ans. Human papillomavirus vaccines should not be given to anyone who has experienced a severe allergic reaction after a previous HPV vaccine dose, or to a component of the vaccine.

Q53. Are better HPV vaccines in the pipeline?

Ans. The present vaccines have a type-specific protection and a high production cost for public use. The next generation HPV vaccines using capsomere or minor capsid HPV L2 protein are undergoing evaluation. L2 is the minor HPV capsid protein increases the formation of cross-neutralizing antibodies. However, L2-based vaccines obtain transient and lower antibody titers than L1-based vaccines. This is being overcome by the use of newer adjuvants. Chimeric L1-L2 VLP vaccines are being evaluated. This combines the immunogenicity of L1-based vaccines and the broad cross-protection property of L2 vaccines.

■ SUGGESTED READING

1. Bruni L, Albero G, Serrano B, Mena M, Gómez D, Muñoz J, et al. ICO/IARC; Information Centre on HPV and Cancer (HPV Information Centre). Human Papillomavirus and Related Diseases in India. Summary Report 10. Barcelona: HPV Information Centre; 2019.
2. Centers for Disease Control and Prevention. Human Papillomavirus (HPV) Vaccine. [online] Available from http://www.cdc.gov/vaccinesafety/vaccines/HPV/Index.html. [Last accessed October, 2020].
3. Ferlay J, Shin HR, Bray F. GLOBOCAN 2008: Cancer Incidence and Mortality Worldwide. IARC Cancer Base No. 10. Lyon: IARC Press; 2010.
4. IAP. (2020). IAP Guidebook on Immunization 2018-19. [online] Available from https://iapindia.org/pdf/124587-IAP-GUIDE-BOOK-ON-IMMUNIZATION-18-19.pdf. [Last accessed October, 2020].

5. ICMR, NCDIR, National Cancer Registry Program. Three-year report of population based cancer registries: 2012–14. Bangalore, India: NCDIR-NCRP; 2016.
6. Joura EA, Giuliano AR, Iversen OE, Bouchard C, Mao C, Mehlsen J, et al. A 9-Valent HPV Vaccine against Infection and Intraepithelial Neoplasia in Women. N Engl J Med. 2015;372:711-23.
7. Paavonen J, Naud P, Salmeron J, Wheeler CM, Chow SN, Apter D, et al. Efficacy of human papillomavirus (HPV)-16/18 AS04-adjuvanted vaccine against cervical infection and precancer caused by oncogenic HPV types (PATRICIA): final analysis of a double-blind, randomized study in young women. Lancet. 2009;374(9686):301-14.
8. WHO. Global Advisory Committee on Vaccine Safety, 12–13 June 2013. Weekly Epidemiol Rec. 2013;88(29):301-12.
9. World Health Organization. Human Papillomavirus Vaccines: WHO position paper. Wkly Epidemiol Rec. 2017;92(9):241-68.

CHAPTER 26

Rabies Vaccines

Arun Wadhwa

Q1. What is Rabies?

Ans. Rabies is a viral disease transmitted by animals to humans. The agent is a single-stranded bullet-shaped ribonucleic acid (RNA) *Lyssavirus* of the Rhabdovirus family.

Q2. What is the scenario of rabies in India?

Ans. There are an estimated 25 million stray dogs within India. India reports about 18,000–20,000 cases of rabies a year and about 36% of the world's deaths from the disease. In India, rabies affects mainly people of lower socioeconomic status and children between the ages of 5 and 15 years. Children are more often affected as the smaller stature of the child makes them more vulnerable to be bitten on face and neck. Also, children tend to report less to parents fearing injections. Small bites and licks may go un-noticed.

Q3. How does the disease spread?

Ans. The virus invades the nervous system of mammals. It is primarily transmitted from the rabid animal's saliva when it bites or scratches someone. Licks to wounds or grazed broken skin, or to the lining of the mouth and nose can also transmit the disease.

Q4. Which animals can transmit rabies?

Ans. Potentially, all mammals can develop rabies and transmit it to humans.

About 96% of human rabies cases are caused by dog bites and 2% by cat bites. Human rabies has also been reported due to bites of monkeys, mongooses, jackals, foxes, wolves, and other carnivorous animals. Horses, donkeys, cattle, and buffaloes can also transmit rabies. Exposure to these animals warrants consideration of postexposure prophylaxis. Although rabies following exposure to bats has been reported in the world literature, bat transmitted rabies has not been reported from India.

Squirrel, rabbit, and domestic rats do not transmit rabies and do not warrant consideration of postexposure prophylaxis.

Human-to-human transmission of rabies may occur following corneal or other organ transplantation. This is rare but possible.

Q5. Why are children more susceptible to rabies?

Ans. Approximately 40% of cases in children aged <15 years. Children are more often affected as their inquisitive nature makes them more susceptible to bites, smaller stature of the child makes them more vulnerable to be bitten on face and neck. Also, children tend to report less to parents fearing injections. Small bites and licks may go un-noticed.

Q6. What are the factors which contribute to the development of the disease?

Ans. Factors that influence development of disease include type of exposure, severity of the bite, amount of rabies virus introduced, the animal responsible for the bite, the immune status of the victim and the site of the bite—head and neck wounds as well as wounds in highly innervated areas such as fingers.

Q7. What are the features of rabies in dogs?

Ans. Dog rabies is characterized by biting without any provocation, eating abnormal items such as sticks, nails, feces, etc., running for no apparent reason, a change in sound, e.g., hoarse barking and growling or inability to make a sound, excessive salivation or foaming at the angles of the mouth.

Q8. What are the signs of disease in humans?

Ans. Rabies in humans can be frantic type or paralytic type the former being more common. It is characterized by pain or itching at the site of the bite wound (in 80% of cases), fever, malaise, headache lasting for 2–4 days, hydrophobia (fear of water), intolerance to noise, bright light or air, fear of impending death, anger, irritability and depression, and hyperactivity. In late stage, sight of water may provoke spasms in the neck and throat. The duration of illness is usually 2–3 days, but might stretch to 5–6 days or more when receiving intensive care support. Rabies is 100% fatal. Only seven recorded cases of survival in the world. No specific treatment, except making the patient comfortable by giving diazepam, morphine, intravenous (IV) nutrition, and other supportive measures.

Q9. How long does it take to show signs of rabies after being exposed?

Ans. The incubation period of rabies in humans is generally 20–60 days. However, fulminant disease can become symptomatic within 5–6 days; in 1–3% of cases the incubation period is >6 months. Confirmed rabies has occurred as long as 7 years after exposure.

Q10. What is the immediate first aid which we all should know?

Ans. As early as possible the wound should be cleaned with soap and running water for 15 minutes. Then apply a viricidal agent such as povidone-iodine. This itself takes care of >50% of the rabies virus.

Q11. What are the various vaccines available and how do they compare with each other?

Ans. The vaccines available initially but now discontinued because of their side effects were the tissue culture vaccine and embryonated egg origin vaccine. The newer vaccines are the human diploid cell vaccine (HDCV), purified chick embryo cell vaccine (PCECV), purified Vero cell vaccine (PVCV), and purified duck embryo vaccine (PDEV). The last one is not in commercial production these days. There is no major difference among the three products available commercially. The Vero cell-derived vaccines are usually 0.5 mL in volume so less painful for small children.

Q12. Is there a "one dose" vaccine?

Ans. No. There is nothing as a single dose antirabies vaccine.

Q13. What are the different classes of bites and when should immunoglobulin be used?

Ans. The animal bites are classified according to the degree of bite:
- *Category I*: Touching or feeding animals. Licks on intact skin. Contact of intact skin with secretions or excretions of a rabid animal or human case.
- *Category II*: Nibbling of uncovered skin. Minor scratches or abrasions without bleeding. This category needs wound hygiene + vaccine.
- *Category III*: Single or multiple transdermal bites or scratches. Licks on broken skin. Contamination of mucous membrane with saliva (i.e., licks) exposure to bats. This category needs wound hygiene + rabies immunoglobulins (RIG)/monoclonal antibodies (MAbs) + vaccine.

All category III bites, all wild animal bites and class II bites in immunocompromised should be given RIG or MAbs. RIG/MAb is not necessary if the patient has received a complete course of postexposure prophylaxis (PEP) or pre-exposure prophylaxis (PrEP) previously.

Q14. What are the latest WHO guidelines on PrEP, PEP, and re-exposure prophylaxis?

Ans. The World Health Organization (WHO) in its position paper published in April 2018 has made certain significant changes (**Tables 1 and 2**).

For re-exposure, vaccination is not recommended if complete PrEP/PEP already received within <3 months previously.

If received >3 months previously: 1-site IM on days 0 and 3, *or* 1-site ID on days 0 and 3, *or* 4-sites ID on day 0.

It should be mentioned that the Drugs Controller General of India (DCGI) has not approved the revised schedule in India due to lack of data from India. Government institutions still follow the older schedule.

CHAPTER 26: Rabies Vaccines

Table 1: Two-sites intradermal (ID) vaccine administered on days 0 and 7.

Dose	Old Day	2018 Day
1	0	0
2	7	7
3	21–28	XXX

Pre-exposure prophylaxis (PrEP):
Intramuscular
Site: Deltoid or anterolateral thigh

Table 2: Two-sites intramuscular (IM) on days 0 and one-site IM on days 7, 21 or two-sites intradermal (ID) on days 0, 3, and 7.

Dose	Day	Day
1	0	0
2	3	3
3	7	7
4	14	14–28
5	28	XXX

Post-exposure prophylaxis (PEP):
Intramuscular
Site: Deltoid or anterolateral thigh
Schedule: Essen

Q15. Should RIG/MAbs be given to all dog bite cases?

Ans. Rabies immunoglobulins/monoclonal antibodies should be administered to all class III bites by a suspected rabid animal. Even class II bites in the immunocompromised should receive RIG/MAbs.

Q16. What is the schedule to administer RIGs/MAbs?

Ans.
- Immediately or within 24 hours of animal bite along with the first dose of the vaccine.
- If vaccine alone was started, then till 7 days after starting the first dose of the vaccine, it can be given.
- It can be administered even a week or more later if the person has not received any vaccine.

Human rabies immunoglobulin (HRIG) is available in 2 mL vials with a strength of 150 IU/mL and the dose is 20 IU/kg body weight (BW) to a maximum of 1,500 IU.

Equine rabies immunoglobulin (ERIG) is available in 5 mL vials with a strength of 300 IU/mL and the dose is 40 IU/kg BW to a maximum of 3,000 IU.

As per latest recommendations from the WHO, skin testing prior to ERIG administration is not recommended as skin tests do not accurately predict anaphylaxis risk and ERIG can be given whatever the result of the test with due precautions.

As much as possible should be infiltrated around the wound and below it. There is no recommendation for intramuscular (IM) administration of remaining RIG. If volume is less, it can be diluted with normal saline (NS) to the desired volume. The calculated dosage should not be exceeded.

Q17. Are the newly launched monoclonal antibodies equally effective?

Ans. A single monoclonal antibody (mAb) product against rabies, which was licensed in India in 2017, has been demonstrated to be safe and effective in clinical trials. This mAb neutralizes a broad panel of globally prevalent reservoir for rabies virus (RABV) isolates. The comparative advantages of mAb products include large-scale production with standardized quality, greater effectiveness than RIG, elimination of the use of animals in the production process, and reduction in the risk of adverse events. *If available, the use of mAb products instead of RIG is encouraged.* —*(WHO PP 2018)*

Rabishield™, which is a human immunoglobulin G1 (IgG1) monoclonal antibody that binds to the G glycoprotein, has been demonstrated to neutralize 25 different isolates of wild-type or street isolates of rabies virus. The recommended dose of Rabishield™ is 3.33 IU/kg body weight. The usage guidelines are similar to HRIG/ERIG outlined above.

Twinrab™, which is a combination of two MAbs, docaravimab and miromavimab, has been recently licensed. These are murine antibodies against the G protein. It is recommended in a dose of 40 IU/kg of body weight.

Q18. Can wound suturing be done for large lacerations?

Ans. Suturing should be done after infiltration of wound with RIG/MAb. The sutures should be loose and not interfere with free bleeding and drainage. Secondary suturing should be preferred where feasible.

Q19. Who should receive "pre-exposure prophylaxis"? Are there any IAP guidelines regarding PrEP?

Ans. Pre-exposure prophylaxis is recommended for subjects at risk of occupational or vocational exposure to rabies. These include diagnosticians, laboratory and vaccine workers, veterinarians, postmen, etc. Indian Academy of Pediatrics (IAP) guidelines say that all children at high risk of being bitten by stray dogs and children with pets at home should be vaccinated.

The main advantage of PrEP is that it simplifies postexposure management. There is no need for RIG/MAb following subsequent class III exposures.

CHAPTER 26: Rabies Vaccines

Q20. What are the guidelines regarding intradermal rabies vaccination?

Ans. In government set-up intradermal (ID) vaccines are given routinely for cost and dose sparing. For the ID route one dose is 0.1 mL of cell culture and embryonated egg-based vaccines (CCEEV) (irrespective of the vaccine brand). The vaccine in one vial can therefore be fractionated to provide 5–10 doses for ID administration depending on the vial size (0.5 mL or 1.0 mL).

A systematic review of vaccine potency has shown that current vaccines (>2.5 IU/IM dose), when administered by the ID route for either PEP or PrEP, have efficacy equivalent to or higher than that of the same vaccine administered by the IM route.

This route of administration is generally not recommended in office practice.

Q21. I just got up in the morning today and noticed slight bleeding from the index finger of my 3-year-old son?

Ans. If you see one or two small specs of blood on finger most likely it is a rodent bite. House rat bites generally do not require PEP.

Q22. Any harm if I still give rabies vaccine?

Ans. In that case, since you actually do not need it, you can utilize the opportunity to give preventive three injection series. These three shots are given over a period of 3 weeks on 0, 7, and 21 days. New WHO recommendations advice only two doses on days 0 and 7. In this case, anytime in his life if the child is bitten by a suspected rabid animal you will need to give only two shots on 0 and 3 days.

Q23. Do I need a tetanus shot also?

Ans. No. All children who are completely vaccinated by routine vaccines do not need a tetanus shot.

Q24. Do I need to give an antibiotic?

Ans. No, unless it is a deep penetrating bite. Normally, cleaning of wound and application of a local antibiotic is sufficient.

Q25. A 5-year-old boy had an abrasion with some bleeding, following exposure to a stray dog 2 months back. Nothing was done. Now the mother gets the news that the dog was suspected rabid and was killed by the people. What should be done?

Ans. It should be categorized as a fresh class III exposure and RIG/MAb administered with four doses of vaccine.

Q26. My friend has a pet rabbit. Should I tell her to do something for her children's protection?

Ans. Normally, rabbits do not bite. They will bite only as self-defense if they are cornered. Ask her to teach her children not to irritate the animal. It is a good idea to vaccinate the children by the preventive two-dose vaccine series as the family is probably animal lovers and would be interacting with other pets too.

Q27. Once a friend staying in a farmhouse discovered a cow dead. On autopsy, the cow was found to have died of rabies. There was history of a dog bite 5 days ago. The family members have been drinking that cow's milk all these days. Should they take the vaccine?

Ans. Rabies is a very heat labile virus. Heating it at 60°C for 30 seconds kills the virus. So, PEP will be required only if they were drinking raw milk. Latest WHO position paper 2018 mentions that even raw milk is unlikely to transmit rabies virus.

Q28. A worker had handled the urine and feces of the dead animal. Should he take five doses?

Ans. Handling of infected urine and feces does not transmit the virus. For extraprecaution, we can give five doses.

Q29. A patient got a stray dog bite on Sunday and got the first vaccine done from a nearby nursing home. The sister gave the vaccine in the gluteal region. Should I count it as first dose or continue second dose on day 3?

Ans. Any rabies vaccine given in the gluteal region is considered as an invalid dose because of erratic absorption of vaccine administered in the gluteal region. Restart the schedule counting today as day 0.

Q30. A patient got first dose of HDCV in another town but now you do not have the same vaccine. Will you wait for arranging the same brand or give whatever you have as the next dose is due today?

Ans. It is always advised to continue with the same brand but if not available give whatever available. Do not disrupt or discontinue the schedule.

Q31. A child received the first dose of PEP at a health center by the ID route. He is brought to my clinic for the second dose. Can I continue the schedule by the IM route?

Ans. Yes. Evidence suggests that a change in the route of administration or in vaccine product during a PEP or PrEP course is safe and immunogenic.

Q32. A lady 10 weeks pregnant gets bitten by a stray dog. Can she take the vaccine? Has the fetus to be monitored for abnormalities later on?

Ans. The vaccine is safe to be used in pregnancy and no further monitoring of fetus required.

Q33. A 3-week-old infant gets bitten by their unvaccinated family dog. Can an infant receive the vaccine? Same dose or half dose?

Ans. The vaccine is safe and can be given to an infant also. The dose remains the same as the inoculum of the virus does not depend on the weight of the patient.

Q34. A wild animal bites a child on a jungle safari. There is no RIG available and cannot be arranged for next 5 days. Can anything else be done?

Ans. In such a situation give double dose of vaccine, one in each side. If RIG is available within 7 days, give RIG also.

Q35. I had given preventive three doses prophylaxis 6 months ago but now the child has had another dog bite. Should I give five doses now?

Ans. After giving three doses of PrEP, if there is a dog bite within 3 months no further doses are required. In this case as 6 months have elapsed, two doses on days 0 and 3 will be required.

Q36. A patient comes late for her second dose. Will you shift the schedule or give on dates as prescribed originally?

Ans. Give the dose today and complete the schedule on the dates calculated initially.

Q37. A child on induction phase of chemotherapy for acute leukemia gets a class II exposure by a stray dog. What is the schedule to be followed?

Ans. In immunocompromised all bites are class III and are to be treated by RIG and five doses of vaccine. Also, antirabies antibody level should be checked after 1 month of completion of course.

Q38. Can the disease be totally eradicated like small pox? Are there any target programs for rabies elimination?

Ans. The disease can be eradicated by universal preventive vaccination, control and vaccination of stray canine population. The target of eliminating the disease has been fixed as the year 2030. Each year "September 28" is observed as the "world rabies day" to increase awareness about the disease.

Q39. Has the disease been eliminated anywhere in the world?

Ans. The rabies virus can be found everywhere except in some countries and territories of the developed world (e.g., Japan and New Zealand) and the developing world (e.g., Barbados, Fiji, Maldives, and Seychelles) and in parts of Europe (e.g., Greece, Portugal, Sweden, and Norway) and Latin America (e.g., Uruguay and Chile). In the United States, Western Europe, Canada, and much of Latin America, rabies has been nearly eliminated from domestic dogs, but still occurs in the wildlife population.

■ CONCLUSION

Rabies is a very serious disease with almost 100% mortality. Immediate cleaning of wound with soap and water for 15 minutes should be strongly emphasized. In class III bites RIG or monoclonal antibodies must be given. As early as possible vaccination should be started and ensure that the injections are taken on days mentioned. Children and adults should be encouraged to take preventive antirabies vaccine.

■ SUGGESTED READING

1. Association for Prevention and Control of Rabies in India (APCRI). (1998). A vision to make "India Rabies Free by 2020". [online] Available from www.apcri.org. [Last accessed November, 2020].
2. Directorate of Health Service, Swasthya Sadan, Government of Himachal Pradesh. (2019). Guidelines for Rabies Prophylaxis and Intradermal Rabies Vaccination in Himachal Pradesh, 3rd edition, June 2019. [online] Available from http://www.nrhmhp.gov.in/sites/default/files/files/Approved%20%20HP-IDRV%2017-6-2019%20%20Rabies%20Guidelines.pdf. [Last accessed November, 2020].
3. Government of India. (2015). National Rabies Control Programme, National Guidelines on Rabies Prophylaxis, National Centre for Disease Control, 2015, Delhi, India. [online] Available from http://clinicalestablishments.gov.in/WriteReadData/238.pdf [Last accessed November, 2020].
4. Immunization Action Coalition. (2020). Vaccine Information You Need. [online] Available from www.vaccineinformation.org; www.immunize.org [Last accessed November, 2020].
5. World Health Organization. (2018). WHO Expert Consultation on Rabies, Technical Report Series, 1012, 2018, Geneva, Switzerland. [online] Available from https://apps.who.int/iris/bitstream/handle/10665/272364/9789241210218-eng.pdf [Last accessed November, 2020].
6. World Health Organization. Rabies vaccines: WHO position paper—April, 2018. Wkly epidemiol rec. 2018;93:201-20.

CHAPTER 27: Meningococcal Vaccines

M Surendranath

Q1. What are the diseases caused by *N. meningitidis*?

Ans. Meningococcal disease is caused by gram-negative diplococcus bacteria *Neisseria meningitidis*. Meningococcus bacteria is commensal organism in the upper respiratory tract of 10% of population. Humans are the only reservoir for meningococcus bacteria. Usually, disease occurs in dry season in endemic areas. It can present as acute illness and rarely chronic illness. Meningococcus can cause meningitis, septicemia, pneumonia, myocarditis, pericarditis, arthritis, and conjunctivitis. Occasionally, it can present as shock known as "Waterhouse-Friderichsen syndrome". *N. meningitidis* is the third most common cause of meningitis in children <5 years in India after *S. pneumoniae* and *H. influenza* b.

Q2. What are the serogroups?

Ans. There are 12 serogroups. 90% of disease is caused by six serogroups, A, B, C, X, Y, and W. In the African meningitis belt, disease is caused by serogroup A and W. Outbreaks in Haj pilgrims are caused by A and W serogroups. In developed countries, disease is caused by B, C, and Y serogroups. Incidence of endemicity in India is low but periodic epidemics have been reported in the past 100 years. Larger epidemics have occurred in large cities of northern and eastern India and are usually caused by serogroup A.

Q3. What are the guidelines for introduction of MCV in the NIP of any country and are these criteria satisfied in India?

Ans. The World Health Organization (WHO) classifies endemic zones into low, intermediate, or high depending on number of cases per lakh population per year. Less than 2 is low, 2–10 is intermediate and >10 is high. The WHO says if the country is high or intermediate endemic or if there are frequent epidemics the vaccine should be introduced in national immunization program (NIP). The exact incidence in India is not known. India falls under the low-endemic zone. Hence, meningococcal vaccines do not qualify to be included in the NIP in India.

Q4. What is the correlate of protection for meningococcal vaccines?

Ans. Serologic assessments of meningococcal vaccine immunogenicity rely on measurements of complement-mediated serum bactericidal activity (SBA). A titer of 1:128 or greater measured with rabbit complement or >1:8 using human serum correlates with protection.

Q5. What are the vaccines available for prevention?

Ans. There two types of vaccines:
1. *Polysaccharide vaccine*: Polysaccharide vaccines are not given below 2 years of age as they have poor immunogenicity and being T-cell independent do not produce memory cells.
    Two formulations are/were marketed in India:
    i. Quadrivalent A, C, Y, and W
    ii. Bivalent A and C.
    Quadrivalent A, C, Y, and W vaccine contains 50 mcg each of the polysaccharide of A, C, Y, and W. Thiomersal is added as a preservative.
2. *Conjugate vaccines*: Conjugate vaccines can be given in infancy, they produce memory cells, giving better and long-lasting immunity. Conjugate vaccines are available in different formulations:
    - Monovalent A serotype
    - Meningococcal serogroup C (MenC) with *Haemophilus influenzae* type B (Hib) combination
    - Meningococcal serogroup B (MenB) monovalent type B serogroup
    - Bivalent A and C serogroups
    - Quadrivalent A, C, W, and Y.
    Of these only two formulations of quadrivalent A, C, W, and Y are marketed in India.
    Monovalent A serotype vaccine has 10 µg of polysaccharide antigen conjugated to 10–33 µg of tetanus toxoid with alum as adjuvant and thiomersal as preservative. Meningococcal conjugate vaccine (MCV)-A is recommended as a single dose in age group 1–29 years in all countries in the African meningitis belt. It can be administered along with other childhood vaccines.
    Quadrivalent MenACWY-D (Menactra®) vaccine contains 4 µg of polysaccharide antigen conjugated to 48 µg of diphtheria toxoid in 0.5 mL liquid form.
    Quadrivalent MenACWY-CRM[197] (Menveo®) has lyophilized MenA component with liquid MenCWY component. Each 0.5 mL contains 10 of meningococcal serogroup A and 5 µg of each of capsular polysaccharide of serogroups C, W, and Y conjugated to CRM[197].

Q6. What is the efficacy of the polysaccharide vaccine?

Ans. Antibody response to each serogroup is specific and independent. Protective level of antibodies is achieved within 10–14 days. Infants as young as 3 months can mount an antibody response to serogroup A, but response is lower than adults. Adult levels of immune response occur only after 4 years of age. Serogroup C is poorly immunogenic in children <2 years of age. Serogroups A and C vaccines elicit good immunogenicity with clinical rates of 85% or higher in children above 5 years of age and adults. Serogroup Y and W-135 polysaccharide are immunogenic in older children and adults but clinical protection has not been documented. In children below 5 years, antibodies against A and C serogroups decrease substantially in 3 years after administering single dose of vaccine. Repeat dose is known to cause hyporesponsiveness.

Presently polysaccharide vaccines are not available in India.

Q7. What is the immunogenicity of MCV-DT?

Ans. Meningococcal conjugate vaccine-diphtheria toxoid (MCV-DT) was licensed based on noninferiority to meningococcal polysaccharide vaccine (MPSV-4), the meningococcal polysaccharide vaccine. MCV-DT recipients showed a more than fourfold increase in SBA titers (range: 80.1–96.7%) to the four serogroups. Booster responses to MCV-4 consistent with immune memory was also demonstrated.

Q8. What is the immunogenicity of MCV-CRM?

Ans. Meningococcal conjugate vaccines (MCV)-4-CRM was studied with MCV-DT as a comparator vaccine in children 2–5 years, 6–10 years, and 11–18 years. It showed noninferiority to MCV-DT to all serogroups in the 11–18 years group. In 2–5 years and 6–10 years groups, noninferiority could not be demonstrated against serogroup A. In general, in pooled cohort of 2–10 years and 11–18 years age group, non-inferiority of MENVEO to MenACWY-DT (Menactra–Sanofi Pasteur Inc) was demonstrated for all serogroups. Persistence of antibodies were demonstrated in children and adolescents up to 5 years post-vaccination.

Q9. What are the efficacy studies of meningococcal conjugate vaccine, done in India?

Ans. All conjugate vaccines are highly immunogenic (>90%). Antibodies are not long lasting and booster may be required. There is no cross protection between serogroups. In a study done in India, 300 healthy vaccine naïve participants (100 children aged 2–11 years, 100 adolescents aged 12–17 years, and 100 adults aged 18–55 years) were administered a single dose of MCV-DT. The percentage of participants (95% CI) with protective serum bactericidal antibody titer for A, C, Y, and W serogroups respectively for child group 96%, 91.9%, 100%, and 97% for adolescent group 96.9%, 96.9%, 100%, and 100%, and for adult groups 99%, 99%, 100%, and 100%, respectively.

Safety and immunogenicity study of MenACWY-CRM vaccine was studied in healthy Indian subjects aged 2–75 years by Sanjay Lalwani et al. (2015).

This has shown that percentage of subjects having postvaccination hSBA titers > 8 were 72%, 95%, 94%, and 90% for serogroups A, C, W, and Y. Geometric mean titers rose sevenfold to 42-fold against four serogroups. Similar immune response was for the age subgroups 2–10 years, 11–18 years, and 19–75 years. Seroresponse rates at 1 month following vaccination were 72%, 88%, 55%, and 71% for serogroups A, C, W, and Y, respectively.

Q10. What are adverse events following immunization (AEFI) with meningococcal vaccines?

Ans. No immediate adverse reactions or adverse events were reported. Grade one severity of local injection site reactions such as redness, pain is reported which will resolve within 3 days. Minor side effects noted are diarrhea, vomiting, pyrexia, nasopharyngitis, upper respiratory tract infection (URTI), cough, and muscle or joint pain. There are a few reports of the association of Guillain-Barré (GB) syndrome after receipt of this vaccine. There is not enough data to suggest vaccine as the cause of GB syndrome.

Q11. What are the IAP recommendations for vaccination?

Ans. With the current epidemiology and burden of the disease, meningococcal vaccine is recommended only for children with certain high-risk conditions listed below:
- During disease outbreaks. Can be given along with prophylaxis if close contact with a patient as a single dose.
- High-risk children:
  - Children with congenital or acquired immunodeficiencies, particularly children with terminal complement component deficiencies (C3, C5–C9, properdin, and factor D and factor H).
  - Those with functional or anatomic asplenia, including sickle-cell disease. Administer two primary doses of either MCV with at least 8 weeks between doses for individuals aged 24 months through 55 years. Vaccination should ideally be started 2 weeks prior to splenectomy.
- Children with HIV. Administer two doses at least 8 weeks interval:
  - *Laboratory personnel and healthcare workers*: Who are exposed routinely to *Neisseria meningitides* in solutions that may be aerosolized should be considered for vaccination. A single dose of MCV is recommended. A booster dose should be administered every 5 years if exposure is ongoing.
  - *Adjunct to chemoprophylaxis*: In close contacts of patients with MD (healthcare workers in contact with secretions, household contacts, and day-care contacts), single dose of appropriate group MCV is recommended.
- *International travelers*:
  (i) *Students going for study abroad* (mandatory in most universities in the USA): Some institutions have policies requiring vaccination

CHAPTER 27: Meningococcal Vaccines

against meningococcal disease as a condition of enrollment. Persons aged <21 years should have documentation of receipt of a MCV not >5 years before enrollment. In the United States, the Advisory Committee on Immunization Practices (ACIP) recommends routine vaccination of all adolescents with single dose of MCV-4 at age 11–12 years with a booster dose at the age of 16 years.

(ii) *Hajj pilgrims:* Vaccination is required for all travelers to Mecca during the annual Hajj. The quadrivalent vaccine is preferred for Hajj pilgrims and international travelers as it provides added protection against emerging W-135 and Y disease in these areas. A single dose of 0.5 mL IM is recommended in age group 2–55 years. The conjugate vaccine is valid for 5 years while the polysaccharide vaccine is valid for 3 years.

(iii) *Travelers to countries in the African meningitis belt:* A single dose of monovalent or quadrivalent vaccine is recommended. Conjugate vaccine is preferred to polysaccharide vaccine. A booster dose of MCV is needed if the last dose was administered 5 or more years previously.

Q12. What is IAP recommended schedule of conjugate meningococcal vaccines?

Ans.
- In children 9 through 23 months of age, Menactra˙ is given as a two-dose series 3 months apart.
- Individuals 2 through 55 years of age, single dose.
- Presently, Menveo˙ is licensed for use above the age of 2 years as a single dose.
- *Booster vaccination:*
  - A single booster dose may be given to individuals 15 through 55 years of age at continued risk for meningococcal disease, if at least 5 years have elapsed since the prior dose.
  - For the immunocompromised, high-risk groups, a two-dose primary series of MCV administered 8–12 weeks apart is recommended for persons aged 24 months through 55 years. A booster dose should be administered every 5 years. Children who receive the primary series before their seventh birthday should receive the first booster dose in 3 years and subsequent doses every 5 years.
  - Each country has different schedule of vaccination depending on their respective epidemiological data.

Q13. How do you compare the two brands of MCV-4 available in India?

Ans. There are two MCV-4 conjugate vaccines available in the market. MCV-DT (Sanofi) is available as a ready to use form and licenced for use above 9 months of age. MCV^{CRM} (GSK) is available in lyophilized form and as of now in India it has been licenced for use only above 2 years of age. Both can be used keeping the age factor in mind.

Q14. A child staying in Mumbai has his grandparents in Delhi and travels 1–2 times a year to Delhi. Will you proactively recommend MCV to this child?

Ans. Generally, a child traveling to a probable intermediate zone need not take the vaccine.

Q15. What is the recommendation for MenB vaccine?

Ans. At present it is not available in India. Two serogroup B vaccines are currently licenced in the United States of America. MenB-FHbp (Trumenba®), MenB-4C (Bexsero®) are two vaccines licenced for use in persons aged 10–25 years in the united states. Preferable age is 16–18 years. These vaccines are given as three dose schedule 0, 1–2, and 6 months for persons at increased risk of meningococcal diseases and for use during serogroup B meningococcal outbreaks. Two-dose schedule 0 and 6 months is recommended for healthy persons. Either of the brands can be used but they are not interchangeable. MenB offers only short-term protection, protective antibodies decrease quickly, within 1–2 years after MenB vaccination.

Q16. What are the precautions and contraindication for this vaccine?

Ans. Children above 2 years with functional or anatomical asplenia or HIV should not receive Menactra® and PCV13 at the same time. They should either receive Menveo® or receive Menactra® 4 weeks after PCV13.

Children can receive Menactra® before or same time with DTaP vaccine. Menactra® should not be given after DTaP as there may interference with immunological response of the meningococcal vaccine antigens. Alternatively, Menveo® can be given.

Contraindications: Any severe allergic reaction such as anaphylaxis after previous dose or any severe allergy to any component of vaccine. If indicated pregnancy and breastfeeding in not a contraindication for meningococcal vaccination.

■ SUGGESTED READING

1. Centers for Disease Control and Prevention. Morbidity and Mortality Weekly Report (MMWR). MMWR Weekly: Past Volume (2014). 2014;63(24):521-36.
2. Centers for Disease Control and Prevention. Morbidity and Mortality Weekly Report (MMWR). MMWR Weekly: Past Volume (2014). 2014;63(43):969-88; ND 593-606.
3. Centers for Disease Control and Prevention. Morbidity and Mortality Weekly Report (MMWR). Healthy and Safe Swimming Week—May 22-28, 2017. Using Molecular Characterization to Support Investigations of Aquatic Facility-Associated Outbreaks of Cryptosporidiosis—Alabama, Arizona, and Ohio, 2016. MMWR. 2017;66(19):493-517.
4. Javadekar B, Ghosh A, Kompithra RZ, Awasthi S, Perminova O, Romanenko V, et al. Safety and immunogenicity of two doses of quadrivalent meningococcal

polysaccharide diphtheria toxoid conjugate vaccine in Indian and Russian children aged 9 to 17 months. Indian Pediatr. 2018;55:1050-5.
5. John TJ, Gupta S, Chitkara AJ, Dutta AK, Borrow R. An overview of meningococcal disease in India: Knowledge gaps and potential solutions. Vaccine. 2013;31:2731-7.
6. Lalwani S, Agarkhedkar S, Gogtay N, Palkar S, Agarkhedkar S, Thatte U, et al. Safety and immunogenicity of investigational meningococcal ACWY-CRM conjugate vaccine (MenACWY-CRM) in healthy Indian subjects aged 2–75 years. Int J Infect Dis. 2015;38:36-42.
7. Meningococcal vaccines: WHO position paper, November 2011. Wkly Epidemiol Rec. 2011;86(47):521-39.
8. World Health Organization (2015). WHO position paper, meningococcal A conjugate vaccine: updated guidance, February 2015. [online] Available from: https://www.who.int/immunization/policy/position_papers/pp_menA_2015_presentation.pdf. [Last accessed October, 2020].
9. Yadav S, Manglani MV, Narayan DA, Sharma S, Ravish HS, Arora R, et al. Safety and immunogenicity of a quadrivalent meningococcal conjugate vaccine (MenACYW-DT): a multicenter, open-label, non-randomized, phase III clinical trial. Indian Pediatr. 2014;51:451-6.

CHAPTER 28: Japanese Encephalitis Vaccines

Pravin Mehta

Q1. What is Japanese encephalitis?

Ans. Japanese encephalitis (JE) is a neurological disease mainly affecting central nervous system (CNS). JE is caused by Japanese encephalitis virus (JEV) which is a flavivirus belonging to family of flaviviridae, which is transmitted to humans by mosquito bites mainly by *Culex tritaeniorhynchus* type of mosquitos. It is a ribonucleic acid (RNA) virus. Pigs and wading birds are main reservoirs of the virus. JE can cause severe complications, seizures, and even death. JE forms an important cause for acute encephalitis syndrome (AES).

Japanese encephalitis is predominantly, although not exclusively, a rural disease.

Japanese encephalitis virus is not transmitted from person-to-person. The incubation period is usually 5-15 days. The case fatality rate can be as high as 30% among those with disease symptoms with young children (<10 years) having a greater risk of severe disease and a higher case-fatality rate; 20-30% of those who survive suffer permanent neuropsychiatric sequelae. In areas where the JE virus is common, encephalitis occurs mainly in young children because older children and adults have already been infected and are immune.

Q2. What is acute encephalitis syndrome (AES)?

Ans. Clinically, a case of acute encephalitis syndrome (AES) is defined as a person of any age with acute onset of fever and a change in mental status (including symptoms such as confusion, disorientation, coma, or inability to talk) and/or new onset of seizures (excluding simple febrile seizures), occuring at any time of the year. Other early clinical findings may include an increase in irritability, somnolence or abnormal behavior greater than that seen with usual febrile illness [the World Health Organization (WHO)]. AES including JE is a group of clinically similar neurological manifestations caused by several different viruses, bacteria, fungus, parasites, spirochetes, chemical/toxins, etc. Some other causes of AES could be tuberculosis, meningitis, viral encephalitis, cerebral malaria, etc. Clinically, it is difficult to distinguish JE from other cases of AES.

Q3. What is the disease burden of JE worldwide?

Ans. The World Health Organization (WHO) figures suggest that nearly 50,000 cases of JE occur worldwide out of which 15,000 people die. Japanese encephalitis is one of the most important forms of epidemic and sporadic encephalitis in the tropical regions of Asia, including Japan, China, Taiwan, Korea, Philippines, all of South eastern Asia, and India. Countries with proven epidemics of JE include India, Pakistan, Nepal, Sri Lanka, Burma, Laos, Vietnam, Malaysia, Singapore, Philippines, Indonesia, China, maritime Siberia, Korea, and Japan. In the past 50 years, the geographic areas affected by JEV have expanded and are still expanding.

Q4. Who is at high risk to get JE?

Ans. Long-term travelers, persons involved in outdoor recreational activities are at risk, especially those visiting rural areas, farms, rice fields and irrigation areas, children and young adults residing in endemic areas. Children under 15 years of age seem to particularly susceptible to the infection. Outbreaks typically occur during or shortly after the rainy season in temperate regions and year-round in tropical regions (peak transmission during summer months). In the temperate regions of China, Japan, the Korean peninsula and eastern parts of the Russian Federation, transmission occurs primarily during the summer and autumn.

Q5. What is the disease burden in India?

Ans. Japanese encephalitis is reported from 268 districts of India from 23 states. Infection is present throughout the country with the exception of: Dadra and Nagar Haveli, Daman and Diu, Gujarat, Himachal Pradesh, Jammu and Kashmir, Lakshadweep, Meghalaya, Punjab, Rajasthan, and Sikkim. In northern India, transmission occurs from May to October and generally all year in southern India. In India, a number of JE cases have increased from 555 in the year 2010 to 2,044 in the year 2017. In 2019, India reported 2,496 JE cases with 240 deaths.

Q6. Why has vaccination been prioritized in JE control?

Ans. The consensus statements from Global JE meetings held in 1995, 1998, and 2002 have clearly stated that *"Human vaccination is the only effective long-term control measure* against JE. All at-risk residents should receive a safe and efficacious vaccine as part of their national immunization program."

In 1994, the WHO stated that "where affordable, JE vaccination should be extended to all endemic areas where JE is considered as a public health problem".

Q7. Who should be vaccinated?

Ans. This vaccine is not an outbreak response vaccine. It is recommended for universal vaccination in endemic areas. All children from 1–18 years should be vaccinated in endemic area. As JE vaccination does not induce herd immunity, high vaccination coverage should be achieved and sustained in populations at risk of the disease.

Q8. Why have adults been included in the JE vaccine program in the NIP?

Ans. Following mass vaccination campaigns with live-attenuated SA-14-14-2 JE vaccine among pediatric age group, adult JE cases have outnumbered pediatric cases in some JE endemic states, including Assam. Recently, National Vector Borne Disease Control Program (NVBDCP) has identified 20 high burden districts in three states–Assam, Uttar Pradesh, and West Bengal for adult JE vaccination (>15–65 years). Till now, eight districts have been covered by the adult vaccination program. As per the data from the Indian Council of Medical Research (ICMR) established virus research diagnostic laboratories (VRDLs), of the 1,231 JE cases diagnosed between January 2014 to April 2017, >40% cases were in age group of >15 years.

Q9. Why has the program been extended to urban areas in endemic districts?

Ans. The increased risk of suburban or periurban areas has been documented in multiple Asian countries (South Korea, China, Singapore, and Taiwan). This change may be due to changes in pig rearing practices or changes in the vector capacity to penetrate areas distant to sites of origin. This shift suggests that JE should not be considered only a disease of rural or farming areas.

Recent list of JE endemic districts includes many urban regions (state capitals); Kolkata, Patna, Lucknow, Goa, Thiruvananthapuram (or Trivandrum), Chennai, Ranga Reddy district (Part of Hyderabad), etc. Cases have been reported from Delhi and Bhopal. As per recent ICMR data 25% of JE cases reported from urban regions, there is indicative of risk of JE in both rural and urban regions.

Q10. What are the recommendations on vaccination for travelers?

Ans. Japanese encephalitis vaccine is recommended for persons moving to a JE-endemic country to live longer-term (e.g., 1 month or longer) and frequent travelers to JE-endemic areas. JE vaccine also should be considered for shorter-term (e.g., <1 month) travelers with an increased risk of JE based on planned travel duration, season, location, activities, and accommodations. Vaccination also should be considered for travelers to endemic areas who are uncertain of specific duration of travel, destinations, or activities.

Japanese encephalitis vaccine is not recommended for travelers with very low-risk itineraries, such as shorter-term travel limited to urban areas or travel that occurs outside of a well-defined JE virus transmission season.

The schedule should be completed at least 1 week before travel.

Q11. What are the vaccines available for prevention of JE?

Ans.
I. Inactivated mouse brain derived
   - Uncertain protection
   - Multiple doses
   - Unacceptable neurological adverse events
   - Production ceased
II. Live JE vaccines: Live-attenuated SA 14-14-2
III. Killed JE vaccines: JEEV™ and JENVAC™
IV. Live-attenuated recombinant SA 14-14-2 chimeric vaccine

Q12. What are the salient features of the live-attenuated SA-14-14-2 vaccine?

Ans. This was the first vaccine used in campaign mode in India in 2006. Minimum age is 8 months. Two dose schedule: 9 months and 18 months. This vaccine is not available in private market for office use.

This vaccine is based on the genetically stable, neuroattenuated SA 14-14-2 strain of the JEV, which elicits broad immunity against heterologous JEVs. Reversion to neurovirulence is considered highly unlikely. WHO technical specifications have been established for the vaccine production. Chengdu Institute of Biological Products is the only manufacturer authorized to export this vaccine from China. This live-attenuated vaccine was licensed in China in 1989. Since then, >300 million doses have been produced and >200 million children have been vaccinated. Currently, >50 million doses of this vaccine are produced annually. Extensive use of this and other vaccines has significantly contributed to reducing the burden of JE in China from 2.5/100,000 in 1990 to <0.5/100,000 in 2004. This vaccine is also licensed for use in Nepal (since 1999); South Korea (since 2001); India (since 2006); Thailand (since 2007); and Sri Lanka. The price per dose of the vaccine is comparable to the expanded program on immunization (EPI) measles vaccine.

Q13. What is the Indian experience with this vaccine?

Ans. In India, one dose of SA 14-14-2 imported from China is being used since 2006 and children between the age group of 1 and 15 years were vaccinated with a single dose of the vaccine. Following the campaigns targeting all children in the age group of 1–15 years in the high-risk districts, the vaccine is integrated into the universal immunization program (UIP) of endemic districts. A small case-control study from Lucknow, India found an efficacy of 94.5% (95% CI, 81.5-98.9) after a single dose of this vaccine within 6 months after its administration. However, data from postmarketing surveillance (PMS) in India showed that protective efficacy of the vaccine in India is not as high as that seen in Nepal. PMS study showed that virus neutralizing antibodies were seen in 45.7% of children before vaccination. Seroconversion against Indian strains 28 days after vaccination was 73.9% and 67.2% in all individuals and in those who were nonimmune prevaccination, respectively. The protective efficacy of the vaccine at 1 year was 43.1% overall and 35% for those who were nonimmune prevaccination, respectively. Preliminary results of a recent case control study carried out by ICMR on impact of JE vaccine shows an unadjusted protective effect of 62.5% in those with any report of vaccination. According to this report, the JE vaccine efficacy has been around 60% in Uttar Pradesh and around 70% in Assam. Following this report, the ICMR has recommended a study on the impact of two doses versus single dose of SA 14-14-2 vaccine in Assam.

Q14. What is the safety profile of this vaccine?

Ans. An estimated 300 million children have been immunized with this vaccine without apparent complication. WHO's Global Advisory Committee on Vaccine Safety acknowledged the vaccine's "excellent" safety profile. Transient fever may occur in 5–10%, local reactions, rash, or irritability in 1–3%. Neither acute encephalitis nor hypersensitivity reactions have been associated with the use of this vaccine.

Q15. Which are the killed JE vaccines available in India?

Ans. Two of them are available for office use in India:
1. Inactivated SA-14-14-2 strain, propagated on Vero-cell culture marketed internationally by Intercell and it is the only United States Food and Drug Administration (US-FDA) approved JE vaccine, marketed in India as JEEV™.
2. Inactivated Vero-cell culture-derived Kolar strain, 821564XY JE vaccine, JENVAC™.

Q16. What are the salient features of JEEV™?

Ans. This is the result of a technology transfer of the inactivated Vero-cell derived, purified, adjuvanted IC51 vaccine, from Intercell. The IC51 vaccine has been licensed in several countries based on the similar safety and immune profile compared to the inactivated mouse-brain derived vaccine which is known to be effective against JE.

Q17. What is the Indian data on IC51 by BE (JEEV™)?

Ans. In 2011, the Biological E Ltd., India, conducted a multicentric open label randomized controlled phase II/III study to evaluate safety and immunogenicity of vaccine in 450 children (≥1 to <3 years old) and compared to control Korean Green Cross Mouse Brain Inactivated (KGCC) vaccine. This study demonstrated seroconversion rate (SCR) of 56.28% on day 28 and 92.42% on day 56 in IC51 by BE vaccinated group. Noninferiority of this vaccine established against control in terms of proportion of subjects seroconverted. Geometric mean titers (GMTs) in IC51 by BE group were significantly higher than GMTs achieved in KGCC-JE vaccine group (218 vs 126). There was no significant difference between the groups in proportion of subjects seroprotected and in proportion of subjects reporting adverse events between groups. IC51 by BE has been licensed by Drug Controller General of India (DCGI) for use in prevention of JEV infection in children and adult population on the basis of its ability to induce JEV neutralizing antibodies as a surrogate for protection.

This is a formalin-inactivated vaccine.

The adult preparation, 0.5 mL, contains 6 μg of SA 14-14-2, corresponding to a potency of <90 ID_{50}.

The pediatric preparation, 0.25 mL, contains 3 μg of SA 14-14-2, corresponding to a potency of <90 ID_{50}.

The vaccine is produced in Vero cells and has aluminum hydroxide 0.25 mg as an adjuvant.

It is to be stored at +2°C to +8°C and should be discarded if frozen.

Q18. What are the salient features of the Kolar strain (JENVAC™) vaccine?

Ans. 821564XY is a Vero cell culture-derived, inactivated, adjuvanted, and thiomersal-containing vaccine developed by Bharat Biotech International Ltd. (BBIL). Original virus strain used in the vaccine was isolated from a patient in the endemic zone in Kolar, Karnataka, India by National Institute of Virology (NIV), Pune, and later transferred to Bharat Biotech for vaccine development.

A phase II/III, randomized, single-blinded, active controlled study to evaluate the immunogenicity and safety of the vaccine was conducted among 644 healthy subjects between the ages 1 and 50 years. Subjects received two doses of the test vaccine or a single dose of a reference vaccine (live-attenuated, SA 14-14-2 Chinese vaccine) as the first dose and a placebo as the second dose. The results revealed that even a single dose of the test vaccine was sufficient to elicit the immune response. On 28th day, the subjects who had received a single dose were 98.67% seroprotected and 93.14% seroconverted (fourfold) for ≤50 to ≥1 years, whereas the corresponding figures for the reference vaccine were 77.56% and 57.69%, respectively (p-value < 0.001). There was no statistically significant difference in all the three groups. The seroconversion (93.14% and 96.90%) and seroprotection (98.67% and 99.78%) percentages on the 28th and 56th day were not significantly different and similarly, no statistically significant difference in these rates was noted among different age groups. Higher GMTs were achieved in younger age groups. After the second dose of the test vaccine, the GMTs increased exponentially from day 28 (145) to day 56 (460.5) in ≤50 to ≥1 years. However, there was waning of both seroconversion and GMTs in both the test vaccine and reference vaccine groups at 18 months. All the subjects were followed up for 56 ± 2 days. There was no serious adverse event or adverse event of any special interest noted in the study.

Table 1: Comparative results between commercially available vaccines.

Vaccine	GMTs			% seroconversion	
	Day 0	Day 28	Day 56	Day 0–28	Day 0–56
Jenvac™	6.1	145	460.53	93.14	96.91
JEEV™	9.7	27.2	217.97	56.68	92.42

In a phase IV immunogenicity clinical trial with a single dose of JENVAC™, the seroprotection rates were 92.4% (28 days), 92.5% (56 days), 92.4% (60 days), 88.9% (180 days), 81.7% (360 days) and 88.5% (720 days). On basis of this study, the DCGI has licensed this vaccine in a single-dose schedule. However, The Indian Academy of Pediatrics (IAP) and the Government of India (GOI) still recommend a two-dose schedule.

Each dose of 0.5 mL contains:
- Purified, inactivated JEV protein (JEV strain 821564-XY): NLT 5.0 µg
- Aluminum (Al) as aluminum phosphate: 0.25 mg
- Thiomersal IP (as preservative): 0.025 mg
- Phosphate buffered saline: q.s. to 0.5 mL

It is to be stored at +2°C to +8°C and should be discarded, if frozen.

Q19. How do the two inactivated vaccines compare regarding immunogenicity?

Ans. Comparison of the two inactivated vaccines regarding immunogenicity has been shown in **Table 1**.

Q20. What are the salient features of the live-attenuated recombinant SA 14-14-2 chimeric vaccine?

Ans. This vaccine is not available in India.

This vaccine, known as ChimeriVax™ or Imojev, is a live-attenuated recombinant, chimeric virus vaccine based on the live-attenuated Yellow fever vaccine (YFV17D). The genomic sequences encoding the Pr and M proteins of the YFV17D has been replaced by the Pr and M proteins of the SA 14-14-2 strain.

It is highly protective with seroconversion rate of >97% after a single dose. It is licensed for use in Australia.

Q21. What are the IAP recommendations for JE vaccine use?

Ans. Storage of these vaccines should be at temperature between 2 and 8°C.

Routine vaccination: Recommended only for individuals living in endemic districts. Both rural and urban children in the district should be vaccinated.

Live-attenuated, Cell culture-derived SA-14-14-2
- *Minimum age:* 8 months.

- *Two-dose schedule*: First dose at 9 months along with measles and rubella (MR) vaccine and second at 16-18 months along with diphtheria, tetanus toxoids, and pertussis (DTP) booster.
- Not available in private market for office use.

Inactivated cell culture-derived SA 14-14-2 (IC51 by BE India)
- *Minimum age*: 1 year [US Food and Drug Administration (FDA): 2 months].
- *Primary immunization schedule*: Two doses of 0.25 mL each administered intramuscularly on days 0 and 28 for children aged ≥1 to ≤3 years. Two doses of 0.5 mL for children >3 years and adults aged ≥18 years.
- Need of boosters still undetermined.

Inactivated Vero cell culture-derived Kolar strain, 821564XY, JE vaccine (by Bharat Biotech International Limited)
- *Minimum age*: 1 year.
- *Primary immunization schedule*: Two doses of 0.5 mL each administered intramuscularly at 4 weeks interval.
- Need of boosters still undetermined.

Catch-up vaccination: All susceptible children up to 15 years should be administered during disease outbreak or ahead of anticipated outbreak in campaigns.

Q22. What are the recommendations regarding booster doses?

Ans. The Centers for Disease Control and Prevention (CDC) recommends that a booster dose may be given if the primary two-dose vaccination series were given 1 year or more previously and there is continued risk of exposure.

The IAP mentions that the need for boosters is uncertain. There are limited data on duration of protection in children and from endemic settings. In a study in Asia, after the primary series, given to children aged ≥2 months to <17 years, the seroprotection rate after 3 years was 90%.

Q23. Are the vaccines interchangeable?

Ans. The live-attenuated JE vaccine (SA-14-14-2) can be administered interchangeably with JEEV™ as well as JENVAC™ vaccine in the interest of the immunization program.

However, there is a need to generate data on the interchangeability of JE vaccines.

SUGGESTED READING

1. Advisory Committee on Vaccines and Immunization Practices (ACVIP), Vashishtha VM, Choudhury P, Bansal CP, Yewale VN, Agarwal R. (2014). IAP guidebook on Immunization 2013-2014. [online] Available from: https://iapindia.org/pdf/IAP-Guidebook-on-Immunization-2013-14.pdf. [Last accessed November, 2020].

2. Advisory Committee on Vaccines and Immunization Practices, Indian Academy of Pediatrics. (2020). IAP guidebook on Immunization 2018–2019. [online] Available from: https://iapindia.org/pdf/124587-IAP-GUIDE-BOOK-ON-IMMUNIZATION-18-19.pdf. [Last accessed November, 2020].
3. Centre for Health Informatics (CHI), set up at National Institute of Health and Family Welfare (NIHFW), by the Ministry of Health and Family Welfare (MoHFW), Government of India. (2018). Universal Immunisation Programme. [online] Available from: https://www.nhp.gov.in/universal-immunisation-programme_pg. [Last accessed November, 2020].
4. Government of India, Ministry of Health & Family Welfare, Directorate General of Health Services. (2014). National Programme for Prevention and Control of Japanese Encephalitis/Acute Encephalitis Syndrome. [online] Available from: https://nvbdcp.gov.in/Doc/JE-AES-Prevention-Control(NPPCJA).pdf. [Last accessed November, 2020].
5. Kanagasabai K, Joshua V, Ravi M, Sabarinathan R, Kirubakaran BK, Ramachandran V, et al. Epidemiology of Japanese encephalitis in India: analysis of laboratory surveillance data, 2014–17. J Infect. 2018;76(3):317-20.
6. The Centers for Disease Control and Prevention (CDC). (2019). Japanese Encephalitis: CDC on JE Vaccine Information Statement Vaccine information. [online] Available from: https://www.cdc.gov/japaneseencephalitis/vaccine/index.html. [Last accessed November, 2020].
7. U.S. Department of Health and Human Services (HHS). (2020). Japanese Encephalitis (JE). [online] Available from: https://www.vaccines.gov/diseases/je [Last accessed November, 2020].
8. World Health Organization. (2015). WHO position paper on JE vaccine 2015. [online] Available from: https://www.who.int/immunization/policy/position_papers/japanese_encephalitis/en/ [Last accessed November, 2020].

CHAPTER 29

Cholera Vaccines

Arun Kumar Manglik

Q1. What is cholera and how much does it affect us?

Ans. Cholera is an intestinal infection caused by a bacterium *Vibrio cholerae* (*V. cholerae*) serogroups O1 and O139. It causes very rapid dehydration when severe, with a mortality of over 40% in the prerehydration therapy era. Being a water-borne disease, good sanitation and availability of potable water have significantly reduced the incidence. Worldwide annual reported incidence has varied widely with about 1–3 million cases and about 50,000–95,000 deaths, though in 2015, only 172,454 cases were reported to WHO with 1,304 deaths. There is a fair possibility of significant under reporting. Asia and Africa are the predominantly affected regions. In India, during the 10-year period 1997–2006, 222,038 cases were reported, while over a 5-year period 2010–2015, the cumulative incidence was 27,615 cases with West Bengal, Assam, Jammu and Kashmir, Punjab, and Karnataka among the most affected states.

Q2. What are the various cholera vaccines?

Ans. Two types of vaccines are known injectable and oral.

Presently, all over the world, only the oral cholera vaccines (OCVs) are in clinical usage.

There are three OCVs:
1. *A killed WC-rCTB* (killed whole-cell with cholera toxin subunit B) containing killed whole cells of *Vibrio cholerae* plus recombinant cholera toxin B subunit developed in Sweden and in market since 1990. This vaccine is WHO prequalified. It is marketed as Dukoral™. This is not marketed in India.
2. *A live CVD103-HgR* used in the Americas is available since 1994 and was withdrawn for commercial reasons. Vaxchora™ was redeveloped and produced and is approved in the United States of America for use in adults aged 18–64 years traveling to cholera-affected areas.
3. And, a *killed whole-cell-bivalent vaccine* effective against both *Vibrio cholerae* O1 and O139 is presently available in India. It was licensed in India in 2009, and received WHO prequalification in 2011. The same formulation is available in other countries as Euvichol® and mORCVAX™.

Q3. What is the composition of the presently used "oral cholera" vaccine in India?

Ans. The killed whole-cell-bivalent vaccine available in India is unique in its bivalent character (both strain O1 and O139). The vaccine contains:

(a) 600 enzyme-linked immunosorbent assay (ELISA) units of lipopolysaccharide (LPS) of formalin killed V. Cholerae O1 El Tor Inaba (strain Phil 6973)
(b) 300 ELISA units of LPS of heat killed *V. cholerae* O1 classical Ogawa (strain Cairo 50)
(c) 300 ELISA units of LPS of formalin killed *V. cholerae* O1 classical Ogawa (strain Cairo 50)
(d) 300 ELISA units of LPS of heat killed *V. cholerae* O1 classical Ogawa (strain Cairo 48), and
(e) 600 units of formalin killed *V. cholerae* O139 (strain 4260B).

It contains minimal amounts of thiomersal. The vaccine is free of any cholera toxin and comes as 1.5 mL liquid suspension.

Q4. What are the presentation, doses, and storage criteria with the oral vaccines?

Ans. Killed oral whole-cell-bivalent vaccine is given in two doses 2 weeks apart. Revaccination is recommended where there is continued risk of *V. cholera*e infection. For the killed WC vaccines, revaccination is recommended after 3 years. It comes as a 1.5 mL ready to use liquid suspension in a glass bottle, to be stored at 2–8°C, and must not be frozen. This is the only vaccine currently available in India.

Dose: Given as two doses 2 weeks apart.

In a study in Bangladesh, the vaccine was found to maintain its efficacy even when exposed to temperatures up to 42°C for 14 days, but that is not recommended as a practice. The bottle needs to be vigorously shaken and then administered directly into the mouth of the vaccine recipient.

Q5. How immunogenic or protective are these newer oral vaccines?

Ans. There is no definite known serologic correlate nor a serological surrogate of protection. Various parameters measured include (i) serum anti-vibriocidal, (ii) serum antitoxin antibodies, (iii) serum antiliposaccharide antibodies, and (iv) intestinal immunoglobulin A (IgA) antibodies. Immune response is widely measured by serum vibriocidal antibody titer. Studies have shown that the risk of cholera declines with rising titers of serum vibriocidal antibody.

The *killed oral whole-cell-bivalent* vaccine available in India induces anti-O1 vibriocidal antibody titers up to sixfold (as seen in a large trial involving 69,328 persons aged 1 year and above in Kolkata), and thus titers are better than the WC-rCTB vaccines. The anti-O139 vibriocidal titers are only twofold. The second dose of this vaccine did not add to the antibody titer levels, thus studies are on to consider giving only a single dose of this vaccine. Postvaccination there is a 65% protection for 5 years with the highest rates in those >15 years of age, but only 42% in children below 5 years of age. This clinical protection existed during the postvaccine surveillance period despite the anti-vibriocidal antibody titers showing a fall after 1 year of postvaccination.

Q6. What are the adverse effects or contraindications of the vaccines?

Ans. Killed whole-cell-bivalent vaccine is quite safe. Nausea, vomiting, diarrhea, weakness, dryness of mouth, vertigo, oral ulcers, and yellowish urine are some of the known side effects. In human immunodeficiency virus (HIV) positive individuals, safety of the vaccine has not been evaluated, but should be safe in view of vaccine containing no live organisms. Of course, the efficacy may be compromised in immunodeficient persons.

Q7. What are ACVIP (IAP) schedules and recommendations of cholera vaccines?

Ans. Cholera vaccines are recommended for use only in special situations, e.g., travel to or residence in a highly endemic area or where there is a risk of outbreaks, e.g., "Kumbh Mela". The schedule should be completed two weeks prior to travel.

Q8. What is the impact of cholera vaccines on public health?

Ans. The killed whole-cell-bivalent vaccine is currently stockpiled by the World Health Organization (WHO) for exigencies. In view of the good efficacy and safety of the current cholera vaccines the WHO suggests to consider the following: (i) the risk of cholera in the targeted populations, (ii) risk of geographical spread, (iii) the programmatic capability to cover as many eligible persons as possible, and (iv) and that no such program had been carried out in the last 3 years, as then a renewed program may not be needed.

The WHO also suggests that in view of the short-term protection data available, only a single dose strategy may be considered to control outbreaks. A fair degree of herd immunity developing following vaccine coverage at even 60% has been demonstrated in Bangladesh on use of whole-cell-bivalent vaccine. Obviously, vaccination without other sanitation measures will be meaningless.

■ SUGGESTED READING

1. Advisory Committee on Vaccines and Immunization Practices, Indian Academy of Pediatrics. IAP Guidebook on Immunizations, 2018-2019, 3rd edition. New Delhi: Jaypee Brothers Medical Publishers (P) Ltd.; 2020. pp. 1-516.
2. Bhattacharya SK, Sur D, Ali M, Kanungo S, You YA, Manna B, et al. 5-year efficacy of a bivalent killed whole-cell oral cholera vaccine in Kolkata, India: a cluster-randomised, double-blind, placebo-controlled trial. Lancet Infect Dis. 2013;13:1050-6.
3. World Health Organization. Cholera vaccines: WHO position paper—August 2017. Weekly epidemiological record No. 34. 2017;92:477-500.

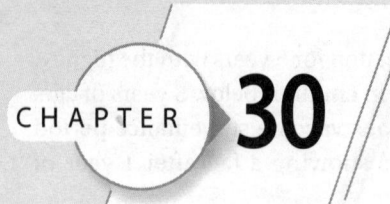

CHAPTER 30: Yellow Fever Vaccine

Rupesh Masand

Q1. What is yellow fever?

Ans. Yellow fever is an acute hemorrhagic disease caused by a ribonucleic acid (RNA) virus of genus *Flavivirus* and transmitted by the bite of infected *Aedes* and *Haemagogus* mosquitoes in Africa and South America, respectively. The "yellow" in the name refers to the jaundice that affects some patients. The mosquitoes either breed around houses (domestic), in the jungle (wild) or in both habitats (semidomestic). It carries the virus from one host to another, primarily between monkeys, from monkeys to humans, and from person to person **(Fig. 1)**.

Q2. Name the countries in which yellow fever is endemic or has prevailed as an epidemic.

Ans. Yellow fever is endemic in the tropical and subtropical parts of Africa, South America, and Central America. The following 43 countries have high incidence of yellow fever cases:

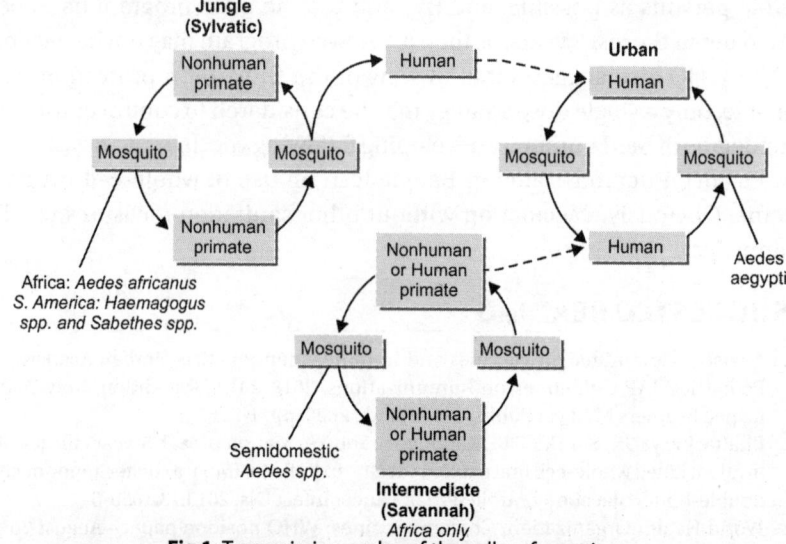

Fig 1: Transmission cycles of the yellow fever virus.
(*Courtesy:* Centre for disease control and prevention)

Africa: Angola, Benin, Burkina Faso, Burundi, Cameroon, Cape Verde, Central African Republic, Chad, Congo, Côte d'Ivoire, Democratic Republic of the Congo, Equatorial Guinea, Ethiopia, Gabon, Gambia, Ghana, Guinea, Guinea-Bissau, Kenya, Liberia, Mali, Niger, Nigeria, Rwanda, Sao tome and Principe, Senegal, Sierra Leone, Sudan, Togo, and Uganda.

Americas: Argentina, Bolivia, Brazil, Colombia, Ecuador, French Guiana, Guyana, Panama, Paraguay, Peru, Suriname, Trinidad and Tobago, and Venezuela.

The notified countries are altered by the World Health Organization (WHO), from time to time. Hence, a traveler should consult the latest guidelines to assess the need for yellow fever vaccine.

As evident, yellow fever cases have not been observed or reported in India.

Q3. If India does not feature in the list of affected countries, then why health authorities in India need to be cautious regarding yellow fever?

Ans. The health authorities in India need to be cautious regarding prevention of yellow fever in the country due to the following reasons:
- Presence of vector for the yellow fever virus—*Aedes Aegypti* is widespread in India.
- Conducive environmental conditions.
- Possibility of the spread of the virus by its carriage in unvaccinated and affected travelers from endemic countries to India.
- Difficulty in recognition of imported cases as clinical manifestations mimics dengue and other similar flaviviral infections.
- Poor surveillance mechanisms to handle situations of epidemic magnitude.

Therefore, strict regulations have been enforced to prevent entry of unvaccinated travelers visiting India from yellow fever endemic countries. Similarly, vaccination is mandatory for Indian citizens travelling to these countries.

Q4. What are the clinical features of yellow fever?

Ans. The clinical manifestations of yellow fever range from an asymptomatic infection to multiorgan failure and death. Majority of the infections are asymptomatic. Most symptomatic cases commonly experience a self-limiting febrile illness associated with myalgia, back pain, and prostration. The fever, which lasts about 4 days, is accompanied by high levels of viremia, thus increasing the risk for mosquito infection during its blood meal.

Approximately 15–25% of infected individuals progress to develop a multisystem disease dominated by hepatorenal failure, profound jaundice, and bleeding manifestations after a brief remission of fever. Death has been observed in 20–50% of these cases, usually 7–10 days after onset of the disease. Morbidity in survivors is significant with a prolonged convalescent phase characterized by weakness and fatigue.

Q5. What is the treatment of yellow fever?

Ans. There is no specific drug available for treatment of yellow fever. Symptomatic management involves bed rest, fluids, antipyretics or analgesics. Further progression to multiorgan involvement may necessitate hospitalization and intensive care. Certain medications need to be avoided, e.g., aspirin and nonsteroidal anti-inflammatory drugs (NSAIDs) as they increase the risk of bleeding.

Q6. What are the preventive measures applicable for yellow fever?

Ans. Yellow fever can be prevented by following methods:
- *Vaccination*: The current commercially available vaccine is a freeze-dried, live attenuated viral vaccine from the 17D lineage, developed more than 80 years ago by empirical passage of a wild-type yellow fever virus (isolated in Ghana in 1927) in tissue culture, principally chicken 140 embryo cells. Numerous mutations in the viral structural and nonstructural genes have led to the attenuated variant 17D, which is nontransmissible by mosquitoes. The currently available vaccine has been considered most effective and safe for prevention of yellow fever. Each dose must contain at least 1,000 international units (IUs) and there is no maximum quantity of virus in a dose. Usually a dose contains anywhere from 4,000 to 1 million IUs.
- Use of insect repellants.
- Wearing full sleeves shirts and full-length trousers all through the day.

Q7. Who should receive the Yellow fever vaccine?

Ans. This vaccine is not meant for routine vaccination in India. The vaccine is indicated in the following groups:
- All travelers of age > 9 months and travelling to/from yellow fever endemic zones
- All children of age 9–12 months and above in yellow fever endemic countries.
- In the event of an outbreak in these countries, all unvaccinated infants of age 6–8 months are also vaccinated. All unvaccinated children ≥ 9 months of age should be vaccinated as usual.
  The WHO recommends that all endemic countries should introduce yellow fever vaccine into their routine immunization programs.

Q8. How is the yellow fever vaccine administered and stored?

Ans. This vaccine is administered as a single dose of 0.5 mL subcutaneously or intramuscularly in lateral aspect of the upper arm or the anterolateral aspect of the thigh in babies and young children.

The freeze-dried vaccine is available in single and multidose vials, which should be stored at 2–8°C along with sterile saline as diluent. As the reconstituted vaccine is heat-labile, it must protected from sunlight, stored at the same temperature, and discarded within 1 hour of reconstitution.

Q9. What is the procedure for validation of vaccination for travelers to countries endemic for yellow fever?

Ans. The following are the guidelines:
- An International Certificate of Vaccination or Prophylaxis (ICVP) duly dated, stamped, and signed by the center administering the vaccine, is issued to each vaccinee as per International Health Regulations (IHR).
- All travelers must visit the embassy of their destination country (endemic for yellow fever) and submit the ICVP before departure.
- In May 2014, the World Health Assembly adopted an amendment to Annex 7 of the IHR (2005), which stipulated that the period of protection afforded by yellow fever vaccination, and the term of validity of the ICVP has changed from 10 years to the duration of the life of the person vaccinated.
- On 11 July 2016, the amended IHR Annex 7 entered into force and is legally binding upon all IHR States Parties. Thus, *from 11 July 2016, the ICVP against yellow fever is valid for the life of the person vaccinated.* This lifetime validity applies automatically to all existing and new certificates, beginning 10 days after the date of vaccination.
- Accordingly, as of 11 July 2016, revaccination or a booster dose of yellow fever vaccine will not be required for international travelers as a condition of entry into a State Party, regardless of the date that their international certificate of vaccination was initially issued.
- If the above procedure for validation is not followed, then travelers may be quarantined, denied entry or can be revaccinated in their destination country at the point of entry (airport/seaport).
- If due to medical contraindications, the physician at the vaccination center can issue a waiver by filling out and signing the Medical Contraindications to Vaccination section of the ICVP. However, the traveler must be advised that the issued waiver may not be acceptable to the destination country leading to their quarantine, refusal of entry or even vaccination at their airport.
- Under the IHR, any changes, deletions, erasures, or additions may cause an ICVP to be rendered invalid.
- Further specific guidelines in relation to yellow fever for international travelers are available on the WHO International Travel and Health website: Annexure 1 and country list and the Pan American Health Organization (PAHO) yellow fever website.

Q10. What are the guidelines for travelers entering India from countries endemic for yellow fever?

Ans. Any traveler with the exception of infants <9 months old, arriving by air or sea to India without a certificate is detained (quarantined) in isolation for up to 6 days if that person:
- Arrives within 6 days of departure from a residential area in a country with risk of yellow fever virus transmission.
- Has actually visited that area while in transit (except those passengers and members of flight crew who, while in transit through an airport in a country with risk of yellow fever virus transmission, remained in the airport during their entire stay and the health officer agrees to such an exemption).
- Arrives on a ship that started from or touched at any port in a country with risk of yellow fever virus transmission up to 30 days before its arrival in India, unless such a ship has been disinfected in accordance with the procedure recommended by WHO, or
- Arrives on an aircraft that has been in a country with risk of yellow fever virus transmission and has not been disinfected in accordance with the Indian Aircraft Public Health Rules, 1954, or as recommended by WHO.

Q11. What are the contraindications and precautions observed in relation with yellow fever vaccination?

Ans. These are as follows:

Contraindications	Precautions
Allergy to vaccine component	Age 6–8 months
Age < 6 months	Age ≥ 60 years
Symptomatic human immunodeficiency virus (HIV) infection or CD4 T lymphocyte count < 200/mm^3 (or less than 15% of the total in <6-year-old child	Asymptomatic HIV infection and CD4 T lymphocyte count 200–499/mm^3 (or between 15 and 24% of the total in <6-year-old child
Thymus disorder associated with abnormal immune cell function	Pregnancy
Primary immunodeficiency	Breastfeeding
Malignant neoplasm	
Transplantation	
Immunosuppressive therapy	

Q12. What is the immunogenicity and efficacy profile of yellow fever vaccine?

Ans. Immunogenicity and efficacy are greater than 90%. Clinical trials have found that 80–100% of vaccine recipients develop protective levels of neutralizing antibodies within 10 days and 99% do so within 30 days. Protection appears to last at least 20–35 years and probably for life.

Since the introduction of yellow fever vaccination in the 1930s, and following the administration of >540 million doses of vaccine since then, only 12 suspected cases of yellow fever disease postvaccination have been identified. All 12 cases involved vaccine recipients who developed symptoms within 5 years of vaccination, and were therefore highly unlikely to reflect secondary vaccine failures due to waning immunity. Factors that have been associated with failure to respond immunologically to yellow fever vaccine include human immunodeficiency virus (HIV) infection, pregnancy, and malnutrition.

Q13. What are the adverse effects of the yellow fever vaccine?

Ans. The mild adverse effects of the yellow fever vaccine are headache, myalgia, low-grade fever, discomfort at the injection site, pruritus, urticaria, and rash, which may be observed in 10–30% of vaccinees lasting up to 5–10 days after vaccination. Female vaccinees report more local adverse events than males, while the incidence of systemic adverse events is higher in males.

The severe adverse events following immunization fall into three categories are as follows:
1. Anaphylactic reactions have been estimated to occur in 0.8 per 100,000 vaccinations, most commonly in children allergic to eggs or gelatin.
2. Yellow fever vaccine-associated neurologic disease (YEL-AND) is due to either direct viral invasion of the central nervous system by the vaccine virus resulting in meningitis or encephalitis, or to an autoimmune reaction resulting in Guillain–Barré syndrome or acute disseminated encephalomyelitis. It usually appears 3–28 days after vaccination in first time vaccinees and is rarely fatal. The reported rate for YEL-AND is 0.25–0.8 per 100,000 vaccine doses. It is higher in the elderly aged > 60 years.
3. Yellow fever vaccine-associated viscerotropic disease (YEL-AVD) is due to replication and dissemination of the vaccine virus in a manner similar to the natural virus. YEL-AVD cases typically develop organ system dysfunction or failure in >60% of cases and have been observed to be fatal. The reported rate of YEL-AVD is 0.25–0.4 per 100,000 vaccine doses.

Q14. Where can one get vaccinated for yellow fever in India?

Ans. As of March 2017, there are total 41 yellow fever vaccination centers in India. Out of these, 17 (41.46%) are in West zone, 9 each (21.95%) are in the North and South zone, and 3 each (7.32%) in Central and East Zone. The complete address and contact details of each authorized yellow fever vaccination center can be accessed online at *https://mohfw.gov.in*. The vaccination charges as approved by the Ministry of Health and Family Welfare, Government of India is INR 300 per dose.

Q15. How long a woman should wait to conceive after receiving the yellow fever vaccine?

Ans. Yellow fever vaccine, being a live virus vaccine has not been found to be associated with any fetal anomalies when administered inadvertently or out of necessity during the first trimester of pregnancy. However, owing to a theoretical risk, a 2-week delay between yellow fever vaccination and conception has been advocated rather than a 1-month delay as suggested by some. A risk-benefit assessment has been recommended in all pregnant and lactating mothers.

Q16. After having received yellow fever vaccination, is it mandatory to avoid contact with an immunocompromised family member?

Ans. There is no evidence that the recipients of the yellow fever vaccination shed the yellow fever virus in their body secretions. Therefore, there is no need to avoid any kind of contact with an immunocompromised person.

Q17. Which vaccines may be coadministered with the yellow fever vaccine?

Ans. Yellow fever vaccine may be administered simultaneously with all other vaccines. As a general rule, any live vaccine may be given either simultaneously or at an interval of 4 weeks. The most notable exception was identified in a study of simultaneous administration of yellow fever vaccine and the combined measles, mumps, and rubella vaccine (MMR) in children 12–23 months of age, which observed a significant decrease in the seroconversion rates and geometric mean titers obtained against yellow fever, mumps, and rubella in the recipients. However, no decrease in response was observed against measles. Separating MMR and yellow fever vaccine administration by 30 days mitigated the effect.

Q18. Where is the yellow fever vaccine produced in India?

Ans. The yellow fever vaccine is produced in the country by Central Research Institute (CRI), Kasauli and supplied to various recognized yellow fever vaccination centers. In case of emergency or breakdown of vaccine production/supply, vaccine procurement by CRI, Kasauli is done through WHO and then supplied to various vaccination centers.

■ SUGGESTED READING

1. CDC. (2010). Yellow Fever Vaccine: Recommendations of the Advisory Committee on Immunization Practices (ACIP). [online] Available from https://www.cdc.gov/mmwr/preview/mmwrhtml/rr5907a1.htm. [Last accessed October, 2020].
2. Guduru VK. Yellow fever vaccine. In: Balasubramanian S, Shastri DD, Shah AK, Chatterjee P, Pemde HK, S Shivananda, Guduru VK (Eds). IAP Guidebook on Immunization 2018-2019, 3rd edition. New Delhi: Jaypee Brothers Medical Publishers (P) Ltd; 2019. pp. 387-95.

3. MoHFW. (2017). List of Authorized Yellow fever Vaccine Centres in India as on 10th March, 2017. [online] Available from https://main.mohfw.gov.in/sites/default/files/List%20of%20Authorised%20Yellow%20fever%20Vaccination%20centres.pdf. [Last accessed October, 2020].
4. Vaccines and vaccination against yellow fever; WHO Position Paper—June 2013. Wkly Epidemiol Rec. 2013;88:269-84.
5. World Health Organization (WHO). (2016). New yellow fever vaccination requirements for travelers. [online] Available from https://www.who.int/ith/updates/20160727/en/. [Last accessed October, 2020].

CHAPTER 31

Zoster Vaccines

Srinivas G Kasi

Q1. What is zoster (shingles)?

Ans. Herpes zoster (HZ) is caused by the reactivation of the varicella zoster virus (VZV), generally in an individual with a past infection with varicella. The clinical manifestation in an immune competent individual is a unilateral vesicular rash, restricted to a single dermatome, which is usually accompanied by radicular pain along that dermatome. Characteristic features include significant pain, burning at the site of reactivation. Postherpetic pain or neuralgia and discomfort may last for weeks, months or even years in severe cases, diminishing the quality of life.

Q2. Who is at risk for developing zoster?

Ans. The risk of developing shingles increases with age and is increased in people who are immunocompromised. There is an exponential increase in incidence after the age of 50 years, which correlates with aging-related decline in cell-mediated immunity (CMI). The risk of developing postherpetic neuralgia (PHN) also increases with age and is highest in adults over 70 years of age. There are no population-based studies from India, on the incidence of zoster. About 15% of zoster cases occur in children who are immune compromised or are exposed to varicella in utero. Immune compromised hosts tend to develop severe zoster with multiple dermatomal involvement, progressive illness, and recurrent episodes of zoster.

Q3. What are the complications of zoster?

Ans. In the majority, zoster is a self-limiting infection lasting for 10–15 days. PHN is the most common serious complication of HZ. PHN is defined as pain that persists for more than 90 days after rash onset. PHN, which is difficult to treat, may have a significant effect on the quality of life.

About 20% of patients with HZ will develop PHN. The most important risk factor for development of PHN is age, with most cases occurring in adults over 40 years of age and adults over 70 years having a four times increased risk of PHN than those younger than 60 years. Other serious complications include pneumonia; hearing loss; ocular zoster with blepharitis, ocular palsy, corneal ulceration, and blindness; encephalitis; strokes;

transient ischemic attacks (TIAs); or even death. Studies from India have shown that the incidence of PHN varies from 10.2 to 14.5% overall with the highest incidence in those >60 years, being 31.25–77%.

Q4. Is there any treatment for zoster?

Ans. Prompt antiviral therapy, if initiated within 72 hours of rash onset, may favorably modify the course of illness and reduce the incidence of PHN, in healthy as well as immunocompromised patients. Treatment is usually given for 7 days in the absence of complications of HZ. For immunocompromised persons who require hospitalization and in case of severe neurologic complications intravenous acyclovir is recommended. Management of acute pain associated with HZ may be treated with nonsteroidal anti-inflammatory drugs (NSAIDs) or opioids. Acyclovir, valacyclovir, and famciclovir are the antivirals used for treatment.

Q5. What are the vaccines available against zoster?

Ans. There are two different vaccines available to prevent zoster:
1. Live zoster vaccine (ZVL; Zostavax, Merck), which is a live attenuated vaccine.
2. Recombinant zoster vaccine (RZV; Shingrix, GlaxoSmithKline) contains a single genetically engineered protein, glycoprotein E (gE) that is essential for replication and intercellular spread of the virus and which is a target for the specific immune response. This vaccine is adjuvanted with AS01B that induces innate immunity as well enhances CMI and humoral response. This is not a live vaccine.

Q6. What are the characteristics of the ZVL?

Ans. This vaccine is a lyophilized preparation of the Oka/Merck strain of live, attenuated VZV, propagated in human diploid cell cultures (WI-38). Each 0.65 mL dose contains minimum of 19,400 plaque-forming units (PFU) of Oka/Merck VZV, which is 14 times the minimum potency of Oka/Merck varicella vaccine.

Each dose also contains 41.05 mg of sucrose, 20.53 mg of hydrolyzed porcine gelatin, 8.55 mg of urea, 5.25 mg of sodium chloride, 0.82 mg of monosodium L-glutamate, 0.75 mg of sodium phosphate dibasic, 0.13 mg of potassium phosphate monobasic, and 0.13 mg of potassium chloride; residual components of Medical Research Council cell strain 5 (MRC-5) cells including deoxyribonucleic acid (DNA) and protein; and trace quantities of neomycin and bovine calf serum. The product contains no preservatives.

Q7. What are the recommendations for its clinical usage?

Ans. This vaccine is recommended for subcutaneous administration, in a single dose, for prevention of HZ (shingles), prevention of PHN and reduction of acute and chronic zoster-associated pain [burden of disease (BoD)], in individuals 50 years of age and older, regardless of a prior episode of HZ.

Zostavax is contraindicated in those with history of anaphylactic/anaphylactoid reaction to gelatin, neomycin, or any other component of the vaccine, those who are immunosuppressed, in pregnant women, and those with active untreated tuberculosis. ZVL and pneumococcal polysaccharide vaccine should not be given concomitantly because concomitant use resulted in reduced immunogenicity of ZVL as the antiglycoprotein enzyme-linked immunosorbent assay (gpELISA) geometric mean titer (GMT) 4 weeks postvaccination are 30% lower if given concomitantly with PPSV23 compared to when given 4 weeks apart. Hence, they should be given at least 4 weeks apart. Pregnancy should be avoided for at least 3 months following ZLV administration.

Q8. How is ZVL stored?

Ans. Zoster vaccine live should be stored at a temperature of 2–8°C until it is reconstituted for injection. The diluent should be stored separately in the refrigerator (2–8°C, 36–46°F). It should be protected from light.

The reconstituted vaccine should be used within 30 minutes, otherwise it should be discarded. The reconstituted vaccine should not be frozen again.

Q9. What is the immunogenicity of this vaccine?

Ans. The magnitude of the vaccine-induced boost in antibody and VZV-CMI responses is also a function of age, and overall the boost in immune response was significantly less in persons 70 years of age or older than in younger vaccinees.

The peak boost in VZV-CMI occurs at 1–3 weeks after zoster vaccination. The magnitude of the boost in VZV-CMI declined by 40–50% in the first year postvaccination and then remained constant in the second and third year.

In the Zostavax Efficacy and Safety Trial (ZEST) study, VZV antibody levels (GMT), as measured by gpELISA, 6 weeks postvaccination, were increased 2.3-fold [95% confidence interval (CI): 2.2, 2.4] in the group of subjects who received Zostavax compared to subjects who received placebo; the specific antibody level that correlates with protection from zoster has not been established.

Shingles Prevention Study (SPS) was done in >60-year-old subjects. Immune responses to vaccination were evaluated in a subset of 1,395 subjects. Immune response in form of gpELISA 6 weeks postvaccination increased 1.7-fold (95% CI: 1.6–1.8) in vaccinees compared to placebo.

Zoster vaccine live was given in three different double-blind placebo-controlled studies; in first study ZVL or a placebo was studied in persons with past history of shingles, in second study ZVL or a placebo was given to subjects receiving 5–20 mg of oral prednisolone for a period of at least 2 weeks prior to and 6 weeks after the vaccination, and in the third study two doses of

ZVL or placebo were given 6 weeks apart to human immunodeficiency virus (HIV) infected subjects who were on antiretroviral therapy (ART) with CD4+ counts of >200/cumm. In all these three studies the anti-gpELISA GMT were higher in vaccinees compared to placebo. It was 2.1-fold higher compared to placebo when ZVL is given to subjects with past history of shingles, 2.1-fold higher with ZVL compared to placebo in subjects on steroids and 1.8-fold higher following first as well as second dose of ZVL compared to placebo when given to HIV-infected subjects on ART with CD4+ counts of >200/cumm.

Q10. What is the efficacy of this vaccine?

Ans. The efficacy of this vaccine was highest in those <60 years and lowest in those >80 years. **Table 1** shows short-term and 5-year long-term efficacy data from the ZEST and the SPS studies.

Q11. Is there any effectiveness data on ZVL?

Ans. Zoster vaccine live was licensed in USA in 2006 for those >60 years and in 2011 for those 50–59 years for prevention of shingles. Vaccine effectiveness was studied over 8 years from 2007 to 2014 at Kaiser Permanente, Northern California. 1.4 million people were age eligible for the vaccine during the study period. 392,677 (29%) actually received the zoster vaccine. During 5.8 million person-years of follow-up, 48,889 cases of shingles were observed, including 5,766 among vaccinees. Vaccine efficacy (VE) was 49.1% (95% CI: 47.5, 50.6) across 8 years of follow-up, 67.5% (95% CI: 65.4, 69.5) in the first year, 47.2% (95% CI: 44.1, 50.1) in the second year and then waned gradually through year 8, when VE was 31.8% (95% CI: 15.1, 45.2).

Table 1: Short-term and long-term efficacy data.

	Vaccine efficacy% (VE) with CIs		Long-term effectiveness study	
	Against HZ incidence	Against PHN incidence	Against HZ	Against PHN fifth year
50–59 years	69.8 (54.1–80.6) 1.3 years median FU		36% (95% CI: –55, 73) third year	
60–69 years	65.5 (51.5–75.5) 3.1 year median FU	5% (–107%, 56%)	34% (95% CI: 25, 42) fifth year	61% (95% CI: 33, 77)
70–79 years	41% (28%, 52%) 3.1 year median FU	55% (18%, 76%)	29% (95% CI: 18, 38) fifth year	69% (95% CI: 44, 82)
>80 years	18% (–29%, 48%) 3.1 years median FU	26% (–69%, 68%)	36% (95% CI: 12, 53) fifth year	34% (95% CI: –49, 71)

(CI: confidence interval; FU: follow-up; HZ: herpes zoster; PHN: postherpetic neuralgia)

Q12. What is the adverse effects profile of this vaccine?

Ans. In ZEST study, the overall incidence of vaccine-related injection-site adverse reactions within 5 days postvaccination was greater for subjects vaccinated with Zostavax (63.6%) as compared to subjects who received placebo (14.0%) and when compared to the placebo included mainly pain (53.9% vs. 9%), redness (48.1% vs. 4.3%), and swelling (40.4% vs. 2.8%). The overall incidence of systemic adverse experiences reported during days 1–42 was higher for Zostavax (35.4%) than for placebo (33.5%).

In SPS, the overall injection site side effects were more with Zostavax (48%) compared to the placebo (17%) and mainly included redness (35.6% vs. 6.9%), pain (34.3% vs. 8.3%) and swelling (26.1% vs. 4.5%). Most of the systemic side effects such as headache or fever were similar between Zostavax and placebo.

In all the three studies as outlined above, side effect profile was similar to that seen in SPS. In another study, a second dose of ZVL was given at 6 weeks following first dose. Again the side effect profile was similar to that seen in SPS study.

Q13. Can ZLV lead to rash?

Ans. In ZEST study, nonvaccine site zoster like rash developed within 42 days of the vaccine or placebo in 19/11,094 vaccinees and 15/11,116 placebo and none of these were due to vaccine virus. Varicella like rash developed within 42 days in 69/11,094 vaccinees and 55/11,116 placebo and again none of them was because of vaccine virus.

Q14. What are the characteristics of the RZV (Shingrix™)?

Ans. This vaccine is not available in India at present. The active antigen, which is recombinant surface gE antigen, is supplied in a freeze-dried form. This has to be reconstituted at the time of use with the accompanying vial of AS01B adjuvant suspension component. The gE antigen is obtained by culturing genetically engineered Chinese hamster ovary cells, which carry a truncated gE gene.

The liquid part for reconstitution comprises the adjuvant AS01B which is composed of 3-O-desacyl-4'-monophosphoryl lipid A (MPL) from *Salmonella minnesota* and QS-21, a saponin purified from plant extract *Quillaja saponaria* Molina, combined in a liposomal formulation.

After reconstitution, each 0.5-mL dose contains 50 µg of the recombinant gE antigen, 50 µg of MPL, and 50 µg of QS-21. The other constituents are 20 mg of sucrose (as stabilizer), 4.385 mg of sodium chloride, 1 mg of 1,2-Dioleoyl-sn-glycero-3-phosphocholine (DOPC), 0.54 mg of potassium dihydrogen phosphate, 0.25 mg of cholesterol, 0.160 mg of sodium dihydrogen phosphate dihydrate, 0.15 mg of disodium phosphate anhydrous, 0.116 mg of dipotassium phosphate, and 0.08 mg of polysorbate 80.

Q15. What is the immunogenicity data with RZV?

Ans. The gE-specific cell-mediated immune response was 3.8 times higher than the prevaccination value (477.3 vs. 119.4 activated gE-specific CD4+ T cells per 106 cells), and the anti-gE antibody concentration was 7.3 times higher than the prevaccination value (8,159.0 vs. 1,121.3 mIU/mL). It is indicated for prevention of HZ (shingles) in adults aged 50 years and older.

Q16. What is the schedule and route of administration of RZV?

Ans. The schedule is to administer two doses (0.5 mL each) at 0 and 2–6 months. However, if more than 6 months have passed since first dose there is no need to restart vaccination schedule. If second dose is given <4 weeks after the first dose, the dose is considered as invalid. It is given intramuscularly. Advisory Committee on Immunization Practices (ACIP)/USA recommends to give one dose of RZV to all those who have taken ZVL in past, minimum gap between ZVL and RZV should be 2 months. It is equally immunogenic when given subcutaneously but more reactogenic. Hence, intramuscular (IM) route is preferred. After reconstitution, the vaccine should be administered immediately or stored between 2 and 8°C (36 and 46°F) and use within 6 hours. If not used within 6 hours, the vaccine is to be discarded. It does not contain any preservative.

Q17. Can RZV be coadministered with other vaccines?

Ans. Recombinant zoster vaccine can be coadministered with influenza vaccine. In certain European countries, it is also approved for coadministration with PPSV23 and Tdap.

Q18. What are the contraindications for RZV?

Ans. The vaccine is contraindicated in those with a history of severe allergic reaction (e.g., anaphylaxis) to any component of the vaccine or after a previous dose of RZV. RZV is not indicated during pregnancy, lactation or in pediatric age group.

Q19. What is the efficacy of this vaccine?

Ans. The efficacy of this vaccine was studied in two studies, randomized, placebo-controlled, and observer-blind clinical study conducted in 18 countries. First study was conducted in >50 years old and second study was in those >70 years of age **(Table 2)**. Subjects were followed for the development of HZ and PHN for a median of 3.1 years (range: 0–3.7 years). The VE in the fourth year was 93.1% (95% CI: 81.3, 98.2).

Among all subjects aged 50 years or older in the modified total vaccinated cohort (mTVC), no cases of PHN were reported in the vaccine group compared with 18 cases reported in the placebo group.

In second study on subjects >70 years, VE against PHN was 85.5% (95% CI: 58.5, 96.3).

Table 2: Age-wise vaccine efficacy.

Age group	Vaccine efficacy (%)
Study 1 results	
>50 years—overall	97.2 (93.7, 99.0)
50–59 years	96.6 (89.6, 99.3)
60–69 years	97.4 (90.1, 99.7)
Combined study 1 and 2 results in >70 years old subjects	
>70 years—overall	91.3 (86.9, 94.5)
70–79 years	91.3 (86.0, 94.9)
>80 years	91.4 (80.2, 96.9)

Q20. What is the adverse effects profile of this vaccine?

Ans. Solicited local adverse reaction and each solicited general adverse event following administration of RZV (both doses combined) seen in two main efficacy trials were pain (78.0%), redness (38.1%), and swelling (25.9%); and myalgia (44.7%), fatigue (44.5%), headache (37.7%), shivering (26.8%), fever (20.5%), and gastrointestinal symptoms (17.3%), respectively. These figures were statistically higher than the placebo figures. The incidence of solicited local and general symptoms was lower in subjects aged 70 years and older compared with those aged 50–69 years. There is no difference in side effects when the second dose is given at 2 months compared to when given at 6 months.

Q21. What is the data on long-term immunogenicity and efficacy?

Ans. At 72 months of follow-up, the gE-specific cell-mediated immune response was 3.8 times higher than the prevaccination value (477.3 vs. 119.4 activated gE-specific CD4+ T cells per 106 cells), and the anti-gE antibody concentration was 7.3 times higher than the prevaccination value (8,159.0 vs. 1,121.3 mIU/mL). However, there was a drop of 25% in both T cell and humoral response between 36 and 72 months, yet it was significantly more than prevaccine status. Recently in 2018, the subjects were followed up at 9 years since the first vaccination and were still found to have both T cell and humoral responses that were significantly higher than the prevaccine values. It is estimated that the immune response will remain elevated for at least 15 years.

Extended term efficacy data of this vaccine in the pivotal efficacy trials is expected to be available soon.

Q22. What about data in immune compromised hosts?

Ans. There are six studies looking at safety and immunogenicity or efficacy of RZV in immune compromised hosts (where ZVL is contraindicated as discussed above). These studies are conducted in HIV patients, stem cell transplant recipients, renal transplant patients, patients with malignancies, etc. RZV has been found to be safe and immunogenic in these studies and hence has these conditions on label in some European countries.

Q23. Can you administer RZV in subjects who have received ZVL in past?

Ans. As there is waning of immune response between 3 and 7 years with ZVL and as the efficacy drops significantly with time after 3 years with ZVL, a study was conducted to see whether these subjects can be vaccinated with RZV. The study compared one dose of RZV in subjects >65 years old who had received ZVL >5 years before this study with those >65 years old who had not received ZVL in past. The result showed that the immune response was noninferior in group who had received ZVL in past as compared to ZVL naive subjects. Hence, ACIP, USA recommends to use two doses of RZV in those who have received ZVL in past starting after a minimum gap of 2 months since ZVL.

Q24. How will you compare the two vaccines?

Ans. Overall, the estimates of efficacy against HZ and PHN (CIs overlap) were higher with RZV than those for ZVL. Waning of efficacy occurs more rapidly with ZVL than with RZV. RZV is estimated to prevent more HZ and PHN compared with ZVL. RZV is the preferred vaccine for protection against HZ.

Q25. What are the recommendations regarding the use of zoster vaccines?

Ans. There are no published recommendations for use of zoster vaccines from India.

In 2018, the ACIP published the following recommendations:
- RZV may be used in adults aged ≥50 years, irrespective of prior receipt of varicella vaccine or ZVL, and does not require screening for a history of chickenpox.
- ZVL remains a recommended vaccine for prevention of HZ in immunocompetent adults aged ≥60 years (however more and more countries and physicians are inclined to use RZV preferentially).
- Following the first dose of RZV, the second dose should be given 2–6 months later.
- The vaccine series need not be restarted if more than 6 months have elapsed since the first dose.
- If the second dose of RZV is given less than 4 weeks after the first, the second dose should be repeated.
- Two doses of the vaccine are necessary regardless of prior history of HZ or prior receipt of ZVL.
- RZV should not be given <2 months after receipt of ZVL.
- RZV can be administered concomitantly, at different anatomic sites, with other adult vaccines.

- Adults with a history of HZ should receive RZV.
- Adults with chronic medical conditions should receive RZV.
- The use of RZV is recommended in persons taking low-dose immunosuppressive therapy (e.g., <20 mg/day of prednisone or equivalent or using inhaled or topical steroids) and persons anticipating immunosuppression or who have recovered from an immunocompromising illness.

■ SUGGESTED READING

1. Baxter R, Bartlett J, Fireman B, Marks M, Hansen J, Lewis E, et al. Long-Term Effectiveness of the Live Zoster Vaccine in Preventing Shingles: A Cohort Study. Am J Epidemiol. 2017;187(1):161-9.
2. Cunningham AL, Lal H, Kovac M, Chlibek R, Hwang S-J, Díez-Domingo J, et al. Efficacy of the Herpes Zoster Subunit Vaccine in Adults 70 Years of Age or Older. N Engl J Med. 2016;375:1019-32.
3. Dooling KL, Guo A, Patel M, Lee GM, Moore K, Belongia EA, Harpaz R. Recommendations of the Advisory Committee on Immunization Practices for Use of Herpes Zoster Vaccines. MMWR Morb Mortal Wkly Rep. 2018;67:103-8.
4. Lal H, Cunnigham L, Godeaux O, Chlibek R, Diez-Domingo J, Hwang S-J, et al. Efficacy of an Adjuvanted Herpes Zoster Subunit Vaccine in Older Adults. N Engl J Med. 2015;372:2087-96.
5. Oxman MN, Levin MJ, Shingles Prevention Study Group. Vaccination against Herpes Zoster and postherpetic neuralgia. J Infect Dis. 2008;197(s2):S228-36.
6. Plotkin S, Orenstein W, Offit P, Edwards K. Zoster vaccines. Plotkin's Vaccines, 7th edition. Amsterdam, Netherlands: Elsevier; 2017.
7. Schmader KE, Levin MJ, Gnann JW, McNeil SA, Vesikari T, Betts RF, et al. Efficacy, safety, and tolerability of Herpes Zoster vaccine in persons aged 50–59 years. Clin Infect Dis. 2012;54(7):922-8.
8. Vashishtha VM, Kalra A. Zoster vaccines. In: Vipin M Vashishtha, Ajay Kalra (Eds). IAP Textbook of vaccines, 2nd edition. New Delhi: Jaypee Brothers Medical Publishers (P) Ltd.; 2020. pp. 431-41.

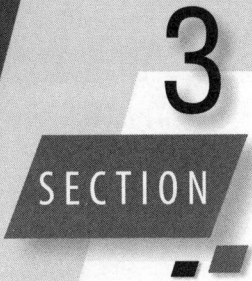

SECTION 3

Vaccination in Special Groups

○ **Adolescent Vaccination**
Mohit Vohra

○ **Adult Vaccination**
Srinivas G Kasi

○ **Vaccinations for Travelers**
Alok Gupta

CHAPTER 32: Adolescent Vaccination

Mohit Vohra

Q1. What is the significance of adolescent immunization?

Ans. The adolescent age particularly needs attention due to high burden of disease, high morbidity and mortality rates, engagement in high-risk activities, decreased contact with physicians, and increase in hospitalization rates and deaths due to communicable diseases which can be significantly decreased by effective immunization.

Q2. Why do adolescents need immunizations?

Ans. The waning immunity induced by vaccines administered during infancy/early childhood (measles, pertussis, tetanus, diphtheria, etc.) need boosting. Moreover, with improved sanitation hygiene and provision of safe drinking water and extensive coverage by the Expanded Program on Immunization (EPI) vaccines, there is an epidemiological rightward shift of childhood diseases, leading to a surge of vaccine-preventable disease (VPD) such as diphtheria, pertussis, tetanus, measles, chickenpox, and hepatitis A in adolescents and young adults. Some of these VPDs (hepatitis A and varicella) carry higher morbidity and mortality in adolescents.

Diseases like cervical cancer, which appear in adulthood, can be prevented by vaccination in the adolescent age group.

It is also possible that certain vaccines were not available to these adolescents during their early infancy and childhood.

Q3. What is the current status of adolescent immunization in India?

Ans. Vaccination coverage in adolescents is "dismal". Specific data on immunization coverage or incidence of VPDs in adolescents is almost nonexistent. Till recently, tetanus toxoid (TT) was the only vaccine recommended for adolescent in the National Immunization Program (NIP).

Presently, tetanus and diphtheria (Td) is the only vaccine recommended for adolescents in the NIP, while the Japanese encephalitis (JE) vaccine is offered in hyperendemic areas. In campaign mode, measles-rubella (MR) vaccine is offered till 15 years of age. Even in the private sector, coverage with the "exclusive adolescent vaccines" is very poor.

Q4. What is the status of VPDs among adolescents in India?

Ans. There is a lack of systematic epidemiological data defining the exact burden of various diseases. However, some sporadic and local data are available.

Diphtheria: Among countries with the top 10 case counts since 2000, India has the largest number of reported diphtheria cases (~92%). In a recent study done in 2016, 41% of cases occurred in those >10 years of age. In a study done in 2,400 school children aged 6–17 years studying in the various government schools in Hyderabad, only 56% were found to be seroprotected with immunoglobulin G (IgG) antidiphtheria titers of >0.1 IU/mL.

Pertussis: The incidence of pertussis in adolescents is unknown. In a recently published article titled "prospective multinational serosurveillance study of *Bordetella pertussis* infection among 10–18 years subjects from 8 Asian countries", with 200 subjects from India, high titers of anti-pertussis toxin (PT) IgG > 62.5 IU/mL indicative of *B. pertussis* infection within 12 months prior was found in 18% of subjects.

Tetanus: In 2016, 3,781 cases were reported from India including 227 cases of neonatal tetanus. In a serosurvey of schoolchildren 7–17 years in Hyderabad, only 64% were immune to tetanus.

In a serosurvey of students from Manipal University, the prevalence of serological susceptibility to measles was 9.5%, mumps 32%, rubella 16.6%, and varicella 25.8%.

Involvement of adolescents has been reported in mumps outbreaks in Rajasthan and Odisha. Susceptibility to rubella has been reported in 7–66% of adolescent females.

In a multicenter serosurvey, about 20–30% of adolescents and young adults were found susceptible to varicella at age 11–20 years.

The shifting epidemiology of hepatitis A infections has increased the incidence of this infection in adolescents with greater morbidity.

Q5. Which are "exclusive" adolescents' vaccines?

Ans. Tdap and human papillomavirus (HPV) vaccines are the *"exclusive"* adolescents' vaccines.

Q6. What are the recommendations for use of Tdap in adolescents?

Ans. Tdap is recommended as a single dose between 10 and 12 years of age, with catch-up till 18 years of age. If the previous diphtheria, pertussis, and tetanus (DPT) vaccination was not given or is unknown, the vaccines should be administered in a three-dose schedule of 0–1–6 months and the first of the series should be Tdap followed by two doses of Td.

It needs to be mentioned that the effectiveness of Tdap against pertussis wanes rapidly, with effectiveness reducing to 12% in the fourth year and 8.9% beyond 4 years.

Q7. What are the recommendations for use of HPV vaccines in adolescents?

Ans. For those 9–14 years of age, HPV vaccines are recommended in a two-dose schedule of 0–6 months. The interval between doses should not be <5 months. Beyond 15 years, HPV vaccines are recommended in a three-dose schedule, 0–1–6 months for bivalent HPV (BHPV) and 0–2–6 months for quadrivalent HPV (qHPV). All immunocompromised, irrespective of age, should receive the three-dose schedule.

Q8. What is Indian Academy of Pediatrics (IAP) view of use of measles, mumps, and rubella (MMR) vaccine in adolescents?

Ans. The IAP recommends two doses of MMR at 4–8 weeks interval for adolescents who have not received MMR vaccine earlier. The incidence of mumps in India is seen in rising trend in children mostly in the adolescent age group. A dose of mumps/MMR given at 4–6 years may not be effective in preventing outbreaks amongst older adolescents 15–18 years due to the waning immunity of the mumps component. So far, there is no recommendation for an additional dose in adolescents.

Q9. What are the IAP recommendations on hepatitis A vaccination in adolescents?

Ans. Due to the shifting epidemiology of hepatitis A infections, studies in India have shown a higher attack rate in adolescents. Hence, hepatitis A vaccination is strongly recommended for adolescents, without a past history of documented jaundice or vaccination against Hepatitis A. Prior serological testing for immunity against hepatitis A may be considered.

Q10. What are the IAP recommendations regarding meningococcal vaccination for adolescents?

Ans. Meningococcal vaccines are not for routine use. They are recommended for adolescents in special situations, during outbreaks of meningococcal disease, international travelers proceeding to the "meningitis belt" in sub-Saharan Africa, Hajj pilgrims and students proceeding to certain western countries for studies. In these situations, the meningococcal conjugate vaccine (MCV4), in a single dose, may be administered, with a booster dose after 5 years, for those who remain at increased risk. The polysaccharide vaccine can be administered as a single dose, with a second dose after 3 years, if indicated.

Q11. What are the IAP recommendations regarding hepatitis B vaccination for adolescents?

Ans. A three-dose schedule of 0–1–6 months is recommended for all adolescents with no/unknown history of vaccination.

SECTION 3: Vaccination in Special Groups

Q12. What are the IAP recommendations for catch-up immunization in adolescents?

Ans.

Vaccine	Schedule
MMR	Two doses at 4–8 weeks interval
Hepatitis B	Three doses at 0, 1, and 6 months
Hepatitis A	Two doses at 0 and 6 months (prior check for anti-HAV IgG may be considered)
Typhoid TCV	Single dose
Varicella	Two doses 4–8 weeks apart

(HAV: hepatitis A virus; IgG: immunoglobulin G; MMR: measles, mumps, and rubella; TCV: typhoid conjugate vaccine)

Q13. What are the IAP recommendations for vaccination of adolescents in special situations?

Ans.

Vaccine	Age recommended
Influenza	One dose every year
Japanese encephalitis	Catch-up up to 18 years (only in endemic areas)
Pneumococcal vaccines	One dose of PCV13 PPSV23, 8 weeks later PPSV23, 5 years after dose one
Rabies 1, 3, 7, and 14–28 days	As soon as possible after exposure

Q14. What are the IAP recommendations for adolescent travelers?

Ans.

Vaccine	Place of travel	Recommendations
Meningococcal vaccines	USA/UK/endemic areas/ Saudi Arabia, Africa	qMCV, single dose, repeat after 5 years
Yellow fever	Yellow fever endemic zones	Single dose At least 10 days before travel Lifelong validity
Oral cholera vaccine	Endemic area or area with outbreak	Two doses 2 weeks apart
JE vaccine	Endemic areas	Up to 18 years
Rabies PrEP	For adolescents going on treks	Two doses, 1 each on 0–7 days

(JE: Japanese encephalitis; PrEP: pre-exposure prophylaxis; qMCV: quadrivalent meningococcal conjugate vaccine)

Q15. What are the barriers for a successful adolescent vaccination program?

Ans. Poor immunization coverage in adolescents is a universal phenomenon, in both high-income and low-income countries. Due to an emphasis on curative services only, adolescents have fewer contacts with healthcare services. Low perceived threat due to the disease, fear of adverse effects, belief that scientific data about the vaccine is insufficient, and the vaccine had not been on the market "long enough" are some of the reasons for poor uptake of vaccines. Misinformation about vaccines in the internet and media is another major cause for vaccine hesitancy. Concerns about vaccine safety are another important barrier against immunization.

■ SUGGESTED READING

1. Arankalle V, Mitra M, Bhave S, Ghosh A, Balasubramanian S, Chatterjee S, et al. Changing epidemiology of hepatitis A virus in Indian children. Vaccine Develop Ther. 2014;4:7-13.
2. Arunkumar G, Vandana KE, Nalini S. Prevalence of measles, mumps, rubella and varicella susceptibility among health science students in a University in India. Am J Ind Med. 2013;56(1):58-64.
3. Balasubramanian S, Shah A, Pemde HK, Chatterjee P, Shivananda S, Guduru VK, et al. Indian Academy of Pediatrics (IAP) Advisory Committee on Vaccines and Immunization Practices (ACVIP) Recommended Immunization Schedule (2018-19) and Update on Immunization for Children Aged 0 Through 18 Years. Indian Pediatr. 2018;55:1066-74.
4. HPV Information Centre. (2019). Human papillomavirus and related diseases report. [online] Available from https://hpvcentre.net/statistics/reports/IND.pdf. [Last accessed October, 2020].
5. Kjaer SK, Sigurdsson K, Iversen O-E, Hernandez-Avila M, Wheeler CM, Perez G, et al. A Pooled Analysis of Continued Prophylactic Efficacy of Quadrivalent Human Papillomavirus (Types 6/11/16/18) Vaccine against High-grade Cervical and External Genital Lesions. Cancer Prev Res. 2009;2:868-88.
6. Klein NP, Bartlett J, Fireman B, Baxter R. Waning Tdap effectiveness in adolescents. Pediatrics. 2016;137:e20153326.
7. Lehtinen M, Paavonen J, Wheeler CM, Jaisamrarn U, Garland SM, Castellsague X, et al. Overall efficacy of HPV-16/18 AS04-adjuvanted vaccine against grade 3 or greater cervical intraepithelial neoplasia: 4-year end-of-study analysis of the randomised, double-blind PATRICIA trial. Lancet Oncol. 2012;13(1):89-99.
8. Murhekar MV, Bitragunta S, Hutin Y, Ckakravarty A, Sharma HJ, Gupte MD. Immunization coverage and immunity to diphtheria and tetanus among children in Hyderabad, India. J Infect. 2009;58(3):191-6.
9. Murhekar MV. Epidemiology of Diphtheria in India, 1996-2016: Implications for Prevention and Control. Am J Trop Med Hyg. 2017;97(2):313-8.
10. Son S, Thamlikitkul V, Chokephaibulkit K, Perera J, Jayatilleke K, Hsueh P-R, et al. Prospective multinational serosurveillance study of *Bordetella pertussis* infection among 10- to 18-year-old Asian children and adolescents. Clin Microbiol Infect. 2019;25:250.e1-250.e7.
11. Verma R, Khanna P, Chawla S. Adolescent vaccines: Need special focus in India. Hum Vaccin Immunother. 2015;11:2880-2.

CHAPTER 33: Adult Vaccination

Srinivas G Kasi

Q1. Why do adults need vaccines?

Ans. Adults need vaccines for the following reasons:
- Adults are 100 times more likely than children to die of vaccine preventable diseases (VPDs).
- Vaccine-induced immunity can wane over time.
- Some adults were never vaccinated as children.
- Newer vaccines were not available when some adults were children.
- Advancing age renders them to be more susceptible to serious disease caused by common infections (e.g., flu and pneumococcus).

Q2. What is the scenario of adult vaccination in India?

Ans. At best, the scenario is dismal! In the National Immunization Program (NIP), tetanus and diphtheria (Td) is the only vaccine recommended for adults (pregnant women). Healthcare providers as well as patients may lack knowledge about the need for vaccinating both high-risk and healthy adults.

Many adults do not visit a clinician regularly, except when they are sick, at which time medical management of acute and chronic illnesses usually receives priority over preventive services.

One of the most important reasons adults identify for not receiving a vaccine is the lack of a provider recommendation for the vaccine.

Q3. What is the scenario of VPDs in adults in India?

Ans. There are no population level surveillance data on VPDs in adults in India. However, available data suggests a significant burden of VPDs in adults in India.

Diphtheria: During 2001–2015, nearly half of the diphtheria cases reported globally were from India. Several outbreaks have been reported in recent times involving adults as well. In outbreaks in Kerala between 2015 and 2017, 18.1% of cases were between 20 and 30 years, 10.9% between 30 and 40 years, and 7.5% were >40 years. More recently, an outbreak was reported in a group of medical students in Kalaburgi, Karnataka.

In a serosurvey done in Delhi in 2009, in 255 adults between 20 and 50 years, 53% did not have protective levels of antidiphtheria antibodies.

Pertussis: Very sparse data exists on the prevalence of pertussis in adults. In a seroprevalence survey done in three countries, Malaysia, Thailand, and Taiwan, 5.13% of the 312 chronically coughing adults had serological evidence of pertussis infection within the previous 12 months. In a small serosurvey done among 62 adults in Pune, 21% were seronegative for pertussis.

Tetanus: In a serosurvey study in Pondicherry for protective level of tetanus antibody (>0.15 U/mL), only 50.4% in 21–30 years, 29.4% in 31–40 years, and 2.2% in >41 years had protective titers. In a serosurvey done in Delhi in 2009, in 255 adults between 20 and 50 years, 47% did not have protective levels of antitetanus antibodies.

In a serosurvey for antivaricella antibodies in four Indian cities, about 20% of young adults did not have protective titers. In outbreaks in West Bengal, 63% were >15 years and in rural South India, 24% were >16 years.

Human papillomavirus (HPV) 16/18 prevalence in India, in women with normal cytology is 5.0% (4.6–5.5). Overall chronic hepatitis B surface antigen (HBsAg) positivity rate in India is 2.1%. As far as pneumococcal disease in adults, there are no population-based studies, only hospital-based data. In 30–50% of adults and elderly with spontaneous bacterial peritonitis (SBI), *Strep. pneumoniae* is the causative organism. Case fatality rate is 20–50% in most studies.

In a health utilization survey (HUS) data on the frequency of influenza-like illness (ILI) in a rural community, by age, in Ballabgarh, India, in the year 2011, 55.3% of persons with ILI detected in the community were >15 years.

Q4. Are there any published guidelines for adult immunizations in India?

Ans. The first published guidelines for adult immunizations in India by the Association of Physicians of India (API), was in April 2009. This was an adaptation of the Advisory Committee on Immunization Practices (ACIP) guidelines of that year. These guidelines have been updated. In 2016, the Indian association of nephrologists published guidelines for vaccination in normal adults in India, which were based on the earlier API guidelines, ACIP, and World Health Organization (WHO) guidelines.

Q5. What are the suggested vaccinations for all healthy adults in India?

Ans.
- Td/Tdap every 10 years.
- Annual influenza vaccination is strongly recommended.
- *Zoster (shingles) vaccine*: Licensed above 50 years of age. Strongly recommended above 65 years of age.
- *Strongly recommended above 65 years*: One dose of 13-valent pneumococcal conjugate vaccine (PCV13) followed by 23-valent pneumococcal polysaccharide vaccine (PPSV23) after 6–12 months.

Q6. Which are the vaccines that might be necessary for some adults?

Ans. HPV, hepatitis A, hepatitis B, typhoid, measles, mumps, and rubella (MMR), and chickenpox.

These vaccines are recommended to those adults who have not received these vaccines, do not have evidence of immunity against the corresponding diseases, incomplete schedules or those with no vaccination records.

- *HPV*: 3 doses, 0-1-6 m (BHPV), 0-2-6 m (QHPV), in those <45 years of age.
- *Hepatitis A*: 2 doses of inactivated vaccine, 6 months apart.
- *Hepatitis B*: 3 dose at 0-1-6 m
- *MMR*: 2 doses, 4-8 weeks apart
- *Varicella*: 2 doses, 4-8 weeks apart.
- *TCV*: Single dose in those <45 years of age.

Q7. Which are the adult, special populations, which need specific vaccinations?

Ans. Pregnant women, adults with medical conditions, and travelers have special vaccine needs.

Q8. What is the schedule for administration of Td/Tdap?

Ans. Adults 18-64 years:
- Previously has not receive Tdap at or after age 11 years: 1 dose Tdap, then Td or Tdap every 10 years.
- Previously did not receive primary vaccination series for tetanus, diphtheria, or pertussis: At least 1 dose Tdap followed by 1 dose Td or Tdap at least 4 weeks after Tdap and another dose Td or Tdap 6-12 months after last Td or Tdap (Tdap can be substituted for any Td dose, but preferred as first dose); Td or Tdap every 10 years thereafter.
- For adults who have not received Tdap vaccine and are likely to come in contact with infants suffering from diphtheria or pertussis, a single dose of Tdap vaccine should be given 2 weeks before the contact with the infant if 2 years or more have elapsed since the last dose of Td vaccination.
- Health care personnel, especially those in direct contact with the patients, who have not received Tdap vaccine should receive a single does of Tdap vaccine if 2 years or more have elapsed since the last dose of Td vaccination.

Q9. What are the recommendations for pneumococcal vaccination of adults?

Ans.
- *All Adults aged 65 years or older*: PCV13 followed by PPSV23, 6-12 months later and a second dose of PPSV23, 5 years after first dose.
- Adults aged 19 years through 64 years with:

- *Immunocompromising conditions or anatomical or functional asplenia*: These are very high-risk category. PCV13 followed by PPSV23 8 weeks later. 2nd dose of PPSV23, 5 years after the first dose.
- *Cerebrospinal fluid (CSF) leaks or cochlear implants*: Very high risk. PCV13 followed by PPSV23 8 weeks later.
- *Chronic heart disease (excluding hypertension), chronic lung disease (including. asthma), chronic liver disease, alcoholism, or diabetes mellitus*: Moderate risk. PCV13 followed by PPSV23 1 year later or one dose of PPSV23.
- *Smokers or residents in nursing home or long-term care facilities*: Moderate risk. PCV13 followed by PPSV23 1 year later or one dose of PPSV23.

In 2019, the ACIP of USA, changed the recommendations for PCV13 usage in those >65 years. PCV13 is no longer routinely recommended for all adults aged ≥65 years. Instead, shared clinical decision-making for PCV13 use is recommended for persons aged ≥65 years who do not have an immunocompromising condition, CSF leak, or cochlear implant and who have not previously received PCV13.

The recommendations for PPSV23 remain unchanged. All adults aged ≥65 years should receive one dose of PPSV23. Adults aged ≥65 years who received ≥1 dose of PPSV23 before age 65 years should receive one additional dose of PPSV23 at age ≥65 years, at least 5 years after the previous PPSV23 dose.

The incidence of PCV13-type invasive pneumococcal disease (IPD) among adults aged ≥65 years declined ninefold during 2000–2014, after introduction of the infant PCV program and before the adult PCV13 program was implemented. However, from 2014 to 2017, no further reduction in PCV13-type IPD incidence was observed among adults aged ≥65 years. Similarly, since 2014, no impact on PCV13-type IPD incidence has been observed among adults aged 19–64 years, a population only experiencing indirect PCV13 effects during this period. Results of the economic analyses were less favorable toward continued PCV13 use for all adults aged ≥65 years compared with PPSV23 alone. This was the reason behind the 2019 recommendations of the ACIP.

The situation in India is very different. Infant immunization coverage in the NIP is restricted to five states and coverage in the private sector doses not contribute significantly to overall coverage. Hence, herd immunity is almost nonexistent. These new recommendations may not be appropriate for the elderly in India.

Q10. Is there a need for HPV vaccines for older and sexually active women?

Ans. HPV vaccines are preventive vaccines and are to be administered before onset of sexual activities. But evidence exists of their beneficial role

Table 1: Vaccine efficacy in the per-protocol population (PPE), intention to treat (ITT), and naïve to relevant type (NRT).

	PPE		ITT		NRT	
	24–34 years	35–45 years	24–34 years	35–45 years	24–34 years	35–45 years
Persistent infection cervical intraepithelial neoplasia (CIN), external genital lesion (EGL) 6, 11, 16, 18	91.3%	83.8%	44.1%	51.2%	83.7%	71.3%
Persistent infection CIN, EGL 16, 18	86%	81.8%	39.4%	43.9%	78.7%	78%

in sexually active women. Moreover, HPV infections have two peaks, the first between 15 and 19 years and the second albeit smaller peak in the fourth and fifth decades of life.

In a study done in 3,819 women between 24 and 45 years of age, who received quadrivalent HPV (qHPV) vaccine, the vaccine efficacy in the per-protocol population (PPE), intention to treat (ITT), and naive to relevant type (NRT) are as shown in **Table 1**.

PPE: Subjects who were seronegative at day 1 and polymerase chain reaction (PCR)-negative (swab and biopsy specimens) from day 1 through month 7 to the relevant vaccine HPV type(s) and did not violate the protocol. The PPE-eligible participants received all three vaccinations within 1 year.

ITT: Subjects who received more than one dose of vaccine or placebo and returned for follow-up. These subjects could have been seropositive and/or PCR-positive to vaccine HPV types at enrolment.

NRT: Subjects who received more than one dose of vaccine or placebo, returned for follow-up, and were deoxyribonucleic acid (DNA) negative at enrolment for the HPV type of interest.

Thus, females who are sexually active may also benefit from vaccination, but they may get less benefit. Very few sexually active young women are infected with all HPV types prevented by the vaccines, so most young women could still get protection by getting vaccinated.

The schedule consists of three doses 0–1–6 m (BHPV) and 0–2–6 m (QHPV).

Q11. What are the recommendations for Herpes Zoster vaccination for adults?

Ans. Recombinant Zoster Vaccine (RZV-Shingrix™) is indicated in adults aged ≥50 years, irrespective of prior receipt of varicella vaccine or Zoster Vaccine Live (ZVL- Zostavax™).

ZVL remains a recommended vaccine for prevention of herpes zoster in immunocompetent adults aged ≥60 years.

Schedules: RZV- 2-dose schedule, following the first dose of RZV, the second dose should be given 2–6 months later. If the second dose of RZV is given less than 4 weeks after the first, the second dose should be repeated.

In those who have received a dose of ZVL, a dose of RZV may be given at least 2 months after the dose of ZVL.

RZV is preferred over ZVL for the prevention of herpes zoster and related complications.

Q12. What is the recommended adult immunization schedule by medical condition and other indications?

Ans.
- Annual inactivated influenza vaccine is recommended for all adults with comorbid medical conditions
- MMR, Varicella and Zoster vaccine live (ZVL) is contraindicated in adults with immunosuppression and HIV infected with CD4 counts < 200/cmm
- Adults with chronic liver disease (e.g., persons with hepatitis B, hepatitis C, cirrhosis, fatty liver disease, alcoholic liver disease, autoimmune hepatitis, alanine aminotransferase [ALT] or aspartate aminotransferase [AST] level greater than twice the upper limit of normal), should be immunized with Hepatitis A and Hepatitis B vaccines, if not administered earlier.
- Adults with asplenia/hyposplenia/surgical splenectomy or complement deficiencies, should be immunized with vaccines against Hib, meningococci, pneumococci and Typhoid.
- In pregnancy, MMR, varicella, HPV and ZVL are contraindicated. All pregnant women should receive the inactivated influenza and Tdap vaccines. Other inactivated vaccines may be administered as per indication.

Q13. What are the special considerations in vaccination of healthcare professionals (HCPs)?

Ans. Vaccination of HCPs is important for two reasons:
1. Susceptible HCPs are at increased risk for occupational acquisition of VPDs.
2. HCPs provide health care to patients, many of whom are at high risk for a serious disease course, complications, or even death because of their age (e.g., neonates, young infants, and elderly) and/or underlying conditions (e.g., pregnant women, immunocompromised patients, and patients with underlying diseases). Unvaccinated, susceptible HCPs can transmit infections to this extremely vulnerable population.

Q14. What are the recommendations for vaccinations of HCPs?

Ans. Hepatitis B: If previously unvaccinated, three doses of a recombinant hepatitis B vaccine in a 0-1-6 months schedule. It is preferable to test for anti-HBs antibody 4–8 weeks after the last dose. Those with past history of vaccinations should have titers estimated and should receive a booster if titers are below threshold levels. Nonresponders to the first series should receive a second three-dose schedule, followed by estimation of antibody titers. If still below threshold levels, the HCP should be labelled as a primary nonresponder.

Influenza: One dose of influenza vaccine annually, inactivated influenza vaccine (IIV) or live attenuated influenza vaccine (LAIV).

MMR: HCP with no documentation of immunity, should receive two doses of MMR at 4–8 weeks interval.

Varicella (chickenpox): For HCP who have no serologic proof of immunity, prior vaccination, or diagnosis or verification of a history of varicella or herpes zoster (shingles) by a healthcare provider, two doses of varicella vaccine, should be administered 4 weeks apart.

Tdap: One dose of Tdap as soon as feasible to all HCP who have not received Tdap previously and to pregnant HCP with each pregnancy. Tdap/Td boosters are to be administered every 10 years thereafter.

Meningococcal: Quadrivalent meningococcal conjugate vaccine (qMCV) is recommended to all HCPs who are routinely exposed to isolates of *Neisseria meningitidis*. A booster is recommended every 5 years, if risk continues.

Rabies: Microbiologists, technicians handling samples from rabies cases, and clinicians working in rabies wards.

Q15. How can adult immunization rates be improved?
Ans.
- Screen for vaccine indications at every visit, whatever the reason for the visit.
- Recommend the vaccines.
- Make the vaccines available in the office.
- Reducing out-of-pocket costs for patients.
- *Expanding access*: Offer immunizations at timings convenient for working adults, evenings or weekends. Have an "express lane" for immunizations and reduce waiting time in clinics.
- Patient reminder and recall system.

SUGGESTED READING

1. Castellsagué X, Muñoz N, Pitisuttithum P, Ferris D, Monsonego J, Ault K, et al. End-of-study safety, immunogenicity, and efficacy of quadrivalent HPV (types 6, 11, 16, 18) recombinant vaccine in adult women 24–45 years of age. Br J Cancer. 2011;105:28-37.
2. Centers for Disease Control and Prevention (CDC). Use of 13-Valent Pneumococcal Conjugate Vaccine and 23-Valent Pneumococcal Polysaccharide Vaccine for Adults

with Immunocompromising Conditions: Recommendations of the Advisory Committee on Immunization Practices (ACIP). MMWR Morb Mortal Wkly Rep. 2012;61(40):816-9.
3. Chandran P, Lilabi MP, Bina T, Thavody J, George S. Re-emergence of diphtheria in Kerala: the need for change in vaccination policy. Int J Community Med Public Health. 2019;6(2):829-35.
4. Expert Group of the Association of Physicians of India on Adult Immunization in India. Executive Summary. The Association of Physicians of India Evidence-Based Clinical Practice Guidelines on Adult Immunization. J Assoc Physicians India. 2009;57:345-56.
5. Guidelines for vaccination in normal adults in India. Indian J Nephrol. 2016;26 (Suppl 1):S7-14.
6. Immunization Action Coalition. (2017). Healthcare Personnel Vaccination Recommendations. [online] Available from www.immunize.org/catg.d/p2017.pdf. [Last accessed October, 2020].
7. Parande MV, Roy S, Mantur BG, Parande AM, Shinde RS. Resurgence of diphtheria in rural areas of North Karnataka, India. Indian J Med Microbiol. 2017;35:247-51.

CHAPTER 34: Vaccinations for Travelers

Alok Gupta

Q1. Who is known as a traveler?

Ans. Traveler is any person (newborn and above) leaving his/her city or town of usual residence for another place or places for a short duration (in days) or for a long duration (in weeks or months). Traveler is different than a person who is relocating from the present place of residence to a new city or town for a longer period for studies or work or as a dependent.

Q2. What precautions should a traveler take against vaccine preventable diseases (VPDs)?

Ans. Every person should be adequately protected as per age and immune status, against VPDs as per recommendations of the country of residence. This is essential for personal protection and transmission of VPDs to the family, the friends, and the community at large.

The traveler must be protected against VPDs for their own protection, as well as to prevent possible transmission of VPDs from them to other persons during travel. It is also important that the traveler does not import back the disease-causing organisms back to his own country or in-transit countries.

Q3. Does a traveler need to be reimmunized with vaccines taken earlier?

Ans. No. Once the vaccine doses have been given adequately at appropriate age, a person may not need those vaccines in future unless they are needed as age-specific boosters or specified in certain places and situations.

Q4. When should the vaccine schedules be completed before travel?

Ans. The vaccines should be taken well before minimum specified time for each vaccine which is usually 2 weeks for most of the vaccines requiring single dose. When two or more doses need to be taken, they should be completed before the travel begins. The traveler may be quarantined if she/he reaches the destination before the minimum time gap specified or may face deportation.

Q5. What are the vaccines that residents of India need before traveling to other countries?

Ans.

General recommendations: The travelers should have completed all age-specific immunizations for their own protection. In addition, one must also be immunized against diseases endemic in the area or country to which one is traveling or steps out of international zone (transit area) in transit, if not immunized earlier as per age. The traveler should go through the travel advisory of the own country, places in transit, and the countries visiting.

Yellow fever vaccine: This is mandatory to visit certain countries where yellow fever (YF) is endemic. The countries of visit where YF vaccine is mandatory are:

- *Africa*: Angola, Benin, Burkina Faso, Burundi, Cameroon, Central African Republic, Chad, Congo, Côte d'Ivoire, Democratic Republic of Congo, Equatorial Guinea, Ethiopia, Gabon, Gambia, Ghana, Guinea, Guinea Bissau, Kenya, Liberia, Mali, Mauritania, Niger, Nigeria, Rwanda, Senegal, Sierra Leone, Sudan, South Sudan, Togo, and Uganda.
- *South America*: Argentina, Bolivia, Brazil, Colombia, Ecuador, French Guyana, Guyana, Suriname, Trinidad (Trinidad only), Venezuela, Panama, Paraguay, and Peru.

(It is necessary to consult the latest WHO guidelines for countries needing mandatory YF vaccination. This is changed periodically.)

Yellow fever vaccine is contraindicated in the following situations:
- Infants aged less than 6 months
- History of severe allergy to egg or to any of the vaccine components
- Hypersensitivity to a previous dose of YF vaccine
- Thymoma or history of thymectomy
- Immunodeficiency from medications, disease or symptomatic human immunodeficiency virus (HIV) infection, and pregnancy.

Dose: 0.5 mL subcutaneously, once above age of 9 months to 60 years (valid for lifetime starting 10 days after vaccination).

Meningococcal meningitis vaccine: It is mandatory for travel for Hajj, study in USA, UK, and other specified countries (ACWY and MenB). Please see requirement of individual place of study or work which is provided in contract.

To travel to countries with hyperendemic or epidemic meningococcal disease, including countries in the African meningitis belt or during the Hajj all pilgrims must have received a single dose of quadrivalent ACWY conjugate vaccine or a single dose of the quadrivalent (ACYW) polysaccharide vaccine and show proof of vaccination on a valid International Certificate of Vaccination or Prophylaxis; Kingdom of Saudi

Arabia (KSA) will not issue visas for Hajj or Umrah without it. Hajjis must receive their meningococcal conjugate vaccination no more than 5 years before arrival. The KSA Ministry of Health currently advises against travel to the Hajj for pregnant women or children; if they choose to travel, however, these groups should receive meningococcal vaccination according to licensed indications for their age.

Dose: 0.5 mL intramuscular (IM), single dose, at least 10 days before travel.
- Quadrivalent (ACWY) conjugate vaccine (valid for 5 years)
- Quadrivalent (ACYW) polysaccharide vaccine (valid for 3 years)

Polio vaccine: It is mandatory for Hajj pilgrims and travelers from Pakistan, Afghanistan, and other notified areas or countries which are still endemic to wild polio virus or are experiencing polio outbreaks. As per the Government of India regulation, people traveling from India to wild polio virus endemic countries (Afghanistan, Nigeria, and Pakistan) and those traveling to countries where polio virus is in circulation following importation (Ethiopia, Kenya, Somalia, and Syria) will require to take a dose of bivalent oral polio vaccine (bOPV) at least 4 weeks before the travel date irrespective of the age. The bOPV vaccination certificate will be issued after this additional dose and it will remain valid for 1 year.

Measles-containing vaccine (MCV) or measles-mumps-rubella (MMR) vaccine: Many countries which had eradicated or eliminated measles are facing serious outbreaks and deaths due to measles. Two doses of MMR given after the age of 12 months at least 4 weeks apart are essential before entry into certain countries. Documentary proof is needed else the point of entry may quarantine the traveler pending antibody titers or vaccination as per their requirement.

Evidence of immunity to measles and rubella for international travelers includes:
- Written documentation of having received the measles and rubella vaccines.
- Laboratory evidence of rubella and measles immunity [a positive serologic test for the measles and rubella-specific immunoglobulin G (IgG) antibodies].

Q6. What are the vaccines travelers to India need before entering India as per immigration requirement?

Ans.
Yellow fever vaccine: For those traveling from or stay in transit in countries endemic for YF as above.

Polio vaccine: Any person of any age residing in any of countries endemic for polio as in question 5 above, traveling to India, will be supposed to take a single dose of bOPV 4 weeks before the travel date.

Travelers arriving from Afghanistan, Democratic Republic of the Congo, Mozambique, Niger, Nigeria, Pakistan, Papua New Guinea, Syria, Myanmar, Yemen, and Somalia should present proof of vaccination with at least one of the following vaccines:
- At least one dose (two drops) of bOPV within the previous 12 months and administered at least 4 weeks prior to arrival, or
- At least one dose (0.5 mL IM) of inactivated polio vaccine (IPV) within the previous 12 months and administered at least 4 weeks prior to arrival.

Travelers arriving from Afghanistan, Nigeria, Pakistan, Papua New Guinea, Syria, Myanmar, Yemen, and Somalia will also receive one dose of bOPV at the border points on entry.

Q7. What are the vaccines that Indian travelers need for domestic travel inside India?

Ans. Indian residents must be fully protected with the age-specific vaccines including age-specific boosters.

Cholera: Endemic in West Bengal and adjacent states, during large religious gatherings as Kumbh melas.

Dose: Killed bivalent oral vaccine (Shanchol). Given at age 12 months and above. Two doses 14 days apart, orally. Where there is continued risk of *Vibrio cholerae* infection, if the WC vaccines (e.g., Shancol) are used then revaccination is recommended after 2 years.

Japanese encephalitis vaccine: Eastern and North-Eastern States of India: The vaccination against Japanese encephalitis (JE) is not recommended for routine use, but only for individuals living in endemic areas. Though occasional cases have been reported from urban areas in a few districts, JE is predominantly a disease of rural areas. Government of India has identified around 231 districts to be endemic for JE in India so far. JE vaccine is also recommended for travelers to JE endemic areas provided they are expected to stay for a minimum of 4 weeks in rural areas in the JE season. Please refer to Indian Academy of Pediatrics (IAP) Immunization Guidebook 2020 for details.

Dose: Inactivated vaccine: JEEV/JENVAC vaccine. 1 year of age and above, two doses 4 weeks apart. One booster after 1 year, if exposure is continued or revisiting.

Q8. Is it better to consult our local doctor or go by this advice?

Ans. It is always better to consult your pediatrician and family doctor well in advance before scheduled travel. It is recommended that travel advisory from country of residence, in-transit countries, and destination countries be checked well before and at weekly intervals to just before travel.

The outbreaks and epidemics occurring in any place may warrant vaccination or protection during any stage of travel.

Q9. Do these recommendations apply to all ages and conditions?

Ans. These are general recommendations. Pregnant women, people with chronic diseases or immunodeficiency should take advice from their local doctor informing of their condition and travel itinerary well before travel (*see* vaccination in special situations also).

Q10. What are the vaccinations advised during pregnancy for traveling abroad?

Ans. The pregnant adolescent or lady should be vaccinated with all vaccines due for age except the live vaccines (measles, mumps, rubella, and varicella). YF vaccine is not recommended routinely in pregnancy, but if travel to endemic area is inevitable that it can be considered giving in the first trimester. Human papillomavirus (HPV) vaccine doses should be postponed till after the pregnancy. Influenza and Tdap vaccine should be specifically given.

Q11. What are the vaccines advised to immunocompromised Indian traveling abroad?

Ans. Immunocompromised persons traveling abroad should be vaccinated as per their medical condition and previous vaccination status.

All age-specific vaccines are advised in immunocompromised person except live influenza, MMR, and varicella vaccines. Rotavirus vaccine should not be given in infants with severe combined immunodeficiency (SCID) disorder.

Q12. Is a doctor's certificate required?

Ans. Whenever essential, e.g., YF, vaccination certificate signed and having seal of appropriate valid issuing authority should be carried along with travel documents and produced when asked for. Failure to do so may lead to quarantine for specific days or deportation. As of now the YF vaccination is valid lifelong if valid documentation is preserved.

Q13. What other health-associated medical requirements are advised during travel?

Ans.
- Vaccination certificates.
- Regular medicines, e.g., for hypertension, hypothyroidism, etc.
- Routine medicines for fever, body aches, oral rehydration solution (ORS), etc.
- Most recent prescriptions of personal doctor.
- Medical travel insurance.

■ SUGGESTED READING

1. Balasubramanian S, Shah A, Pemde HK, Chatterjee P, Shivananda S, Guduru VK, et al. Indian Academy of Pediatrics (IAP) Advisory Committee on Vaccines and Immunization Practices (ACVIP). Recommended Immunization Schedule (2018-19) and Update on Immunization for Children Aged 0 Through 18 Years. Indian Pediatr. 2018;55:1066-74.
2. CDC. (2020). Vaccines and Immunizations. [online] Available from https://www.cdc.gov/vaccines/index.html. [Last accessed October, 2020].
3. NHM. (2018). National Immunization Schedule. [online] Available from https://nhm.gov.in/New_Updates_2018/NHM_Components/Immunization/report/National_Immunization_Schedule.pdf. [Last accessed October, 2020].
4. WHO. (2017). Cholera vaccines: WHO position paper-August 2017. [online] Available from https://apps.who.int/iris/bitstream/handle/10665/258763/WER9234.pdf;jsessionid=73DA2052BEFDB35FC9760AF99AD8FB2F?sequence=1. [Last accessed October, 2020].
5. WHO. (2020). Vaccines. [online] Available from https://www.who.int/travel-advice/vaccines. [Last accessed October, 2020].

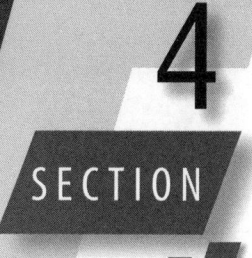

SECTION 4
Newer Technologies and Newer Vaccines

- **Newer Vaccine Technologies**
  NP Singh

- **Newer Vaccines in Pipeline**
  NP Singh

- **Vaccines against Novel Viruses**
  NP Singh

- **Covid-19 Vaccines**
  NP Singh, Srinivas G Kasi

- **Therapeutic Vaccines**
  Dhanya Dharmapalan, NP Singh

CHAPTER 35 / Newer Vaccine Technologies

NP Singh

Q1. What are technical challenges in the development of new vaccines?

Ans. In the 21st century, the technical challenges facing development of new vaccines are twofold: challenges related to the characteristics of the pathogen and challenges related to characteristics of the target population.

Challenging pathogens: Pathogens that make vaccine development challenging are those: that are intracellular (*Mycobacterium tuberculosis*), with complex life cycles (*malaria*), that induce immune dysfunction in the host *[human immunodeficiency virus (HIV)]*, with a latent disease phase [*herpes viruses, M. tuberculosis,* and *human papillomavirus (HPV)*], who undergo continuous evolution process, either slow (*Neisseria meningitides* and *HIV*) or rapid (*influenza*), who have multiple disease-causing serotypes/serogroups whose epidemiology varies regionally and over time (*Streptococcus pneumoniae* and *N. meningitides*), and for whom vaccines have been successfully developed and licensed for use, but their efficacy is suboptimal and/or short-lived (*tuberculosis* and *pertussis*).

Challenging populations: Immunosenescence associated with increasing age, the immunocompromised, individuals with chronic disease, and neonates and infants (particularly *premature infants*) are the populations in whom the present day vaccines result in suboptimal immune responses.

Q2. What are potential solutions of these challenges?

Ans. Multiple approaches exist to address the challenges of pathogen and population. Improved understanding of the functioning of the immune system, the response to pathogens at the molecular level, and utilization of advances in all fields of science and engineering has resulted in new technologies and sophisticated vaccine design for the discovery of more potent and safer vaccines. Approaches for new vaccines development would be related to improvement of both the antigen (vaccine) and the adjuvants.

Q3. What are the antigen-related approaches for new vaccines development?

Ans. These include reverse vaccinology, synthetic peptide vaccines, deoxyribonucleic acid (DNA) vaccines, ribonucleic acid (RNA) vaccines, and viral-vectored vaccines.

Q4. What is reverse vaccinology?

Ans. Reverse vaccinology literally implies a complete change of direction in the development of vaccines. Reverse vaccinology is based on sequencing whole genomes of microorganisms and utilizing bioinformatics for design of vaccines. The Group B meningococcus are the first vaccines to enter clinical usage with this methodology. Reverse vaccinology has now been applied to many other bacterial pathogens as full genome sequencing has advanced, including group B streptococcus, group A Streptococcus, *Streptococcus pneumoniae*, *Staphylococcus aureus*, and *Chlamydia*.

Q5. What are synthetic peptide vaccines?

Ans. Synthetic peptide vaccines are produced by identifying the peptide sequences of the epitopes, that trigger a protective immune response and to use completely synthetic versions of these as the vaccine candidates. This approach is most suitable for T-cell responses as these responses are mediated by linear epitopes. On the other hand, B-cell responses are dependent on nonlinear and often discontinuous epitopes. *Advantages* of this approach include no risk of mutation or reversion, little or no risk of contamination by pathogenic or toxic substances, and chemical manipulation of the peptide structure could possibly increase stability and decrease unwanted side effects seen in the native sequence. Peptide antigens could be rapidly modified to generate strain-specific responses. *Disadvantages* include the need for powerful adjuvants as these peptides are poorly immunogenic. Often the antigenic epitope is not a simple sequence of amino acids, but a structure composed of various parts of the protein sequence coming together to build a three-dimensional structure. Modeling of these structures will be needed to generate the correct antigenic site synthetically.

Q6. What are RNA vaccines?

Ans. Messenger RNA (mRNA) is the intermediate step between the translation of protein-encoding DNA and the production of proteins by ribosomes in the cytoplasm. RNA vaccine consists of an mRNA strand that codes for a disease-specific antigen. Once the mRNA strand in the vaccine is inside the body's cells, the cells use the genetic information to produce the antigen. This antigen is then displayed on the cell surface, where it is recognized by the immune system with elicitation of an immune response. mRNA vaccines result in an intracellular production of antigen with a native conformation which can result in processing of antigen by both major histocompatibility complex (MHC)

Class I and MHC Class II pathways with optimum generation of functional antibodies. There are three types of mRNA vaccine being studied:
1. *Nonreplicating mRNA*: The simplest type of RNA vaccine, mRNA strand is packaged and delivered to the body, where it is taken up by the body's cells to make the antigen. It is the simplest and safest type. However, the duration of expression in cells is transient and results in production of low levels of antibodies.
2. *In vivo self-replicating mRNA*: This is a longer RNA strand which encodes an alphavirus genome, in which the genes encoding the structural proteins are replaced by a cassette of antigens of interest. Self-replicating mRNA vaccines are being developed as a platform that can be used for a wide variety of targets.
3. *In vitro dendritic cell (DC) nonreplicating mRNA vaccine*: In this variety, DCs are extracted from the patient's blood, transfected with the RNA vaccine, then given back to the patient to stimulate an immune reaction.

Q7. What are the benefits of mRNA vaccines and what is its present status in modern vaccinology?

Ans. Messenger RNA vaccines have several benefits over conventional approaches:
- RNA vaccines are not made with pathogen particles or inactivated pathogen, so are noninfectious. RNA does not integrate itself into the host genome and the RNA strand in the vaccine is degraded once the protein is made. So, mRNA vaccines are safe.
- Early clinical trial results indicate that these vaccines generate a reliable immune response, with recruitment of CD4 and CD8 T cells.
- mRNA vaccines are synthetic vaccines with the capacity for rapid development and potential for low-cost manufacture and safe administration.

Early research with mRNA vaccines focused on cancer applications. However, these vaccines are being investigated against a wide variety of infectious pathogens, including influenza virus, Ebola virus, Zika virus, *Streptococcus* species, *Toxoplasma gondii*, and now severe acute respiratory syndrome coronavirus 2 (SARS CoV-2) also.

Q8. What are the basics of DNA vaccine?

Ans. A DNA vaccine contains a nucleotide sequence encoding a key antigenic determinant from a given pathogen that is injected into a host, then translated and transcribed by host cells into a peptide that is foreign to the host. Therefore, the protein is capable of inducing an immune response which may confer protection against the given pathogen. They stimulate a cellular immune response (cell-mediated immunity) in addition to an antibody response (humoral immunity).

The advantages of this approach include improved vaccine stability, the absence of any infectious agent, and the relative ease of large-scale manufacture.

Q9. How do DNA vaccines work?

Ans. Deoxyribonucleic acid vaccines are composed of a bacterial plasmid. Expression plasmids used in DNA-based vaccination normally contain two units: the antigen expression unit composed of promoter/enhancer sequences, followed by antigen-encoding and polyadenylation sequences and the production unit composed of bacterial sequences necessary for plasmid amplification and selection. The construction of bacterial plasmids with vaccine inserts is accomplished using recombinant DNA technology. Once constructed, the vaccine plasmid is transformed into bacteria, where bacterial growth produces multiple plasmid copies. The plasmid DNA is then purified from the bacteria, by separating the circular plasmid from the much larger bacterial DNA and other bacterial impurities. This purifies DNA acts as the vaccine.

The standard method of DNA vaccine administration is intramuscular injection of naked DNA. Delivery by other methods is being investigated including physical, chemical or biological methods.

Q10. What is the present status of DNA vaccine development and what is anticipated in future?

Ans. Despite the promise of initial trials, clinical experience is disappointing. Vaccines currently being developed use not only DNA, but also include adjuncts that assist DNA to enter cells, target it towards specific cells, or that may act as adjuvants in stimulating or directing the immune response. Coformulation with plasmids encoding immune mediators, e.g., cytokines is being investigated. Currently, no DNA vaccines are in human clinical usage. However, in veterinary practice, DNA vaccines against influenza in poultry have been in development since 1993, and recently, the United States Department of Agriculture (USDA) conditionally approved the first DNA vaccine against H5N1 for chickens. Numerous preclinical and clinical trials (phases I and II) against various types of cancer: lymphomas, melanomas, cervical, breast, kidney, and prostate are underway. The Canine Melanoma Vaccine is the first licensed DNA vaccine used to protect dogs from melanoma.

Deoxyribonucleic acid vaccines are being actively investigated as adjuvant therapy for a variety of cancers. Tumor cells express a variety of antigens with potential to produce a tumor-specific immune response. These could be either tumor-associated antigens (TAA) or tumor-specific antigens (TSA). Application of DNA vaccines as a new and novel therapeutic strategy to combat tumor cells has arisen from this property. DNA vaccines are designed to express tumor antigens which are fused to costimulator and/

or cytokine [granulocyte macrophage colony-stimulating factor (GM-CSF) or interleukin-2 (IL-2)] proteins, for the recruitment and activation of DCs.

Q11. What is vector-based vaccine concept?

Ans. The basic concept behind vector-based vaccine is the introduction the antigen of choice via a live attenuated viral vector which when injected may (replication-competent) or may not (replication-defective) replicate depending on the way the virus is attenuated but none the less deliver the antigen it carries for the body to mount an immune response. Several viruses are used as vectors such as adenovirus, measles virus, vesicular stomatitis virus (VSV), and others such as parvovirus, togavirus, poxvirus, etc. Generally the vector viruses backbone is prepared with deletion of genes causing disease or replication or recognition by the host immune cells as infected cells to avoid its elimination and replaced by the concerned antigen cassette (of up to 8 kb size) through homologous recombination or direct cloning so that the same after being injected is then expressed in the host for the immune system to mount immune response. Viral vector vaccines induce strong immune response and do not need adjuvants. These viral vectors are produced on mammalian cell lines that support high yields with much lower production cost.

Q12. What are the examples of viral vector-based vaccines and how are they administered?

Ans. Viral vector-based vaccines can be administered orally, intramuscularly, intranasally or intradermally. Recent example of virus vector-based vaccine includes the recombinant tetravalent dengue vaccine (Dengvaxia^R-Sanofi) where each of the four-dengue virus antigen is expressed in the backbone of attenuated 17D yellow fever vaccine. The other example is Ebola vector-based vaccines using several vectors are used such as adenovirus, VSV or Chimpanzee adenovirus that have entered clinical trials. The Oxford ChAdOx-1 vaccine against SARS CoV-2 is also an example of this strategy.

Q13. What is adjuvant and what is its role in vaccinology?

Ans. Adjuvants are constituents of the vaccines, which enhance the immunogenicity of the antigen and induce a stronger, and longer lasting immune responses. As more purified antigens with lower immunogenicity are selected for modern vaccines, there is a greater need for adjuvants. Adjuvants are currently used clinically to:
- Increase the response to a vaccine in the general population, increasing mean antibody titers, and/or the fraction of subjects that become protectively immunized
- Increase seroconversion rates in populations with reduced responsiveness because of age (both infants and the elderly), disease, or therapeutic interventions

- Facilitate the use of smaller doses of antigen
- Permit immunization with fewer doses of vaccine.

The modern adjuvants additionally:
- Provide functionally appropriate types of immune response (e.g., T helper 1 [Th1] cell versus Th2 cell, CD8+ versus CD4+ T cells, and specific antibody isotypes)
- Increase the generation of memory—especially T-cell memory
- Increase speed of initial response, which may be critical in a pandemic outbreak of infection
- Alter the breadth, specificity, or affinity of the response.

Examples of some of the novel adjuvants in clinical usage are:
- *MF59* (an oil-in-water emulsion of squalene oil) in *influenza vaccine.*
- *CpG-ODN* (short synthetic single-stranded DNA molecules containing unmethylated CpG dinucleotides which are TLR9 agonists) in Heplisav (*hepatitis B vaccine*).
- *Virosomes:* Hepatitis and influenza vaccines.
- *AS04*: (*3-deacyl-monophosphoryl lipid A*) derived from lipopolysaccharides (LPS) from *Salmonella minnesota and aluminum salts* in HPV vaccine.
- *AS03*: Vitamin E (α-*tocopherol*), surfactant polysorbate 80, and squalene in pandemic influenza vaccines.
- *ISA51*: Mineral oil *(DRAKEOL 6 VR),* surfactant *(mannide monooleate)* in therapeutic vaccines against lung cancer.

Q14. Describe the property and use of some clinically important adjuvants.

Ans. Characteristics of adjuvants used in licensed vaccines are compiled in following table:

Adjuvant	Vaccines where used	Component	Origin	Other Uses
Aluminum	D, T, pertussis, IPV, hepatitis A & B, HPV, meningococcal and pneumococcal	Aluminum as salts mixed with antigen (adsorption)	Naturally occurring present in soil, water, air	Medicines, cosmetics, food industry
Virosomes	Hepatitis and influenza	Vesicles where influenza antigens in aqueous volume are enclosed within a standard phospholipid cell	Natural phospholipids, Seasonal influenza glycoproteins	None

Adjuvant	Vaccines where used	Component	Origin	Other Uses
AS04	Hepatitis B, HPV	(3-deacyl-monophosphoryl lipid A) derived from LPS from Salmonella Minnesota, Aluminum salts	Natural exposure to LPS from Gram-negative bacteria occurs frequently	None
MF59	Influenza-seasonal and pandemic	Squalene	Animal source (shark liver oil). Found naturally in human tissues: skin, adipose tissues, arterial walls, muscles, skeleton, lymph nodes	Cosmetics, moisturizers
AS03	Influenza-pandemic	Vitamin E (α-Tocopherol), Surfactant polysorbate 80, Squalene	Naturally occurring in humans, Surfactant and emulsifier, Animal source (shark liver oil).	Used in foods, Vit., eye drops & intravenous injections
ISA51	Therapeutic vaccine, NSCLC	Mineral oil (DRAKEOL 6 VR), Surfactant (mannide-mono-oleate)	Refined mineral oil of vegetable origin	Food industry
Thermo-reversible oil-in-water	Influenza-pandemic	Squalene	Animal source (shark liver oil).	Naturally occurring

Q15. What is an adjuvant system?

Ans. Adjuvant systems are combinations of immunostimulatory molecules that are designed to allow vaccines to provide better and broader protection than classical formulations containing aluminum salts. Ten different adjuvant system families have been designed, five have been investigated in clinical trials, and three are in vaccines that are licensed, or close to licensure. Adjuvant systems investigated in clinical trials are AS01 (malaria and herpes zoster vaccines), AS02, AS03 [pre-pandemic H5N1 vaccine and pandemic H1N1 influenza vaccines (Arepanrix™, Pandemrix™], AS04 (HPV vaccine-Cervarix™ and hepatitis B for pre- and hemodialysis patients Fendrix™), and AS15.

Q16. What is mucosal vaccination?

Ans. Nasal mucosa intrinsic characteristics favor drug absorption. Nasal-associated lymphoid tissue (NALT) comprises B and T cells, and a dense network of antigen-presenting cells (APCs). Nasal route can mimic the natural infection of pathogens to elicit specific mucosal and systemic immune responses and therefore, constitutes an alternative and promising strategy for drug and vaccine delivery. Two important strategies for improving the effectiveness of mucosal vaccination are mucosal immune cells (M cells and DCs) targeted strategies and mucosal immune-stimulator adjuvants, which include bacterial adjuvants, nucleic acid adjuvants, cytokine adjuvants, and particle adjuvants.

Q17. What is the concept of mucosal vaccine delivery system?

Ans. An optimal mucosal vaccine formulation, including the appropriate combination of antigens and delivery carriers, should be able to induce a comprehensive series of protective immune responses. The expression form of vaccine antigens has an important effect on the type and efficiency of immune response. Soluble antigens generally present less immunogenicity in mucosal vaccines. To ensure durable immunostimulation, antigen delivery carriers are being used to control the release of the antigens to APCs in the small intestine. A promising strategy to surmount this hurdle is the encapsulation of vaccine antigens in an appropriate delivery system. This concept is mainly utilized for mucosal vaccinations. Three common types of vaccine delivery systems are:
1. Liposomal system
2. Biodegradable polymeric particle system
3. Adenoviral system

Q18. What are nanoparticles and what are opportunities and limitations for nanotechnology in vaccinology?

Ans. A nanoparticle or ultrafine particle is usually defined as a particle of matter that is between 1 and 100 nanometers (nm) in diameter. The term is sometimes used for larger particles, up to 500 nm or fibers and tubes that are less than 100 nm in only two directions. Nanoparticles can operate both as a delivery system to enhance antigen processing and as an immunostimulatory adjuvant to induce and amplify protective immunity. Nanoparticles should protect the antigens from premature proteolytic degradation. Enhancement of the immune response is in part because of their ability to activate the inflammasome and induce the maturation of interleukin. Nanoparticles can be excellent adjuvants due to their biocompatibility and their physicochemical properties (e.g., size, shape, and surface charge), which can be tailored to obtain different immunological effects. Nanocarriers composed of lipids, proteins, metals or polymers have already been used to attain some of these attributes.

Nanoparticle covering of adjuvant (*aluminum oxide-based nanocarriers*) possess big advantages over the conventional adjuvant alum and may provide an alternative vaccine adjuvant-delivery system (VADS) for making effective vaccines.

Q19. Give brief accounts of various alternative methods of vaccine delivery.

Ans. In modern vaccinology several alternate methods of vaccine delivery techniques have been applied to improve the acceptance of immunizations and also to improve immunogenicity and effectiveness of vaccination. Examples of the new techniques are microarray patches (MAPs), hollow microneedle array, plant-based edible vaccines, intralymphatic and epicutaneous vaccinations, and most recently immunization by electroporation.

Q20. What are microarray patch and microneedle technologies? What are its considerations for programmatic vaccine deliveries?

Ans. An MAP consists of a cluster of tens to thousands of projections less than one millimeter in length attached to a backing that can be applied to the skin with finger pressure or an applicator. When applied, the projections pierce the stratum corneum to deliver vaccines to the epidermis or dermis, depending on the length of the microprojections. There they encounter a high density of APCs (e.g., dermal DCs), where vaccine delivery can evoke a strong immune response. This technology has potential to transform the way that vaccines are delivered within immunization programs in low and middle-income countries (LMICs), where vaccine delivery faces several challenges.

Q21. What is plant-based vaccine and what is its current status development?

Ans. It has been evident that using plants to produce vaccines would have several advantages. First, plant vaccines would likely have a low production cost and could be easily scaled-up, as has been demonstrated by the biopharmaceutical industry. Indeed, another advantage of this strategy is that plant cells would provide antigen protection due to their rigid cell wall. This is also known as the bioencapsulation effect and could increase bioavailability of antigenic molecules to the gut-associated lymphoid tissues (GALTs) through preserving structural integrity of vaccine components through the stomach to elicit both a mucosal and a systemic immune response. Finally, plant-based oral vaccines are characterized by improved safety relative to traditional recombinant vaccine platforms, especially since contamination from mammalian-specific pathogens can be eliminated. To date, vaccine antigens have been transformed into many edible species including lettuce, tomato, potato, papaya, carrot, quinoa, and tobacco.

SUGGESTED READING

1. Azegami T, Yuki Y, Kiyono H. Plant-Based Mucosal Vaccine Delivery Systems. Mucosal Vaccines. 2020;1:357-70.
2. Chen H. Recent advances in mucosal vaccine development. J Control Release. 2000;67(2-3):117-28.
3. Diaz-Arévalo D, Zeng M. Nanoparticle-based vaccines: opportunities and limitations. Nanopharmaceuticals. 2020;1:135-50.
4. Gruver AL, Hudson LL, Sempowski GD. Immunosenescence of ageing. J Pathol. 2007;211:144-56.
5. Jin Z, Gao S, Cui X, Sun D, Zhao K. Adjuvants and delivery systems based on polymeric nanoparticles for mucosal vaccines. Int J Pharm. 2019;572:118731.
6. Khan KH. DNA vaccines: Roles against diseases. Germs. 2013;3:26-35.
7. Kovaiou RD, Herndler-Brandstetter D, Grubeck-Loebenstein B. Age-related changes in immunity: Implications for vaccination in the elderly. Expert Rev Mol Med. 2007;9:1-17.
8. Leroux-Roels G. Unmet needs in modern vaccinology: Adjuvants to improve the immune response. Vaccine. 2010;28:C25-C36.
9. Longet S, Lundahl MLE, Lavelle EC. Targeted strategies for mucosal vaccination. Bioconjug Chem. 2019;29(3):613-23.
10. Mato YL. Nasal route for vaccine and drug delivery: Features and current opportunities. Int J Pharm. 2019;572:118813.
11. Morel S, Didierlaurent A, Bourguignon P, Delhaye S, Baras B, Jacob V, et al. Adjuvant System AS03 containing α-tocopherol modulates innate immune response and leads to improved adaptive immunity. Vaccine. 2011;29:2461-73.
12. Pasquale AD, Preiss S, Da Silva FT, Garçon N. Vaccine Adjuvants: from 1920 to 2015 and Beyond. Vaccines. 2015;3:320-43.
13. Peyraud N, Zehrung D, Jarrahian C, Frivold C, Orubu T, Giersing B. Potential use of microarray patches for vaccine delivery in low- and middle-income countries. Vaccine. 2019;37:4427-34.
14. Reed SG, Orr MT, Fox CB. Key roles of adjuvants in modern vaccines. Nat Med. 2013;19:1597-608.
15. Stanberry L, Strugnell R. Vaccines of the future. Underst Mod Vaccines Perspect Vaccinol. 2011;1:151-99.
16. Wanga N, Chenb M, Wang T. Liposomes used as a vaccine adjuvant-delivery system: From basics to clinical immunization. J Control Release. 2019;303:130-50.
17. Wilson-Welder JH, Torres MP, Kipper MJ, Mallapragada SK, Wannemuehler MJ, Narasimhan B. Vaccine adjuvants: Current challenges and future approaches. J Pharm Sci. 2009;98:1278-316.
18. Zepp F. Principles of vaccine design-Lessons from nature. Vaccine. 2010;28:C14-C24.

CHAPTER 36

Newer Vaccines in Pipeline

NP Singh

Q1. Which hepatitis B candidate vaccine has undergone most recent clinical trial?

Ans. The third-generation hepatitis B vaccine, Sci-B-Vac® contains three recombinant proteins of hepatitis B virus (HBV) viral envelope: small S, medium pre-S2, and large pre-S1 surface antigens. In a Phase 3 study, this vaccine was found to be safe and elicited superior immune responses to the comparator vaccine Engerix-B [GlaxoSmithKline's (GSK)] in the Phase 3 CONSTANT study. Seroprotection rates were 99% for Sci-B-Vac® and 95% for Engerix-B after completing the full three-dose regimen at the 6-month mark. The investigational vaccine was noninferior following incomplete two-dose course as well. The double-blind, randomized trial, which enrolled 2,800 adults aged 18–45 years, also demonstrated lot-to-lot consistency of Sci-B-Vac®. Applications for regulatory approval in North America and Europe are expected later in 2020. Being more immunogenic, this vaccine may find a place in the vaccination of human immunodeficiency virus (HIV) infected and other immunocompromised conditions.

Q2. What are the vaccine candidates under current clinical trials for group A streptococcus (GAS)?

Ans. Peptide antigens derived from M protein are the most extensively studied vaccine candidates and all current GAS vaccine candidates in clinical trials are designed based on M protein-derived peptides. Various multivalent vaccines derived from the N-terminus of GAS M proteins are in preclinical and clinical trials, among them following two are in advance phases:

	Stage of development		
Name	Preclinical	Phase 1	Phase 2
6-valent vaccine	9 white rabbits intramuscular (IM) injection	28 healthy adults	No further information is available
26-valent vaccine	9 white rabbits IM injection	9 white rabbits IM injection	90 healthy adults IM injection

Q3. Is there a vaccine being developed for hand, foot, and mouth disease (HFMD)?

Ans. Hand, foot, and mouth disease is caused by enterovirus 71 (EV71) infection. Several strategies are currently being applied to develop vaccine candidates, some of which have resulted in commercialization. An inactivated EV71 whole viral candidate vaccine (INV21) was found to be safe and immunogenic in a single center, double blind, placebo controlled, randomized, and dose escalation Phase I study of two dosages in adult volunteers; the first use of this investigational vaccine in humans. Results also showed that the EV71 candidate vaccine produced cross-neutralizing antibodies against the heterologous subgenotypes of EV71 viruses. These observations support its further clinical development as a potential vaccine by initiating a dose-escalation study for determining the dose-dependent safety and immunogenicity of the vaccine in young naïve children. In December 2015, the Food and Drug Administration (FDA) of China approved the first vaccine against EV71, [C4a (H07 strain)] made by the Institute of Medical Biology at the Chinese Academy of Medical Sciences. In January 2016, the Chinese FDA approved a second EV71 vaccine made by Sinovac Biotech [(C4a (*FY7VP5 strain*)].

Q4. Is there any approved malaria vaccine?

Ans. The only approved vaccine as of now is RTS,S/AS01, known by the trade name Mosquirix. In a Phase III study, the following vaccine efficacy (VE) (%) was observed:
- 5–17 months: 0-1-2-20 months schedule: Clinical malaria: with Booster: VE 36.3%, [95% confidence interval (CI) 31.8–40.5], without booster: 28.3%, (23.3–32.9); Severe Malaria: With booster: 32.2% (13.7–46.9), Without booster: (1.1%, –23.0 to 20.5).
- 6–12 weeks: 0-1-2-20 months schedule: Clinical malaria: with Booster: 25.9 (19.9–31.5), without booster: 18.3 (11.7–24.4); Severe Malaria: with booster: 17.3 (–9.4 to 37.5), without booster: 10.3 (–17.9 to 31.8).

It is indicated to be used to vaccinate children aged 6 weeks to 17 months outside the European Union. A World Health Organization (WHO)-led implementation program is piloting the vaccine in three high-malaria countries in Africa in 2019. Research continues into recombinant protein and attenuated whole organism vaccines.

Q5. Which are the other malaria vaccines showing favorable results in clinical trials?

Ans. Several vaccines are under development. Two vaccines showed favorable results. These are:
1. *PfSPZ vaccine*: Developed using radiation-attenuated sporozoites to elicit an immune response. Clinical trials have been promising, with trials taking

place in Africa, Europe, and the US protecting over 80% of volunteers and granted fast track designation by the US FDA in September 2016.
2. *NYVAC-Pf7*: *Multistage vaccine*, trials of which in humans demonstrate cellular immune responses in over 90% of the subjects but *very poor antibody responses*. Despite this following administration of the vaccine, some candidates had complete protection when challenged with *Plasmodium falciparum*. This result has warranted ongoing trials.

Q6. Any other malaria vaccines also under development?

Ans. Some other candidate vaccine agents are also under clinical evaluation. These are:
- *SPf66*: A *synthetic peptide* based vaccine, tested extensively in endemic areas in the 1990s, but clinical trials showed it to be insufficiently effective, 28% efficacy in South America and minimal or no efficacy in Africa.
- *Circumsporozoite protein (CSP vaccine)*: Based on the CSP, but additionally has the recombinant *(R32LR)* protein covalently bound to a purified *Pseudomonas aeruginosa* toxin (A9). Initially appeared promising enough to undergo trials, however at an early stage a complete lack of protective immunity was demonstrated in those inoculated.
- *[NANP]19-5.1*: Consists of the schizont export protein (5.1) and 19 repeats of the sporozoite surface protein [NANP].
- *Nanoparticle enhancement of RTS,S*: Uses repetitive antigen display technology to engineer a nanoparticle that displayed malaria specific B cell and T cell epitopes.
- *FMP01–ALFQ*: Circumsporozoite protein *FMP013-based vaccine* with the adjuvant army liposome formulation containing *QS21* (most recent trial).

Q7. What are the perspectives and future outlook of newer meningococcal vaccine development?

Ans. Vaccination strategies against meningococcal meningitis include polysaccharide, glycoconjugate, combined conjugate, and protein/outer membrane vesicle (OMV)-based vaccines. These vaccines have been proven to be safe and effective against *Neisseria meningitidis* serogroups A, B, C, W, and Y. Glycoconjugate vaccines of the future will likely use approaches such as chemical/chemoenzymatic synthesis, advanced carrier protein characterization, and site-specific conjugation chemistry to obtain homogeneous vaccines. These approaches are already underway in the development of a glycoconjugate vaccine for *N. meningitidis* serogroup X for which there is currently no protective vaccine.

Q8. Is there any trial vaccine candidate for respiratory syncytial virus (RSV) in pipeline?

Ans. About 45 vaccines are currently in development with 18 in clinical trials. ResVax™, an aluminum-adjuvanted RSV fusion (F) protein recombinant nanoparticle vaccine investigated for maternal immunization to prevent RSV disease in infants. In a Phase III trial (Prepare trial), 4,636 pregnant women from 87 sites in 11 countries, received a single intramuscular (IM) dose of this vaccine between 28 and 36 weeks of gestational age. Efficacy against the primary and two secondary endpoints in per-protocol infants with RSV lower respiratory tract infection (LRTI) was: 39.4% against medically significant RSV LRTI (−1% to 64%), 44.4% against RSV LRTI hospitalizations (20–62%), and 48.3% against RSV LRTI with severe hypoxemia (−8% to 75%). Prespecified exploratory analyses of these same VE endpoints, which include additional data ascertained from records, were: 40.9% against medically significant RSV LRTI (95% CI, 16–58%) 41.7% against RSV LRTI hospitalizations (95% CI, 17–59%) 59.6% against RSV LRTI with severe hypoxemia (95% CI, 32–76%). Efficacy against all-cause LRTI data through 180 days with expanded data was: 20.2% (3.5–34) against medically significant RSV LRTI, 25.3% (5.3–41) against RSV LRTI hospitalizations and 39.1% (14.6–56) against RSV LRTI with severe hypoxemia. It is awaiting licensure.

Other adenoviral platform-based vaccine candidates are especially being developed by GSK and Janssen pharmaceuticals for pediatric/neonatal uses. Most of them are in *Phase-2* clinical trials.

Q9. Any new pertussis vaccine under development?

Ans. Acellular pertussis vaccines are less effective than expected over the time necessary for protecting humans against *Bordetella pertussis*. Also, they do not prevent infection and transmission of the causative pertussis agent, therefore, a new vaccine for whooping cough is much needed as a primary and/or boost. A new *live attenuated pertussis vaccine*, BPZE1, in which three toxins, including the pertussis toxin have been genetically modified has been developed. Current studies indicate that upon nasal administration, BPZE1 can prevent colonization, pertussis disease, and ultimately may block transmission, which could halt whooping cough in both young children and adults. If successful in the clinic, global introduction of BPZE1 could, in time, eliminate whooping cough.

Q10. What are oral cholera vaccines in developmental phase?

Ans. Research firm Hilleman Labs and Hyderabad-based vaccine maker Bharat Biotech are coming together for Phase-3 development of an oral cholera vaccine HillChol, which can potentially fill supply gap. It contains a single serotype *Hikojima*, which expresses the antigen *Inaba* and *Ogawa*, resulting in a shorter and simpler manufacturing process as compared with licensed oral cholera vaccines. The vaccine is expected to enter the commercial stage in the next 3 years.

Q11. What is the need for a new rabies vaccine?

Ans. In most cases, rabies vaccines are given to humans after their exposure to a rabid animal and pre-exposure vaccination is largely reserved for humans at high risk for contacts with the virus. With the multiple dose regimens of current rabies vaccines, vaccinations is not cost-effective for most countries particularly for the pre-exposure prophylaxis (PrEP), and this warrants the development of new rabies vaccines, which are as safe as current vaccines, and achieve protective immunity after a single dose, and most importantly, are less costly.

Q12. What are the new rabies vaccine candidates suited for postexposure prophylaxis (PEP), currently under development?

Ans. Following vaccine candidate are suited for PEP:
1. *Adjuvanted rabies vaccines*: PIKA rabies vaccine, containing a second-generation adjuvant based on a Toll-like receptor (TLR)-3 agonist.
2. *Protein vaccines*: Developed by CPL Biologicals (Dholka, Gujarat, India), by infection of insect cells with a recombinant baculovirus expressing a form of the rabies virus glycoprotein. One would assume the vaccine to be safe and immunogenic in humans, but unfortunately none of the trials result have been published.
3. *Genetically modified, inactivated rabies virus*: By reverse genetics a rabies virus genome was constructed that encoded two copies of the glycoprotein.

Q13. What are the rabies vaccine candidates suited for PrEP currently under development?

Ans. The candidate PEP vaccines could also be used for PrEP. To make their use for mass PrEP in endemic remote areas feasible, they would have to be cost-effective to allow for single dose PrEP regimens. Following vaccine candidate are especially suited for PEP:
- *Genetic (DNA and RNA) vaccines*: Production and purification is relatively easy and cheap; vaccines can be formulated to ensure their thermostability. Immune responses are focused on the encoded antigen unlike viral vector vaccines, which also elicit responses to antigens of the carrier, which limits their usefulness for homologous booster immunizations. Genetic vaccines carry their own adjuvant.
- *Viral vector (adenovirus) vaccines*: Advantageous in the sense that they enter cells more efficiently upon binding to cell surface receptors, which as a rule renders them more immunogenic. Disadvantages are that production is more complicated and costly, they can only be used once in an individual as virus neutralizing antibodies (VNAs) induced against the vector backbone will reduce vaccine uptake and thereby expression and immunogenicity of the vaccine antigen upon its use for a boost.

Q14. What is neonatal rotavirus vaccine and what is its developmental status in clinical trials?

Ans. An oral live vaccine candidate has been developed from a naturally-attenuated human strain found in newborns (G3P[6]) that does not cause disease and that replicates well in the newborn gut. This is true even in the presence of maternal antibodies and when an infant is breastfed, thus making it well-adapted to newborns. The vaccine, neonatal RV3-BB has been licensed to PT Biofarma in Indonesia, administered in three doses starting 0–5 days after birth. Vaccine was found in a *Phase 2/3* clinical trial in Indonesia to be well tolerated and to provide better efficacy rates than the same vaccine given in a typical schedule. Efficacy rates also compare favorably with those of globally available vaccines in low- and middle-income countries. Ongoing development of RV3-BB is underway in Indonesia by BioFarma with plans to have the vaccine available to infants in the Indonesian National Immunization Program, and prequalified by WHO.

Q15. What is injectable rotavirus vaccine (IRV) and what is its developmental status in clinical trials?

Ans. Nonreplicating and injectable vaccines [nonreplicating rotavirus vaccine (NRRV)] are either killed rotaviruses or just parts (subunits) of the virus that, unlike current live, oral vaccines, do not require multiplying in the gut to induce immunity. Inspired by the successes of the injectable inactivated polio vaccine (IPV), these vaccines, are given through injection, thereby bypassing the gut. They could potentially be more effective than oral vaccines in low-income settings by avoiding factors that may limit immune responses in the intestine, such as gut inflammation, malnutrition, or coinfections. By avoiding the gut, these vaccines should also reduce the increased risk of intussusception associated with rotavirus vaccination. Two candidate vaccines have undergone clinical trials:

1. A monovalent, parenteral, subunit rotavirus vaccine P2-VP8-P[8] was well tolerated and immunogenic in adults in the USA and in toddlers and infants in South Africa, but elicited poor responses against heterotypic rotavirus strains.
2. Safety and immunogenicity of another parenteral trivalent subunit rotavirus vaccine, P2-P8-P[4]P[6]P[8] is being assessed in a multisite, randomized, double-blind, placebo-controlled trial, and Phase 2 study in South Africa. Result showed that it was well tolerated with promising anti-P2-VP8 immunoglobulin G (IgG) and neutralizing antibody (nAb) responses across the three vaccine P types and these findings support advancing the vaccine to efficacy testing against severe rotavirus disease.

CHAPTER 36: Newer Vaccines in Pipeline

Q16. What strategies are required for development of new tuberculosis (TB) vaccine? What is the current status?

Ans. Alternative vaccines and delivery strategies focusing on *Mycobacterium tuberculosis (Mtb)* antigens and appropriate immune stimulating adjuvants are needed to induce protective immunity targeted to the lungs, the primary sites of infections, and pathology. A comprehensive global TB vaccination strategy should be targeted at both Mtb-uninfected and infected adolescents and adults. About 16 different TB vaccine candidates are currently in clinical trials globally, with a handful approaching or currently in proof-of-concept (*Phase IIb*) studies in the field, and many more in preclinical development. There are currently eight vaccines in Phase II or Phase III trials. These vaccines aim either to prevent infection (pre-exposure) or to prevent primary progression to disease or reactivation of latent TB infection (LTBI-post-exposure). These would have a critical role in India's fight against TB.

Q17. What is Indian Council of Medical Research (ICMR) project regarding developmental trials of new TB vaccines? What are the achievable targets set and what is progress so far?

Ans. Vaccine research is undergoing in different Indian academic laboratories under the project by ICMR with the aim that vaccine candidates under clinical development by different manufacturers will be evaluated for immunogenicity and efficacy in the Indian population. Deliverable target by ICMR are an efficacious antirelapse TB vaccine in 5 years, and an efficacious TB preventative vaccine in 10 years. The landscaping of TB vaccines has identified three vaccine candidates, which can be tested for different endpoints in the immediate future. The three vaccines identified are:
1. *VPM1002*: Live recombinant vaccine from the Serum Institute, India
2. *ID93/GLA-SE*: Combinant protein vaccine, discovered by Infectious Disease Research Institute, Seattle and licensed to Gennova Biopharmaceuticals, India
3. *M72/AS01*: A recombinant protein vaccine by GSK, Belgium, Phase 2b placebo-controlled (efficacy) trial.

Q18. Are any new TB vaccines being tried with mode of delivery other than conventional one?

Ans. Many scientific experiments are being tried to improve the present available vaccine [Bacillus Calmette–Guérin (BCG)] or develop newer agents to replace old one. Two such trials are mentioned below:
1. Intravenous administration of the BCG vaccine improves protection from TB in nonhuman primates. Nine out of 10 macaques were highly protected against TB after intravenous administration of the BCG vaccine. Seven animals immunized intradermally or by aerosols showed significantly higher rates of infection when challenged with Mtb delivered

intrapulmonary 6 months postvaccination. Furthermore, intravenous delivery increased the count and persistence of antigen-responsive CD4+ and CD8+ T cells in the lungs. BCG's effectiveness has been low and variable against pulmonary TB. Moreover, waning immunity has been a problem, especially in resource-limited countries.

2. Since the primary site of disease manifestation of TB is the lungs, selection of mucosal route of administration of vaccine and adjuvant give the advantage of activating local natural killer T (NKT) cells as well in the circulating population. By sublingual delivery, the antigens are absorbed directly into the bloodstream from oral mucosa with limited proteolytic degradation and without induction of anaphylaxis. Based on their immuno-dominant nature, the secreted Mtb proteins Ag85B and ESAT-6 adjuvanted with the glycolipid alpha-galactosylceramide (GalCer), a potent NKT cell agonist have been widely explored as safer candidate subunit vaccines against Mtb. Aerosol/sublingual trial on mice has given satisfactory results and hope for its future implications, especially in newborn and infants.

Q19. Is there any progress towards in the development of vaccines for human cytomegalovirus (CMV) disease?

Ans. Any case of congenital CMV prevented would be a major success for public health. Vaccines preventing persistent infection and also boosting the immune response of seropositive individuals would be highly desirable. Major targets of such a vaccine would be young women and adolescents to prevent congenital CMV (cCMV), as well as toddlers, to prevent transmission to adults and, thus, decrease virus dissemination. Three vaccine candidates are in most recent phases of their clinical trials. These are:

1. *V160 (MSD)*: A conditionally replication defective virus, termed V160, is currently being evaluated in a Phase II clinical trial by MSD. The V160 vaccine has shown promising safety and immunogenicity profiles in a Phase I clinical trial. In seronegative subjects, there was a significant increase in nAb titers against epithelial cell infection after vaccination. At 1 month after the third dose, V160-induced nAb titers were comparable to those elicited by natural infection. The antibody levels remained elevated above the baseline at month 18.
2. *gB/MF59 vaccine (Sanofi)*: Results of 50% protection from pregnancy interval (PI) of seronegative pregnant women receiving the gB/MF59 vaccine, as reported in clinical trials, appear to be a good step forward towards prevention of cCMV. In adolescent girls, overall VE was 43% ($P = .20$). Two doses were sufficient to give a VE of 45% ($P = .08$) in seronegative subjects regardless of age.
3. *Triplex vaccine (City of Hope)*: City of Hope selected a highly attenuated, nonproliferating viral vector referred to as modified vaccinia Ankara (MVA) to insert three immunodominant CMV antigens: pp65, IE-1-exon4,

and IE2-exon5. A test of vaccine-protective efficacy has recently been completed in at-risk hematopoietic cell transplantation (HCT) recipients in a multicenter, randomized, and placebo-controlled Phase II clinical trial. Success in demonstrating tolerability of the triplex vaccine in pediatric HCT recipients (clinicaltrials.gov pending, NCT03354728) would prompt an additional approach to vaccinating the donor as a means to forestall early reactivation events before antiviral prophylaxis using letermovir.

Q20. What are the *Shigella* vaccine candidates under recent clinical?

Ans. Following are the vaccine candidates under most recent trial:
- Polysaccharide-conjugate candidates:
  - *Flexyn2a subunit bioconjugate vaccine*: Conjugates *Shigella* O-antigen to recombinant exotoxin A of *Pseudomonas aeruginosa* recently advanced through a Phase 2 controlled human infection model (CHIM) *study* and found preliminary evidence of efficacy. (Adult trial only)
  - *S. Sonnei O-SP-rEPA and S. flexneri 2a O-SP-rEPA*: Subunit conjugate vaccine in *Phase 3 trials*. (Pediatric trial only)
- Whole-cell candidates:
  - *WRSS1 (live oral S. sonnei) vaccine*: The functional antibody and cytokine responses from a recent Phase 1 and 2 trial in Bangladeshi adults and children were promising. (Pediatric and adult trials)
  - *S. flexneri 2a inactivated (killed) and S. flexneri 2a CVD1208S (live attenuated) vaccines*: Both are currently in Phase 1 trials. (Adult trial only)

Q21. What are the *Shigella* vaccine candidates under most recent preclinical stage?

Ans. Following vaccines are in preclinical stage of development through different approaches:
- *Flexneri 2a Invaplex 50 intranasal vaccine*: Also elicit cross-protective immune responses against *S. sonnei* and *S. flexneri* 3a.
- *InvaplexAR*: Second-generation Invaplex subunit vaccine consisting of a complex of lipopolysaccharide (LPS) extracted from *Shigella* in combination with recombinant forms of IpaB and IpaC.
- *S. sonnei 53G lyophilized CHIM*: Baseline parameters of higher LPS-specific IgA titers and serum bactericidal activity (SBA) titers were associated with disease resistance, supporting other observations and potential immune correlates of protection.

Q22. What are the vaccine candidates for enterotoxigenic *Escherichia coli* (ETEC) are under recent clinical trial?

Ans. Following are five candidate vaccines among many others which are under current clinical trials:

1. *ETEC/rCTB*: Inactivated whole target organism, Phase 3, pediatric trial
2. *ETVAX*: Inactivated whole target organism, Phase 1 and 2, pediatric and adult trials.
3. *ACE527*: Inactivated whole target organism, Phase 2a, adult trial. The first ETEC vaccine containing all necessary cellular components for broad colonization factor and LT-toxin coverage (complete vaccine) to demonstrate protection in humans following a challenge.
4. *Dukoral (cholera vaccine)*: Inactivated whole target organism, Phase 2, adult cholera vaccine booster study trial.
5. *CssBA ± dmLT*: Recombinant [(nonvirus-like particle (VLP)] vaccine, Phase 1, adult trial.

Q23. Is the any promising vaccine candidate against *Staphylococcus Aureus*?

Ans. None of the failed *S. aureus* vaccine trials that targeted the generation of opsonic antibodies had definitive clinical data that clearly supported the role of targeting opsonophagocytosis as a mechanism to improve outcomes against *S. aureus* in human infections. The newer evidences form the basis for a hypothesis that staphylococcal toxins (including *superantigens* and *pore-forming toxins*) are important virulence factors, and targeting the neutralization of these toxins are more likely to provide a therapeutic benefit. Based on the previous preclinical and clinical trial results *rFSAV* is found to be a potentially promising vaccine candidate for defensing against *S. aureus* infection and it can also induce Th1 and Th17 cell immune responses. Although detailed mechanisms are very complicated and undefined, it is necessary to induce comprehensive natural and acquired cellular and humoral immune responses for an effective *S. aureus* vaccine to be most effective.

Q24. What are the new developments in typhoid and paratyphoid vaccines?

Ans. Vi capsular polysaccharide (ViCPS) conjugated vaccines (TT, exoprotein A, DT, and typhoid toxoid), stimulate strong immune response and therefore can protect against typhoid in infants. Moreover, no vaccines are available against *Salmonella paratyphi* infection. Thus, a new formulation capable of providing long-term protection against both the pathogens and safe for all age groups is immediately required. A recombinant, *S. typhi* outer membrane protein STIV (rSTIV) is found to be immunogenic in mice and elicits high serum titers of different immunoglobulin subtypes. Immunization with rSTIV also induces robust cell-mediated immunity, including antigen-specific T cell proliferation and cytotoxic T lymphocyte response. Finally, mice immunized with rSTIV are significantly protected against *S. typhi* and *S. paratyphi* A challenge, with reduced visceral bacterial load. Therefore, there is the potential of rSTIV as a novel vaccine candidate for enteric fever.

SUGGESTED READING

1. Azuar A, Jin W, Mukaida S, Hussein WM, Toth I, Skwarczynski M. Recent Advances in the Development of Peptide Vaccines and Their Delivery Systems Against Group A Streptococcus. Vaccines (Basel). 2019;7:58.
2. Barry E, Cassels F, Riddle M, Walker R, Wierzba T. Vaccines Against Shigella and Enterotoxigenic Escherichia coli: A summary of the 2018 VASE Conference, Vaccine. 2019;37:4768-74.
3. Bines JE, Thobari JA, Satria CD, Handley A, Watts E, Cowley D, et al. Human Neonatal Rotavirus Vaccine (RV3-BB) to Target Rotavirus from Birth. N Engl J Med. 2018;378(8):719-30.
4. Blanco JCG, Boukhvalova MS, Shirey KA, Gregory A. Prince GA, Vogel SN. New insights for development of a safe and protective RSV vaccine. Hum Vaccin. 2010;6:482-92.
5. Brennan MJ. A New Whooping Cough Vaccine That May Prevent Colonization and Transmission. Vaccines. 2017;5:43.
6. Das S, Chowdhury R, Pal A, Okamoto K, Das S. Salmonella Typhi outer membrane protein STIV is a potential candidate for vaccine development against typhoid and paratyphoid fever. Immunobiology. 2019;224(3):371-82.
7. Der Meeren OV, Hatherill M, Nduba V, Wilkinson RJ, Muyoyeta M, Brakel EV, et al. Phase 2b placebo-controlled trial of M72/AS01E candidate vaccine to prevent active tuberculosis in adults. N Engl J Med. 2018;379(17):1621-34.
8. Fooks AR, Banyard AC, Ertl HCJ. New human rabies vaccines in the pipeline. Vaccine. 2019;37 Suppl 1(Suppl 1):A140-A145.
9. Giersing BK, Dastgheyb SS, Modjarrad K, Moorthy V. Status of vaccine research and development of vaccines for Staphylococcus aureus. Vaccine. 2016;34:2962-6.
10. Groome MJ, Koen A, Fix A, Page N, Jose L, Madhi SA, et al. Safety and immunogenicity of a parenteral P2-VP8-P[8] subunit rotavirus vaccine in toddlers and infants in South Africa: a randomised, double-blind, placebo-controlled trial. Lancet Infect Dis. 2017;17(8):843-53.
11. Harro C, Bourgeois AL, Sack D, Walker R, DeNearing B, Brubaker J, et al. Live attenuated enterotoxigenic Escherichia coli (ETEC) vaccine with dmLT adjuvant protects human volunteers against virulent experimental ETEC challenge. Vaccine. 2019;37:1978-86.
12. Human Vaccines & Immunotherapeutics: news. Hum Vaccin Immunother. 2020;16:3:478-9.
13. IMCR. (2017). Vaccine. [online] Available from http://bmi.icmr.org.in/itrc/index.php/projects/portfolio/3-cols-with-sidebar/item/42-vaccines. [Last accessed October, 2020].
14. Khan A, Singh S, Galvan G, Jagannath C, Jagannadha K. Prophylactic Sublingual Immunization with Mycobacterium tuberculosis Subunit Vaccine Incorporating the Natural Killer T Cell Agonist Alpha-Galactosylceramide Enhances Protective Immunity to Limit Pulmonary and Extra-Pulmonary Bacterial Burden in Mice. Vaccines (Basel). 2017;5:47.
15. Malariasite. Accelerating malaria vaccine development. [online] Available from https://www.malariasite.com/malaria-vaccines/. [Last accessed October, 2020].
16. McCarthy PC, Sharyan A, Moghaddam LS. Meningococcal Vaccines: Current Status and Emerging Strategies. Vaccines. 2018;6:12.
17. Mogasale V, Kanungo S, Pati S, Lynch J, Dutta S. The history of OCV in India and barriers remaining to programmatic introduction. Vaccine. 2020;38 Suppl 1:A41-A45.
18. Plotkin SA, Wang D, Oualim A, Diamond DJ, Kotton CN, Mossman S, et al. The Status of Vaccine Development Against the Human Cytomegalovirus. J Infect Dis. 2020;221(Supplement_1):S113-S122.

19. Shaikh H, Lynch J, Kim J, Excler JL. Current and future cholera vaccines. Vaccine. 2020;38 Suppl 1:A118-A126.
20. Tambyah PA, Oon J, Asli R, Kristanto W, Hwa SH, Vang F, et al. An inactivated enterovirus 71 vaccine is safe and immunogenic in healthy adults: A phase I, double blind, randomized, placebo-controlled, study of two dosages. Vaccine. 2019;37(31):4344-53.
21. Weinberg A, Lambert SL, Canniff J, Yu L, Lang N, Esser MT, Falloon J, et al. Antibody and B cell responses to an investigational adjuvanted RSV vaccine for older adults. Hum Vaccin Immunother. 2019;15:2466-74.
22. Wrighton KH. A novel vaccine target for malaria. Nat Rev Drug Discov. 2020;19:386.
23. Yang Y-A, Chong A, Song J. Why Is Eradicating Typhoid Fever So Challenging: Implications for Vaccine and Therapeutic Design. Vaccines. 2018;6:45.

CHAPTER 37

Vaccines against Novel Viruses

NP Singh

Q1. What is novel virus?

Ans. Novel virus refers to a virus not seen before. It can be a virus that is isolated from its natural reservoir or isolated as the result of spread to an animal or human host where the virus had not been identified before. It can be an emergent virus, one that represents a new virus, but it can also be an extant virus, one that has not been previously identified. Viral diseases continue to pose a serious threat to public health. The world has witnessed several viral epidemics in past 20 years that include severe acute respiratory syndrome coronavirus (SARS-CoV-1) in 2003, H1N1 influenza in 2009, the Middle East respiratory syndrome coronavirus (MERS-CoV) in 2012, the 2013 Ebola outbreak in West Africa, and SARS-CoV-2 in 2019.

Q2. What are novel vaccine candidates in the developmental phase under the control of Coalition for Epidemic Preparedness Innovations (CEPI)?

Ans. Coalition for Epidemic Preparedness Innovations, which was launched in January 2017 in Oslo, London and Washington with the aim to prevent future epidemics by the development of new vaccines. Three major targets have been selected for the manufacturing and testing of candidate vaccines: MERS-CoV, Lassa fever virus, and Nipah virus (NiV). CEPI is responsible for vaccine development from preclinical to Phase 2a trial. Several vaccines are being followed up: a Lassa-VSV vaccine, developed by International AIDS Vaccine Initiative (IAVI); a Lassa-deoxyribonucleic acid (DNA) vaccine; a Lassa-measles [measles virus (MV)] vaccine, developed by Themis; a MERS-CoV-MV vaccine, also developed by Themis; and a Nipah glycoprotein (GP) subunit vaccine with adjuvant. Most Phase 1 studies have taken place in 2018–2019 and Phase 2a trials are expected to follow in 2020–2022.

Q3. Is there any Food and Drug Administration (FDA) approved licensed vaccine for the Ebola virus disease?

Ans. ERVEBO™ is the first-licensed vaccine for prevention of Ebola virus disease. The vaccine, originally developed by the Public Health Agency of Canada, is delivered in a single 1 mL dose and has been delivered to >200,000 people in an ongoing 2018–2020 outbreak of disease. Merck licensed the vaccine from NewLink in November 2014 to further develop, manufacture, and distribute it. In vivo efficacy and safety studies have been performed by multiple groups. It is a recombinant and live-attenuated vaccine (LAV) containing recombinant vesicular stomatitis virus (VSV) backbone in which the VSV envelope GP has been replaced with the envelope GP of Ebola virus. ERVEBO® has shown to be safe and protective against the Zaire strain of the Ebola virus and is now approved by FDA for prevention of Ebola virus disease in persons 18 years or older.

Q4. Who are eligible for Ebola virus vaccine?

Ans. Each person to be considered for the expanded access of the vaccine will receive one dose of the vaccine. The persons to be considered include:
- Contacts and contacts of contacts of confirmed Ebola virus disease patients (dead or alive)
- Health care and frontline workers (local and international) in the affected areas
- Health care and frontline workers in areas at risk of spread of the outbreak.

Q5. For how long can the vaccine protect a person from Ebola virus infection?

Ans. We do not have sufficient data to say for how long the vaccine will protect a person from Ebola virus infection. Some studies suggest that persons who were given the Ebola vaccine can be protected for up to 12 months. More research is needed to look into the matter.

Q6. What are other vaccines under developmental process for Ebola virus?

Ans. Multiple investigational Ebola vaccines have been tested in numerous clinical trials around the world. These are shown in **Table 1**.

Table 1: Vaccines under developmental process for Ebola virus.

Vaccine	Status
Chimp adenovirus 3 vectored glycoprotein (cAd3-EBO Z)	Phase III
Human adenovirus 5 vectored 2014 glycoprotein insert (Ad5-EBOV)	Phase I complete
Adenovirus 26 vectored glycoprotein/MVA-BN (Ad26.ZEBOV/MVA-BN)	Phase I complete
Purified glycoprotein	NHP challenge initiated
Rabies vectored glycoprotein and Ebola ΔVP30 H_2O_2 treated	NHP challenge complete

(NHP: nonhuman primates)

Table 2: Zika virus vaccine candidates in most advanced stages of their development.

Vaccine platform	Name	Immunogen	Sponsor	Vaccine candidate	Phase
mRNA	mRNA-1325	prM-E	Moderna Therapeutics	NCT03010489	II
DNA	VRC5283	prM-E	NIAID/VRC	NTC03110770	II

(DNA: deoxyribonucleic acid; NIAID: National Institute of Allergy and Infectious Diseases; mRNA: messenger ribonucleic acid; prM-E: pre-membrane and envelope; VRC: Vaccine Research Center)

Q7. What is Zika virus (ZIKV)? Is there any approved vaccine for ZIKV disease at present?

Ans. Zika virus is a reemerging arbovirus of the *Flavivirus* genus that includes multiple important human pathogens including dengue viruses (DENV), Japanese encephalitis virus (JEV), West Nile virus (WNV), and yellow fever virus (YFV). Similar to other flaviviruses in this family, ZIKV transmission occurs from the bite of an infected *Aedes aegypti* mosquito. Rapid spread of ZIKV worldwide prompted the World Health Organization (WHO) to declare it "Public Health Emergency of International Concern". Efforts to combat ZIKV infections led to the development of several vaccine candidates, including LAVs. Currently, there are no FDA-approved vaccines available. About 45 vaccine candidates are in development and beginning to show promise, of these, two are currently in Phase 2 and more than 15 are in Phase 1 clinical trials. **Table 2** shows two vaccine candidates in most advanced stages of their development.

Q8. What is Nipah viral disease and when was it detected in India?

Ans. Nipah (Nee-pa) viral disease is a zoonotic infection and an emerging disease caused by NiV. Transmitted by specific types of *fruit bats*, the disease was recognized for the first time in 1998 in Nipah village, state of Perak, Malaysia. The causative agent was characterized and since then has been named as "Nipah virus (NiV)". In India, it was detected for the first time in Siliguri, West Bengal, in the year 2001 during an outbreak characterized by febrile illness in association with altered sensorium. Another outbreak was reported from Nadia district, West Bengal in the year 2007. Most recently in the year 2018, Nipah viral disease outbreak has been reported in Kozhikode district, northern Kerala, and during this outbreak, deaths occurred in the infected subjects as well as in healthcare personnel who were involved in treatment of patients.

Q9. Are there any vaccines in the developmental pipeline for prevention of NiV disease?

Ans. Vaccination of humans is an integral part of preventing infection due to NiV. Extensive research involving preclinical studies in a number of animals

Table 3: WNV vaccine candidates in most advanced clinical trial.

Vaccine candidate	Type	Key data to date	Stage
Inactivated WNV	Inactivated using formaldehyde	Neutralizing antibodies after three doses	I/II
ChimeriVax-WN02	Recombinant yellow fever vaccine strain expressing the prM/E-fragment of WNV	Neutralizing antibodies (>90%) in younger and older age groups after one dose	II

(prM/E: pre-membrane and envelope; WNV: West Nile virus)

and nonhuman primates have identified multiple vaccine candidates, including vectored and subunit vaccines, offering protective immunity. Experimental vaccines based on the several viral vectors, including the canarypox virus, vesicular stomatitis virus glycoprotein (VSVDG) and rhabdovirus have been evaluated. A recombinant measles virus (rMV) vaccine that expresses envelope GP of NiV has been found to be promising for use in human.

Q10. What is WNV? What are vaccines in pipelines against it?

Ans. West Nile virus is a widely spread human pathogenic arthropod-borne virus, transmitted primarily by *Culex* mosquitoes, when they feed on infected birds. It can lead to severe, sometimes fatal, neurological disease. Over the last two decades, several vaccine candidates for the protection of humans from WNV have been developed. Some technologies were transferred into clinical testing, but these approaches have not yet led to a licensed product. Following two vaccine candidates are in most advanced clinical trial **(Table 3)**.

Q11. What is the concern with the existing dengue vaccine-Dengvaxia™?

Ans. CYD-TDV (Dengvaxia, Sanofi Pasteur), a tetravalent dengue vaccine based on a YFV backbone, has been licensed in several countries on the basis of a 56–61% vaccine efficacy (VE) against virologically confirmed dengue among children in Asia and Latin America. This vaccine is associated with an increased risk of severe dengue and dengue leading to hospitalization in seronegative persons. As a result, in 2018, the WHO recommended that it be provided only to persons with evidence of past infection.

Q12. Which other dengue vaccine has completed Phase III trials?

Ans. TAK-003 of Takeda Pharmaceuticals Japan is a live tetravalent dengue vaccine that has completed Phase III trials. A live attenuated DENV-2 (TDV-2) virus provides the genetic backbone for all four of the viruses in the vaccine, the other three virus strains (TDV-1, TDV-3, and TDV-4) are chimeras that were generated by replacing the pre-membrane and envelope genes of TDV-2 with those from wild-type DENV-1, DENV-3, and DENV-4 strains.

Q13. What are the results of the Phase III trials of this vaccine?

Ans. The overall VE was 80.2 (73.3–85.3) in the per-protocol population. 27.7% of the per-protocol population was seronegative at baseline. VE in this group was 74.9% (57.0–85.4) and 82.2 (74.5–87.6) in the seropositive group. Efficacy trends varied according to stereotype. Efficacy against DEN-1 was 73.7 (51.7–85.7), DEN-2 was 97.7 (92.7–99.3), DEN-3 was 62.6 (43.3–75.4), and DEN-4 was 63.2 (64.6–91.8). Efficacy against virologically confirmed dengue leading to hospitalization was 94.4 (84.3–98.0) in those who were seropositive and 97.2 (79.1–99.6) in those who were seronegative. The incidence of serious adverse events was similar in the vaccine group and placebo group (3.1% and 3.8%, respectively). No disease enhancement was observed in this study.

Q14. What are other dengue vaccines currently in clinical trials?

Ans. Candidate vaccines under development include additional LAVs, purified inactivated vaccines (PIV), and recombinant protein and plasmid vaccines. All of these dengue vaccine candidates seek to target all four DENV serotypes, and all rely on the DENV structural antigens, prM and E to elicit DENV neutralizing antibodies (nAbs). The US National Institutes of Health (NIH) tetravalent dengue vaccine (*TetraVax-DV*) is in Phase III efficacy trials at the current time.

Q15. What is the status of dengue vaccine development in India?

Ans. Dengvaxia has not been licensed in India as the regulators required additional safety data. India has initiated its own efforts to develop two dengue vaccine candidates. One is a LAV and the other is an indigenously developed protein-based tetravalent dengue subunit vaccine, DSV4. The Indian vaccine producers Panacea Biotec, Serum Institute, and Biological E have secured nonexclusive licenses for the clinical development and commercialization of the dengue vaccine TetraVax-DV developed by the US NIH. Data at hand from the TetraVax-DV Phase I trials as well as upcoming data from the ongoing Phase II and Phase III trials of the NIH vaccine in the Asian countries and in Brazil will serve as a valuable reference for the clinical trial data anticipated to be generated by the Indian companies in the near future. Panacea Biotec Ltd with its tetravalent LAV *(CTRI/2017/02/007923)* has currently in Phase I/II clinical trial.

Q16. What is DSV4? How does DSV4 differ from other LAVs?

Ans. DSV4 is tetravalent dengue subunit vaccine being indigenously developed by the International Centre for Genetic Engineering and Biotechnology (ICGEB) and Sun Pharma. Unlike the four component LAVs, DSV4 is a single-component and nonreplicating vaccine based on a VLP platform [*provided by the hepatitis B virus surface antigen (HBsAg)*], produced using the methylotrophic yeast *Pichia pastoris*. It has been found to be immunogenic in multiple strains of mice, eliciting high levels of nAbs capable of potently blocking the infection by each of the four prevalent DENV serotypes. Importantly, DSV4-elicited antibodies *did not manifest enhancement potential* in an in vivo antibody-dependent enhancement (ADE) model. The lack of ADE is a critical attribute of DSV4 from the viewpoint of vaccine safety. Currently, DSV4 vaccine development work is centered on process development and scale-up as a prelude to efficacy and toxicity studies in small animals before initiating cyclic guanosine monophosphate (cGMP) production for clinical testing in the coming years.

Q17. What is the status of vaccine development against chikungunya virus (CHIKV)?

Ans. Two of the most promising vaccines against CHIKV infection, a *CHIK VLP vaccine* and a *measles-vectored vaccine* expressing CHIK VLPs, have cleared Phase I trials with positive outcomes. These vaccines are overall safe and tolerable, and elicit CHIKV neutralization titers in adults 18–50 years of age. These two candidates are now being tested in healthy adults of 18–60 years of age in five Caribbean island nations. Based on results from Phase I trials, at least two immunizations with the live-vectored or CHIK VLPs are needed for 100% seroconversion and induction of nAbs in healthy adult subjects.

Q18. What are vaccines types under developmental trial for MERS-CoV?

Ans. Currently, a vaccine for MERS-CoV is not available, although several candidates have been developed using a variety of approaches. These are:
- *Subunit vaccines (immunogenically focused)*: They have gained popularity in recent decades due to the relative ease of their production and their reduced risks in vivo compared to other vaccine types.
- *DNA vaccines (efficient protection)*: Administration via *electroporation*, has been tested in clinical trials with immunogenicity comparable to other vaccine types and predominantly low-grade adverse events reported.
- *Viral vector vaccines (optimized delivery)*: Contain one or more immunogenic proteins of the pathogen of interest in the context of an attenuated virus backbone.
- *Live attenuated and inactivated vaccines (situationally useful)*: Resemble the original virus, preserving structural features and a full or nearly full repertoire of immunogenic components.

Q19. What is the current state of MERS-CoV vaccine candidates?

Ans. While development of therapeutic treatment is critical, vaccination carries the promise of mitigating future outbreaks and alleviating disease burden from the most vulnerable populations including the aged, the immunosuppressed. MERS-CoV vaccines have shown encouraging results in preclinical studies and we hope these vaccines stand up to safety

considerations in order to proceed through clinical trials. Among various candidates in developmental states, only three have been there in *Phase I clinical trial*. These are:
1. *pVax1-S* (DNA vaccine),
2. *MVA-S* (viral vector vaccine), and
3. *ChAdOx1-S* (viral vector vaccine).

Q20. Why there is a need for vaccine, even after the huge success of antiretroviral therapy (ART) in the treatment and prevention of human immunodeficiency virus-1 (HIV-1) infections?

Ans. Currently, 36.7 million persons are living with HIV-1 worldwide. However, even in higher income countries, 20–30% of HIV-infected persons are not aware of their infection and these persons are most likely to spread the virus among their contacts, as in the absence of ART higher viral loads increase the probability of HIV transmission. Therefore, in order to prevent transmission, an HIV vaccine is still urgently needed. Effective vaccination would prevent transmission of HIV-1 from donors to recipients irrespective of their serological status. Furthermore, an effective vaccine could substitute the administration of antiviral drugs for prevention of infection in healthy people at risk.

Q21. What are the major challenges in vaccine development against HIV-1?

Ans. Although over 35 years have passed since the discovery that HIV-1 was the etiological agent behind the acquired immunodeficiency syndrome (AIDS) epidemic, a preventive vaccine has not yet been realized. Vaccine development against HIV-1 is one of the major challenges in medical research. There is a bag of tricks of HIV-1 to evade the immune system that hinders vaccine development. These are:
- *Fast rate of replication of virus coupled with high mutability (1–10 mutations/genome/replication cycles)* and recombination rapidly leads to the emergence of *quasispecies of viral clones* that are able to thrive as escape mutants and evade both the cell-mediated and the humoral immune responses of the host.
- *Viral variability* (same as for the influenza viruses).
- *Downregulation of the major histocompatibility complex (MHC) class I antigen presentation* at the surface of the infected cell, allowing for escape from antiviral cytotoxic T-lymphocyte (CTL) responses.
- *Nature of the native Env spikes on the viral surface*: Env-HIV protein is a heavily glycosylated trimeric protein which has formidable defenses that hinder broadly neutralizing antibodies (bnAbs) development, linked to its conformational dynamic and extremely variable sequence.

These evasion tricks of HIV-1 do not only fool our immune system, but also did so with researchers involved in HIV vaccine research for decades.

Q22. What are the experiences of previous clinical human trials?

Ans. The six completed human HIV-1 efficacy (Phase III) and proof of concept (Phase IIb) vaccine trials indicated that the development of an Ab-based vaccine might be more likely than a T-cell-based vaccine. Both T-cell-focused trials, i.e., STEP and Phambili, were stopped due to an increased risk of infection in vaccinated participants. RV144 was the only study that achieved moderate VE of 31.2% after 3.5 years follow-up in a modified intention-to-treat analysis. Collectively, a great wealth of information has been accrued from these studies, with vaccines based on just viral vectors or heterologous viral vector prime protein-boost protocols appearing to perform better than multidose protein-based vaccines.

Q23. What is the prospect of future vaccine development for HIV-1?

Ans. From a historical standpoint, vaccinology has been successful at preventing infections from organisms that express stable/invariant antigenic structures that can be targeted by antibodies. For this reason, the HIV-1 virus has essentially presented vaccine researchers with a "moving target" for which to create a vaccine, necessitating the development of novel vaccine approaches. It is important to understand that, despite the history of failures in HIV vaccine development, the preclinical and early phase clinical vaccine pipeline is rich in both novel and diverse anti-HIV vaccine strategies. This, coupled with the ongoing efficacy trials designed to improve upon RV144, leads many to see a bright future for HIV vaccine development.

Q24. What different development approaches are being tried in recent clinical trials for HIV-1 vaccines?

Ans. Although many vaccine candidates are composed of the whole virus or specific proteins, the use of only a minimal pathogen epitope which can stimulate long-lasting protection is becoming a tendency in vaccine development. Broadly, there are two approaches found to have potentials in clinical trials for developing efficacious vaccine against HIV-1 disease. These are:
- Structure-based reverse vaccinology and epitope vaccines (*peptide-based approach*), and
- Vectored expression of bnAbs (*viral vectors approach*)

Q25. What are two most important parameters that will serve to design and decide strategies for bnAbs-based vaccine for HIV-1?

Ans. Initial vaccine trials were based on soluble monomeric gp120, often derived from culture-adapted HIV-1 strains, as we know today, due to its non-native conformation are *not suited to induce bnAbs*, i.e., antibodies able to neutralize a broad spectrum of primary HIV-1 strains belonging to different subtypes of HIV-1. At best, these vaccines could induce antibodies neutralizing autologous HIV-1 strains. We now have a detailed vision of the obstacles we face, including the discovery and characterization of potent bnAbs isolated from both infected individuals and immunized animals, the description of the structure of the Env trimer, which is the sole target of nAbs and the determination of the course of Ab-virus coevolution in individuals who develop bnAbs responses. These two new parameters serve to design new immunogens and strategies for HIV bnAbs-based vaccines.

Q26. What are the most recent ongoing clinical trials for HIV vaccines?

Ans. A rich array of HIV-1 vaccine clinical trials in pipeline, along with the initiation of HVTN702 (a repeat of the RV144) trial in South Africa, provides much hope that additional correlates of protection will be elucidated and that an HIV-1 vaccine might yet become a reality. The two-viral vector-based vaccine trials, Imbokodo and HVTN702, have resulted from years of scientific testing and clinical development, currently representing the best efforts in HIV vaccine development:

1. HVTN702 (The Uhambo study) is a Phase 2b/3 clinical trial based on the modestly protective RV144 clinical trial. This is the most advanced and largest HIV vaccine clinical trial initiated thus far and is being carried out in South Africa. It enrolls 5,400 healthy and sexually active men and women aged 18–35 years old. Results from the study are expected in late 2020–2021.
2. Imbokodo efficacy trials is a Phase 2b proof of concept study, and the vaccine regimen is based on "mosaic" immunogens in an effort to induce immune responses targeting the diverse global HIV strains, which differs from HVTN 702 study. It enrolled 2,600 HIV-negative women in sub-Saharan Africa. Results are expected in 2021–2022.

■ SUGGESTED READING

1. Arévalo MT, Huang Y, Jones CA, Ross TM. Vaccination with a chikungunya virus-like particle vaccine exacerbates disease in aged mice. PLoS Negl Trop Dis. 2019;13(4):e0007316.
2. Blight J, Alves E, Reyes-Sandova A. Considering Genomic and Immunological Correlates of Protection for a Dengue Intervention. Vaccines (Basel). 2019;7(4):203.
3. Burton DR. Advancing an HIV vaccine; advancing vaccinology. Nat Rev Immunol. 2019;19(2):77-8.
4. Dietrich U. Advances in Antibody-Based HIV-1 Vaccines Development. Vaccines. 2020;8:44.
5. Girard M, Nelson CB, Picot V, Gubler DJ. Arboviruses: A global public health threat. Vaccine. 2020;38(24):3989-94.
6. Mubarak A, Alturaiki W, Hemida MG. Middle East Respiratory Syndrome Coronavirus (MERS-CoV): Infection, Immunological Response, and Vaccine Development. J Immunol Res. 2019;2019:6491738.
7. Saphire EO. A Vaccine against Ebola Virus. Cell. 2020;181(1):6.
8. Singh RK, Dhama K, Chakraborty S, Tiwari R, Natesan SK, Khandia R, et al. Nipah virus: epidemiology, pathology, immunobiology and advances in diagnosis, vaccine designing and control strategies—a comprehensive review. Vet Q. 2019;39:26-55.

9. Steffen T, Hassert M, Hoft SG, Stone ET, Zhang J, Geerling E, et al. Immunogenicity and Efficacy of a Recombinant Human Adenovirus Type 5 Vaccine against Zika Virus. Vaccines. 2020;8:170.
10. Swaminathan S, Khanna N. Dengue vaccine development: Global and Indian scenarios. Int J Infect Dis. 2019;84S:S80-S86.
11. Ulbert S. West Nile virus vaccines—current situation and future directions. Hum Vaccin Immunother. 2019;15(10):2337-42.
12. Wang N, Shang J, Jiang S, Du L. Subunit Vaccines Against Emerging Pathogenic Human Coronaviruses. Front Microbiol. 2020;11:298.
13. Wilder-Smith A, Vannice K, Durbin A, Hombach J, Thomas ST, Thevarjan I, et al. Zika vaccines and therapeutics: landscape analysis and challenges ahead. BMC Med. 2018;16:84.

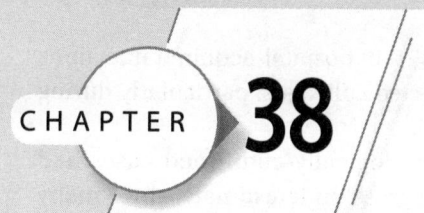

CHAPTER 38: Covid-19 Vaccines

NP Singh, Srinivas G Kasi

Note: Covid vaccines is a rapidly evolving field. The information presented in this chapter is current as of 7 January 2021.

Q1. What is the timeline of COVID-19 events?

Ans.
- On 31 December 2019, the Wuhan Municipal Health Commission released a briefing on its website about a pneumonia outbreak in the city.
- On 11 January 2020, the genome of the virus was sequenced.
- On January 13, the NIH and Moderna's infectious disease research team finalized the sequence for mRNA-1273.
- On 30 January 2020, the World Health Organization declared the COVID-19 outbreak a Public Health Emergency of International Concern.
- On 07 February, the first clinical batch of mRNA-1273 was completed, a total of 25 days from sequence selection to vaccine manufacture. The batch then proceeded to analytical testing for release.
- On 11 Feb 2020, the WHO named the virus as SARS CoV-2 and the disease as COVID-19
- On Feb 24, Moderna shipped the first clinical batch of mRNA-1273 to the NIH for use in their Phase 1 clinical study.
- On 11 March 2020, the WHO declared it as a pandemic.
- Globally, as of, 7 January 2021, there have been 85,929,428 confirmed cases of COVID-19, including 1,876,100 deaths.
- In India, as of 7 January 2021, there have been 10,395,278 confirmed cases of COVID-19 with 150,336 deaths.

Q2. Are healthcare workers (HCWs) at increased risk of COVID-19?

Studies in UK and USA have shown that the healthcare workers (HCWs) are at increased risk of COVID-19. The probable reasons include a shortage of personal protective equipment (PPE), long-time exposure to large numbers of infected patients, inadequate training in infection prevention and control (IPC), and exposure to unrecognized COVID-19 patients. Infection in HCWs may also occur due to contact in non-clinical settings, wherein strict IPC may not be followed. In a study from Oman, 35% of hospital-acquired infections were a result of contact with another infected colleague, particularly during 'break' times.

In a study done in China, 13% of virologically-confirmed cases had asymptomatic infection, which may be a gross underestimate, since many asymptomatic children are unlikely to be tested.

In the USA, as of October 29, 2020, 9% of all cases of COVID-19 reported to the Centers for Disease Control and Prevention (CDC) were among children. Children accounted for 1–3.4% of total reported hospitalizations and between 0.6–6.4% of all child COVID-19 cases resulted in hospitalization.

Therefore, despite the low COVID-19 incidence and severity in children, the pediatricians should not lower his/her guard against the disease.

Q3. What is the difference between traditional vaccine development and development using a pandemic paradigm? Give some example where development of vaccines was done at pandemic speed.

Ans. Over the past decade, scientific community and the vaccine industry have been asked to respond urgently to epidemics of H1N1 influenza, Ebola, Zika, SARS-CoV-1, MERS-CoV, and now SARS-CoV-2.

The normal vaccine development paradigm involves multiple steps, each following the other in a sequential pattern, a process that may take 5–10 years.

To accelerate COVID-19 vaccine development, steps are done in parallel (**Fig. 1**), with production of a vaccine commencing even before the outcome of a clinical trial is known, to ensure readiness for distribution once approval is given. Clinical phases are also happening in parallel, with some beginning before the previous one ends. Creation of the infrastructure for vaccine production is commenced almost coinciding with phase 1–2 trials. Manufacturing of the vaccine is commenced during phase 2–3 trials, even

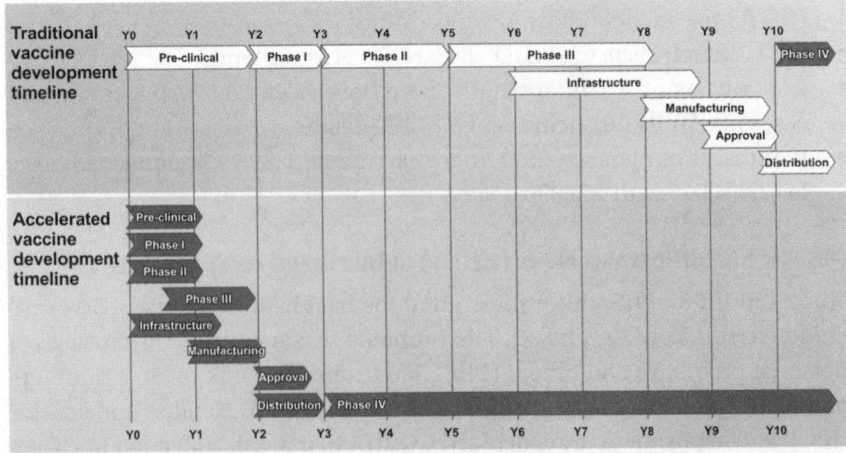

Fig. 1: COVID-19 vaccine accelerated development.

before the results of phase 2–3 studies are known. This pattern of accelerated development is conducted at financial risk to developers and manufacturers, with uncertainty about the success of the vaccine candidate. However, even in this accelerated development paradigm, all the usual safety and efficacy monitoring mechanisms remain in place. There is a critical and essential need for robust phase 4 post-marketing surveillance, to detect the rarer adverse effects.

Q4. What is Antibody Dependent Enhancement (ADE)? How is it an impediment for successful vaccine development against COVID-19?

Ans. Generally, virus-specific antibodies aid in the control of virus infections in a number of ways. In some instances, the presence of specific antibodies can be beneficial to the virus. This activity is known as antibody-dependent enhancement (ADE) of virus infection. The ADE of virus infection is a phenomenon in which virus-specific antibodies enhance the entry of virus, and in some cases the replication of virus, into monocytes/macrophages and granulocytic cells through interaction with Fc and/or complement receptors. Viruses for which ADE has been demonstrated share some common features such as preferential replication in macrophages, ability to establish persistence, and antigenic diversity. ADE effects have been reported in some vaccines against *Dengue* and *Zika* viruses. Although the occurrence of ADE of SARS-CoV-2 has not yet been clearly demonstrated, potential ADE of MERS-CoV and SARS-CoV1 was observed in an in vitro model system.

Q5. What are the WHO recommended target product profile (TPP) for human COVID-19 vaccines?

Ans. Target product profile for a human COVID-19 vaccine must have following key features:
- Favorable benefit/risk profile in the context of observed vaccine efficacy; with no severe adverse events related to vaccination.
- Clear demonstration of efficacy (on population basis) ideally with ~50% point estimate
- Endpoint may be assessed vs. disease, severe disease, and/or shedding/transmission
- No more than two dose regimen
- Confers protection for at least 6 months
- Any route of administration is acceptable, if vaccine is safe and effective.
- Shelf life of at least 6–12 months at as –60°C to –70°C, and demonstration of at least 2-week stability at 2–8°C.
- Minimizes undesired immunopotentiation
- Suitable for adult healthcare workers
- Suitable for adults >60 years old or with underlying diabetes or hypertension
- Suitable for stockpiling

Table 1: COVID-19 vaccine technology platforms in clinical development, December 2020

Platform	Number of candidate vaccines
Inactivated virus	8
Non-replicating viral vector	10
RNA-based	7
Protein subunit	18
DNA-based	8
Virus-like particle (VLP)	2
Replicating viral vector	6
Live attenuated virus	2

Q6. What are the vaccine platforms being explored for COVID-19 vaccines?

Ans. Several platforms are being explored. These include the traditional platforms- inactivated virus, live-attenuated virus, subunit vaccines, VLPs and the newer platforms- viral vectored vaccines and DNA/mRNA vaccines. The newer platforms are first in human vaccines **(Table 1)**.

Q7. What are the current vaccine candidates against COVID-19 in most advanced phase of its development?

Ans. As per the WHO draft landscape of COVID-19 candidate vaccines as on 5 January 2021, there are 60 candidate vaccines in different phases of clinical evaluation and 172 candidates in pre-clinical development. Of the 60 in clinical development stage, 20 are in phase 1, 22 are in phase 1-2, 3 are in phase 2, 4 in phase 2-3 and 11 in phase 3.

Q8. What is the status of vaccine development by Indian manufacturers against COVID-19? Who are in the most advanced stage of development?

Ans. India will play a major role in the development of CoV vaccine. Six Indian companies are working presently on a total of seven vaccine candidates for COVID-19, joining the global race to find a preventive for the deadly infection spreading rapidly across the world. Nearly 100 "vaccine candidates" are being tested and at least three have moved to the human clinical trial stage.

Serum Institute of India and Zydus Cadila is working on two vaccines each, while Bharat Biotech, Biological E, Indian Immunologicals, and Mynvax are developing one vaccine each. Another four or five homegrown vaccines are in early stages of development.

Pune-based Serum Institute of India has partnered with the University of Oxford for the mass production of ChAdOx1 vaccine, which has completed and published the interim analysis of the phase 3 trials.

India's indigenous COVID-19 vaccine by Bharat Biotech is developed in collaboration with the Indian Council of Medical Research (ICMR) - National Institute of Virology (NIV). BBV152 is a whole-virion inactivated SARS-CoV-2 vaccine formulated with a TLR 7/8 agonist molecule adsorbed to alum (Algel-IMDG). The indigenous, inactivated vaccine is developed and manufactured in Bharat Biotech's BSL-3 (Bio-Safety Level 3) high containment facility. After successful completion of the interim analysis from the Phase 1 & 2 clinical trials of COVAXIN, Bharat Biotech received DCGI approval for Phase 3 clinical trials in 26,000 participants in over 25 centers across India. Phase 3 trials have commenced in multiple centers.

ZyCov-D, a Plasmid-DNA vaccine by Zydus vaccines, has completed phase 1 and 2 trials and has been granted authorization for phase 3 trials. This vaccine is administered intradermally in a 0–28–56 days schedule.

BE vaccines is investigating aRBD-S protein vaccine adjuvanted with CpG 1018 which is administered in 2 doses, IM, 0–28 days. Phase 1–2 trials have been approved by DCGI.

In addition, Ohio State Innovation Foundation (OSIF), USA, has licensed novel live attenuated measles virus vectored vaccine candidates against SARS-CoV-2, which were developed by the Ohio State University College of Veterinary Medicine, exclusively to Biological E. Limited (BE).

In phase 1 and 2 studies, Gamaleya'srAd26 and rAd5 vector-based heterologous prime-boost COVID-19 vaccine(Sputnik V), has demonstrated a good safety profile and induced strong humoral and cellular immune responses in participants. This vaccine is being further developed by Dr Reddy's lab, Hyderabad.

Spybiotech's RBD-HBsAg-VLP vaccine is I phase 1 trial in Australia. This vaccine is being jointly developed with Serum Institute of India.

BBL is also working on a nasal live attenuated vaccine Coriflu based on Influenza vaccine backbone. Gennova Biopharmaceuticals Limited of Pune, is developing a mRNA vaccine, which can be stored at +2° C to +8°C.

Live attenuated vaccines, which are attenuated by a patented Codon deoptimization technology, is being jointly developed by Griffith University and Indian Immunol Ltd and a second vaccine by Codagenix and Serum Institute of India.

Q9. Which vaccines are likely to be available in India?

Ans. Covishield of Oxford-Astra-Sii, Covaxin of Bharat Biotech, Sputnik V of Gamaleya Institute, ZyCov-D of Zydus Vaxxicare. India will also be entitled for the Pfizer and Moderna vaccines under the agreement with Covax.

Q10. What is an Emergency Use Authorization (EUA)?

Ans. Vaccines, medicines, diagnostic tests and medical devices, require the approval of a regulatory authority before they can be administered. In India, the regulatory authority is the Central Drugs Standard Control Organisation (CDSCO).

Vaccines and medicines are approval after an assessment of their safety and effectiveness, based on data from trials. The approval process may take a long time and ensures that a medicine or vaccine is safe and effective.

In an emergency situation, like the current COVID-19 pandemic, mechanisms have been developed to grant interim approval to a vaccine, if there is evidence of reasonable efficacy and safety. This is known as Emergency Use Authorization (EUA). For an EUA to be issued for a vaccine, for which there is adequate manufacturing information to ensure quality and consistency, the National Regulatory Authority (NRA) must determine that the known and potential benefits outweigh the known and potential risks of the vaccine.

Marketing approval is granted only after completion of the trials and analysis of full data. EUA permits governmental bodies to use the medicine or the vaccine on the public.

The United States Food and Drug Administration (USFDA) has set guidelines for EUA of vaccines. EUA application can be considered only after sufficient data from phase 3 trials, with a median follow-up of at least 2-months, demonstrate efficacy and safety. Data should include phase 3 safety database of well over 3,000 vaccine recipients, representing a high proportion of participants enrolled in the phase 3 study, who have been followed for serious adverse events and adverse events of special interest for at least one month after completion of the full vaccination regimen.

Q11. Which COVID-19 vaccines have been granted EUA?

Ans.

Astra: UK, India, Argentina

Pfizer: USA, UK, EU

Moderna: UK, US, Israel, Brazil, France

BBIP-CorV (Sinopharm-Inactivated): China, UAE

CoronaVac (Sinovac-Inactivated): China

Gamaleya: Russia

Bharat Biotec/ICMR: India

Q12. Which COVID-19 vaccines have completed phase 3 trials?

Ans.
1. ChAdOx1 nCoV-19 vaccine (AZD1222) of Astra Zeneca
2. BNT162b2 mRNA vaccine of Pfizer-BioNtech
3. mRNA-1273 vaccine of Moderna

Q13. Which COVID-19 vaccines are in phase 3 trials?

Ans.
1. Sinovac: Inactivated
2. Wuhan Institute of Biological Products/Sinopharm: Inactivated
3. Beijing Institute of Biological Products/Sinopharm: Inactivated

4. Bharat Biotech: Inactivated
5. CanSino Biological Inc./Beijing Institute of Biotechnology: Non-Replicating Viral Vector
6. Gamaleya Research Institute: Non-Replicating Viral Vector
7. Janssen Pharmaceutical Companies: Non-Replicating Viral Vector
8. Novavax: Protein subunit
9. Anhui ZhifeiLongcom Biopharmaceutical/Institute of Microbiology, Chinese Academy of Sciences: Protein subunit
10. Medicago Inc.: Plant-derived VLP adjuvanted with AS03.

Q14. What are the results of the Phase 3 studies of ChAdOx1 nCoV-19 vaccine (AZD1222) of Astra Zeneca?

Ans. In symptomatic Covid participants with NAAT +ve test, the overall VE was 70·4% (54·8 to 80·6). In those who received the low-dose (LD) followed by the standard dose (SD), LD/SD, the VE was 90.0% (67.4–97), while it was 60.3% (28.0–78.2) in the SD/SD group. There were no hospitalizations in the vaccine group vs 10 in the control group. The VE was better with a 6 weeks interval between doses.

The vaccine had a good safety profile with serious adverse events and adverse events of special interest balanced across the study arms. One case of transverse myelitis, 14 days after the 2nd dose of vaccine was possibly unrelated to the vaccine. 2 cases of transverse myelitis were observed one each in vaccine and control groups. This was determined to be unrelated by the Independent Safety and Data Monitoring Board (ISDMB).

Q15. What are the results of the Phase 3 studies of BNT162b2 mRNA vaccine of Pfizer-BioNtech?

Ans.
- The efficacy of the vaccine against laboratory-confirmed COVID-19 was 95.0% (90.3–97.6).
- Similar vaccine efficacy (generally 90 to 100%) was observed across subgroups defined by age, sex, race, ethnicity, baseline body-mass index, and the presence of coexisting conditions.
- Among 10 cases of severe COVID-19 with onset after the first dose, 9 occurred in placebo recipients and 1 in a BNT162b2 recipient.
- The VE of 1 dose was 52% (95% CI, 29.5 to 68.4).
- BNT162b2 recipients reported more local reactions than placebo recipients. Pain at the injection site: most commonly reported local reaction, Severe pain was observed in <1%, which was more frequent in younger participants. No participant reported a grade 4 local reaction.
- The most commonly reported systemic events were fatigue and headache, which were more common in the younger participants. Sixty-four vaccine recipients (0.3%) and 6 placebo recipients (<0.1%) reported lymphadenopathy.

- No deaths were considered by the investigators to be related to the vaccine or placebo.

Q16. What are the results of the Phase 3 studies of the mRNA-1273 vaccine of Moderna?

The vaccine efficacy against 94.1% (89.3–96.8). Efficacy was similar in who had evidence of SARS-CoV-2 infection at baseline and in participants 65 years of age or older. Severe COVID-19 occurred in 30 participants, with one fatality; all 30 were in the placebo group. Moderate, transient reactogenicity after vaccination occurred more frequently in the mRNA-1273 group. Serious adverse events were rare, and the incidence was similar in the two groups.

Q17. What are the results of the Phase 3 studies of the Russian Gamaleya institute vaccine (Sputnik V)?

Ans. This is an Adeno-based (rAd26-S+rAd5-S) vaccine utilizing the prime-boost principle.

In a small phase 2–3 study, with 76 subjects, the vaccine demonstrated high anti- RBD-IgG titers and a good T-cell response. Most adverse events were mild and no serious adverse events were detected.

The Russian government granted EUA and subsequently based on the analysis of data on volunteers (n = 18,794) who received both the first and second doses, a VE of 91.4% has been claimed. In India a Phase 2 trial with, 100 subjects has been completed and a phase 3 with 1500 subjects is ongoing.

Q18. What is the data about Covaxin, the vaccine by Bharat Biotech?

Ans. This is a whole-virion inactivated SARS-CoV-2 vaccine formulated with a TLR 7/8 agonist molecule adsorbed to alum (Algel-IMDG). In a phase 1 study, the vaccine elicited high IgG antibodies against the S1 protein, RBD and the Nucleoprotein. Pain at the injection site was the most common local adverse event in the Algel-IMDG groups. The distribution of local and systemic AEs was equal among the vaccine treatment groups when compared to the control arm.

A phase 3 study with 25800 subjects is in the final stages.

This vaccine has been granted EUA.

Q19. What is the data about ZyCov-D, the vaccine by Zydus Vaxxicare?

Ans. This is a plasmid-DNA vaccine. This vaccine is administered in intradermally, 3 doses at 0–28–56 days. Phase 1 is completed. The vaccine is safe.

Phase 2 study was initiated in August 2020, in 1085 subjects in 9 centers. The results are being analyzed. Approval has been granted for the phase 3 study.

Q20. What is the schedule of the COVID-19 vaccines?

Ans. Generally, most are administered in a two dose schedule 21–28 days apart.

Astra-Zeneca: 2 doses IM at 0–28 d

Pfizer: 2 doses IM at 0–21 d

Moderna: 2 doses IM at 0–28 d

Gamaleya: 2 doses IM at 0–21 d

Covaxin (BBIL): 2 doses IM at 0–28 d

Janssen Pharmaceuticals: 2 doses IM at 0–56 d

Q21. Which routes of administration are recommended for different COVID-19 vaccines?

Ans. Most of the COVID-19 vaccines are recommended to be given by IM route, however many other routes are also recommended as follows:
- *Intradermal (ID)*: Inovio Pharmaceuticals/International Vaccine Institute (DNA), Cadila Healthcare Limited (DNA), GeneOne Life Science, Inc (DNA), CORVax (DNA),
- *Subcutaneous (SC)*: IMP CoVac-1 (Protein subunit), aAPC vaccine (Replicating viral vector + APC), LV-SMENP-DC vaccine (Non-Replicating viral vector + APC).
- *Oral*: Vaxart (Non-Replicating viral vector), Symvivo corporation (DNA), ImmunityBio Inc (Non-Replicating viral vector).
- *Intranasal (IN)*: Jiangsu Provincial for Disease Prevention and Control (Replicating viral vector), Codagenix/Serum Institute of India (Live attenuated virus), Center for Genetic Engineering and Biotechnology (Protein Subunit)
- *Intravenous (IV)*: LV-SMENP-DC vaccine (Non-Replicating viral vector + APC).

Q22. How long after vaccination does protection begin?

Ans. Significant protection is observed at least 10 days after the last dose of the vaccine.

Q23. Which COVID-19 vaccines are contraindicated in the immunocompromised?

Ans. All the live attenuated vaccines and replicating viral vector vaccines are to be avoided.

Q24. What are the safety aspects of these new platforms being used for COVID-19 vaccines?

Ans. mRNA vaccines do not contain any infectious materials. Since mRNA vaccines exert their effect in the cytoplasm and never enter the nucleus, there is no risk of integration into the host genome. The multiplication of the vaccine mRNA will not last beyond a few replications. The manufacturing process for mRNA does not require toxic chemicals or cell cultures that could be contaminated with adventitious viruses, mRNA production avoids the common risks associated with other vaccine platforms.

The advantages of Adenovirus-based vectors include broad range of tissue tropism, well-characterized genome, ease of genetic manipulation including acceptance of large transgene DNA insertions, inherent adjuvant properties, ability to induce robust transgene-specific T cell and antibody responses, non-replicative nature in host, and ease of production at large scale. Most adenoviruses cause mild diseases in immunocompetent human adults and by deletion of crucial regions of the viral genome the vectors can be rendered replication-defective, which increases their predictability and reduces unwanted side effects.

The major disadvantage is pre-existing immunity to the viral vector, in humans. This may blunt the response to the vaccine. This is usually overcome by adjusting the dose of the viral vector, using a prime-boost combination with different vectors or by using non-human adenovirus vectors.

Human adenovirus-based drugs have been in use for more than 50 years.

An anti-cancer drug was approved for use among the civilian population in China, and has already been given to more than 30,000 patients.

Adenovectors are being tested in vaccines against HIV, Malaria, Ebola, Zika, Hepatitis C and many other diseases. No major safety issues have been observed.

Q25. What are the cold chain requirements of these vaccines?

Ans. mRNA vaccines have very stringent cold chain requirements. The Pfizer vaccine is should be stored between –60° C and -80°C. The Moderna vaccine should be stored at –20° C for long term storage. For short term storage up to a month, it can be stored between +2° C to + 8°C. The Gamaleya vaccine (Sputnik) has two formulations, the liquid form should be stored at –18°C, while the freeze-dried formulation can be stored at +2° C to + 8°C. The Astra-Zeneca/Oxford vaccine and the Inactivated vaccine of Bharat Biotech, should be stored at +2° C to +8°C.

Gennova Biopharmaceuticals, a Pune based company, has received permission for a phase 1 trial of a mRNA vaccine which can be stored at + 2°C to + 8°C.

Q26. How long after vaccination does protection begin?

Ans. Significant protection is observed at least 10 days after the last dose of the vaccine.

Q27. How long will the vaccine induced protection last?

Ans. These are new vaccines with limited follow up period of 2–3 months. Only follow up of the vaccinees will provide information about the longevity of the immune response. While antibody titers may wane rather rapidly, memory B-cell and memory T-cell responses are expected to provide longer term protection. Generally, protection is expected to last at least for 6–12 months.

Q28. Will everyone get the vaccine?

Ans. As there will be a short supply of vaccines, vaccine administration is to be prioritized to groups that are at greatest risk of morbidity and mortality due to COVID-19 and the frontline workers, whose health and well-being is vital in the response to the COVID-19 pandemic.

Based on the potential availability of vaccines the Government of India has selected the priority groups who will be vaccinated on priority as they are at higher risk.

The first group includes healthcare and frontline workers. The second group to receive COVID-19 vaccine will be persons over 50 years of age and persons under 50 years with comorbid conditions. Those > 50 years will be sub-classified into > 65 years, 60–65 years and 50–60 years in decreasing order of priority.

Q29. What are the recommendations for vaccination of pregnant women and women intending to become pregnant?

Ans. Presently, there is insufficient evidence to recommend routine use of COVID-19 vaccines during pregnancy. Vaccination in pregnancy should be considered where the risk of exposure to Severe Acute Respiratory Syndrome coronavirus 2 (SARS-CoV2) infection is high and cannot be avoided, or where the woman has underlying conditions that put them at very high risk of serious complications of COVID-19. In these circumstances, clinicians should discuss the risks and benefits of vaccination with the woman. This applies only to the inactivated/non-live vaccines. Routine pregnancy testing before receipt of a COVID-19 vaccine is not recommended. Those who are trying to become pregnant do not need to avoid pregnancy after vaccination.

Q30. What are the recommendations for vaccination of lactating women?

Ans. Breastfeeding women may be offered vaccination with the Covid vaccines. the woman should be informed about the absence of safety data for the vaccine in breastfeeding women.

Q31. What are the prospects of vaccination in the pediatric populations?

Ans. None of the vaccines which have gained EUA, have been tested in children. The Pfizer vaccine authorized in the United Kingdom and the United States is for people of age 16 years and older. Also, testing began in October 2020 in children as young as 12 and is expected to take several more months. Moderna, which has become the second COVID-19 vaccine to get greenlit in the US, began enrolling study participants ages 12 to 17 in December 2020, and will track them for a year. Testing in children younger than 12 is expected to start in early 2021.

Bharat Biotech, which received emergency approval for its COVID-19 vaccine only in "clinical trial mode", is allowed to conduct its trials on children who are above the age of 12 years. The vaccine has already been used for children above 12 in the last round and has been found safe.

Q32. Does the mutation of coronavirus affect the capacity of vaccines to prevent disease?

Ans. Generally, No. Most mutations are single gene mutations affecting a very small part of the S-protein or the RBD of the S-protein. All vaccines have employed the RBD or the entire S-protein, which have multiple epitopes. Most vaccines target multiple epitopes and elicit antibodies against multiple epitopes. Unless the virus accumulates a large number of mutations, the antigenic character of the epitope will not be altered. Hence, it is unlikely that these mutations (escape mutants) will affect the efficacy of Covid vaccines.

Q33. Are COVID-19 vaccines necessary for those with past history of Covid?

Ans. Yes. But they will be lower down in the priority list.

Q34. Will vaccination render masking, hand hygiene and physical distancing, redundant?

Ans. NO. They will have to be continued, till the majority of the population is vaccinated.

Q35. What is Covax, Covax facility and the Gavi COVAX AMC?

Ans. COVAX is the vaccine component of three pillars of the Access to COVID-19 Tools (ACT) Accelerator, which was launched in April by the World Health Organization (WHO), the European Commission and France in response to this pandemic. It has brought together governments, global health organizations, manufacturers, scientists, private sector, civil society and philanthropy, with the aim of providing innovative and equitable access to COVID-19 diagnostics, treatments and vaccines.

COVAX is coordinated by Gavi, the Vaccine Alliance, the Coalition for Epidemic Preparedness Innovations (CEPI) and the WHO. COVAX is a platform that will support the research, development and manufacturing of a wide range of COVID-19 vaccine candidates, and negotiate their pricing. All participating countries, regardless of income levels, will have equal access to these vaccines once they are developed. The initial aim is to have 2 billion doses available by the end of 2021, which should be enough to protect high risk and vulnerable people, as well as frontline healthcare workers.

The principal role of the COVAX Facility is to maximize the chances of people in participating countries getting access to COVID-19 vaccines as quickly, fairly and safely as possible. By joining the Facility, participating countries and economies will not only get access to the world's largest and most diverse portfolio of COVID-19 vaccines, but also an actively managed portfolio.

The aim of the Gavi COVAX AMC is to ensure that the 92 middle- and lower-income countries that cannot fully afford to pay for COVID-19 vaccines themselves get equal access to COVID-19 vaccines. Subject to funding availability, funded countries will receive enough doses to vaccinate up to 20 per cent of their population in the longer term. *"No one is safe until everyone is safe"*

Q36. What is CoWIN?

The central government has introduced an application named CoWIN (Covid Vaccine Intelligence Work). It is a digitized platform for the roll-out of the vaccine in the country.

It has the data of over 75 lakhs health officials who will be first in line to get the vaccination. The app will have four modules — User administrator module, beneficiary registration, vaccination and beneficiary acknowledgment, and status updation.

Prior beneficiary registration is mandatory to be eligible for the govt. immunization program.

Q37. What preparations has the Govt. of India made to roll out the vaccines?

Ans. The Govt. of India has set a priority list for vaccination as mentioned in Q.22.

Govt. of India is preparing for the introduction of the Covid vaccines in the country, so that it can be expeditiously rolled out when available.

In this regard, the Govt. of India has constituted the National Expert Group on Vaccine administration for Covid vaccines (NEGVAC). The NEGVAC will guide all aspects of Covid vaccine introduction in India. A "COVID-19 vaccination: Operational Guidelines" has been formulated and published, for training of resource persons for the rollout.

■ SUGGESTED READING

1. Baden LR, El Sahly HM, Essink B, Kotloff K, Frey S, Novak R., et al. Efficacy and Safety of the mRNA-1273 SARS-CoV-2 Vaccine. DOI: 10.1056/NEJMoa2035389
2. Covid-19 vaccines. Operational guidelines. Available at https://main.mohfw.gov.in/newshighlights-31.
3. Draft landscape of Covid-19 candidate vaccines. Available at https://www.who.int/publications/m/item/draft-landscape-of-covid-19-candidate-vaccines. Assessed on 7 January 2021.
4. Polack FP, Thomas SJ, Kitchin N, Absalon J, Gurtman A, Lockhart S, Perez JL, et al. Safety and Efficacy of the BNT162b2 mRNA Covid-19 Vaccine. DOI: 10.1056/NEJMoa2034577.
5. Rauch S, Jasny E, Schmidt KE, Petsch B. New Vaccine Technologies to Combat Outbreak Situations. 2018; Front. Immunol. 9:1963.
6. Situation dashboard. Available at https://covid19.who.int/. Assessed on 7 January 2021.
7. Voysey M, Clemens SAC, Madhi SA, Weckx LY, Folegatti PM, Aley RK, , et al. Safety and efficacy of the ChAdOx1 nCoV-19 vaccine (AZD1222) against SARS-CoV-2: an interim analysis of four randomised controlled trials in Brazil, South Africa, and the UK. https://doi.org/10.1016/ S0140-6736(20)32661-1.

CHAPTER 39

Therapeutic Vaccines

Dhanya Dharmapalan, NP Singh

Q1. What are therapeutic vaccines? How do they differ from preventive vaccines?

Ans. Therapeutic vaccines are given to diseased individuals to reduce the morbidity associated with the disease. These differ from preventive vaccines, which are offered to healthy individuals to prevent a disease. Therapeutic vaccines are administered with the aim of overcoming the suppressed immune response of the recipient, induced either by a variety of pathogens causing chronic infections or by cancer cells and the cancer environment. These vaccines enable the vaccinee to mount a response against the pathogen causing the chronic infection or overcome the immune suppression associated with cancers. Therapeutic vaccines are also targeting some noncommunicable diseases (NCDs) such as allergies, neurological diseases, Alzheimer's disease, atherosclerosis, obesity, hypertension, and some addictions. The chronic infections for which vaccines are in development are hepatitis B, hepatitis C, human papillomavirus (HPV), herpes simplex virus (HSV), cytomegalovirus (CMV), human immunodeficiency virus (HIV), *Helicobacter pylori*, tuberculosis (TB), and malaria.

Q2. How do therapeutic vaccines work?

Ans. Therapeutic vaccines work in diseased condition by overcoming the impaired immune system associated with chronic viral infections or cancers. In cases of NCDs, therapeutic vaccines elicit immune responses against certain proteins associated with these NCDs.

Q3. What is the role of therapeutic vaccines in allergic disorders?

Ans. Therapeutic vaccines aim to provide improvement in the quality of life in those suffering from allergic disorders by inducing unresponsiveness to the relevant antigen responsible for the allergic response. The mechanism involves the induction of allergen-specific regulatory T and B cells resulting in suppression of innate and adaptive effector populations. The route for introduction of multiple allergens is most commonly either subcutaneous immunotherapy (SCIT) or sublingual immunotherapy (SLIT) though various other routes are being explored.

The method is most useful for patients who are known to react to a specific allergen. In this method, repeated introduction of allergen is made, often in increasing doses in a controlled setting followed by a longer maintenance phase until an adequate long-lasting tolerance is reached. Serious adverse effects can occur if the dose exceeds the threshold.

Q4. What are the clinical applications in cancers?

Ans. Therapeutic cancer vaccines can be antigen based, deoxyribonucleic acid (DNA) vaccines, dendritic cell (DC) vaccines or tumor cell vaccines.

There are two types of therapeutic cancer vaccines, which are being studied.
1. Autologous vaccines are personalized vaccine which is made from an individual's own cells which could be either cancer cells or immune system cells
2. Allogenic vaccines, which are majorly cancer vaccines and are made from nonself-cancer cells which are grown in a laboratory.

A large number of mutations occurring in cancer cells, result in the production of neoantigens which are not expressed in normal tissues. These neoantigens are highly immunogenic and can activate CD4+ and CD8+ T cells to generate immune response against the cancer cells. Tumor vaccines targeting neoantigens mainly include nucleic acid, DC-based, tumor cell, and synthetic long peptide (SLP) vaccines. Neoantigen-based vaccines in combination with immune checkpoint inhibition therapy or radiotherapy and chemotherapy have the potential to better therapeutic effects. Currently, several clinical trials have demonstrated the safety and efficacy of these vaccines.

Currently the only United States Food and Drug Administration (USFDA) approved therapeutic vaccine is an autologous cell vaccine, sipuleucel-T. It was approved in April 2010 for the treatment of asymptomatic and minimally symptomatic metastatic castration-resistant prostate cancer (mCRPC). Its approval in April 2010 was mainly based the results of the randomized and double-blind phase III IMPACT trial 50 that showed a median overall survival of 25.8 months in patients treated with sipuleucel-T (n = 341) compared with 21.7 months in those treated with placebo (n = 171). This had corresponded to a relative reduction of 22% in the risk of death.

Talimogene laherparepvec (TVEC) has received approval by the USFDA for inoperable melanoma. This is a genetically engineered herpes virus, in which a gene for human granulocyte-macrophage colony-stimulating factor (GM-CSF) is added. When injected intralesionally it results in the generation of a systemic immune response against the patient's cancer. The final 4-year analysis from the pivotal phase 3 study upon which TVEC was approved by the FDA showed a 31.5% response rate.

The other therapeutic cancers vaccines in phase III development are breast cancers, gliomas, lung cancers, melanoma, colorectal cancers, and follicular lymphoma. Most of the 118 cancer vaccines that have completed phase 3 trials have shown negative results. Thus, most of these trials are using vaccines in combination with other cancer treatment modalities such as chemotherapy, radiotherapy, endocrine therapy, etc.

Q5. How do therapeutic vaccines work against chronic infections?

Ans. Persistent viremia is due to exhaustion of antiviral T cells. Negative signaling pathways like T cell expression of programmed death, cytotoxic T lymphocyte antigen 4 (CTLA-4), and interleukin-10 (IL-10) have also been reported to be potential factors of establishing immune suppression. Blocking these negative pathways could restore the host immune system, enabling it to respond to further stimulation. Humoral immune response lowers the viral antigen load and polyfunctional effector T cell response is directed against continuously expressed viral antigens.

Q6. Can the available HPV vaccine be used as a therapeutic vaccine?

Ans. No. The current vaccine is given at a younger age to prevent HPV infection. A therapeutic vaccine will help older women who are already infected. It can be used as an adjunct to standard therapies. Boosting the specific immune response during treatment may help prevent low-grade disease from progressing or control the metastatic spread or prevent recurrence of cancer after complete treatment. This can be done by the boosted immune response eliminating the HPV oncogenes E6 and E7. The expressions of these two genes are required for growth of warts and cancer cells.

At present two therapeutic vaccines are undergoing clinical trials.
1. *MVA E2*: It is a recombinant Vaccinia viral vaccine MVA E2 composed of modified Vaccinia virus Ankara and the *E2* gene of bovine papillomavirus. In early trials in men, it elicited regression of flat condyloma lesions.
2. *VGX-3100*: It is in phase III trial for the treatment of HPV-induced high-grade squamous intraepithelial carcinoma.

Q7. What are the applications in Epstein–Barr virus (EBV) infection?

Ans. The vaccines aim to eliminate the tumor cells by stimulating T cell responses against EBV antigens. Cancers associated with EBV have tumor cells, which express EBV-coded nuclear antigen EBNA-1 and latent membrane protein LMP2. This vaccine was tested in phase I trial for nasopharyngeal carcinoma and has been found to be safe and immunogenic.

The other potential targets are for conditions such as posttransplant lymphoproliferative disorder (EBNA-1, 2, 3A, 3B, 3C; LMP1; and LMP2) X-linked lymphoproliferative disease (EBNA-1, 2, 3A, 3B, 3C; LMP1; and LMP2), Hodgkin lymphoma (EBNA-1, LMP1, and LMP 2), nasopharyngeal carcinoma (EBNA-1, LMP 1, and LMP 2), and Burkitt lymphoma (EBNA-1).

Q8. What are the candidate therapeutic TB vaccines in recent clinical trials?

Ans. Several inactivated mycobacterial candidate vaccines have been tested as immunotherapeutic adjuncts to TB treatment. These are:

- Vaccae™, derived from *Mycobacterium vaccae* and licensed in China as an immunotherapeutic adjunct to drug treatment of TB in adults, has been tested among drug-sensitive (DS)- and drug-resistant (DR)-TB patients in a number of clinical trials in China. Meta-analysis of 25 studies involving 2,281 Chinese multidrug-resistant-TB (MDR-TB) patients suggested that multidose *M. vaccae* during treatment was associated with faster sputum smear conversion and radiographic disease resolution. A large meta-analysis of more than 4,000 DS- and DR-TB patients in 54 studies, including six conducted in countries other than China, also reported faster sputum smear conversion and radiographic improvement in *M. vaccae* recipients. These encouraging data require confirmation in other populations and epidemic settings.

- A multidose regimen of heat-killed *Mycobacterium indicus pranii (MIP)*, previously known as *Mycobacterium w*, has also been tested for therapeutic potential among 890 retreatment pulmonary TB patients in a randomized, double-blind, placebo-controlled trial in India. MIP vaccinees showed a modest increase in the rate of sputum culture conversion from 4 weeks onward compared to placebo (67% vs. 57%), but the rate of relapse TB disease was not significantly different.

- The inactivated mycobacterial vaccine candidate RUTI, a liposomal formulation of fragmented *M. tuberculosis*, is planned to enter a double-blind, placebo-controlled trial of safety and immunogenicity in 27 DR-TB patients after 12 or 16 weeks of successful intensive phase treatment.

Q9. Do therapeutic vaccines offer any benefit in HIV infections?

Ans. Various therapeutic vaccines using DNA and viral vectors, DC-based vaccines or combination of these have been tried in the treatment of HIV patients. Few studies have shown about a 0.5 to 1 log reduction in plasma viral load. But the clinical success remains unclear. Moreover, it has been found that there is minimal effect on reducing the HIV reservoir or benefit following interruption of antiretroviral treatment. Recent studies have shown that a combination of antiretroviral therapy (ART) and therapeutic vaccines may result in a better outcome than just ART alone. Therapeutic vaccination broadens the host immune response and helps to recognize a wide array of escape variants.

Q10. What are the applications of therapeutic vaccines in chronic hepatitis B infections?

Ans. Therapeutic vaccines are a promising strategy to boost the immune response in patients with chronic hepatitis B infection who have impaired immunity to clear the virus and high antigen load on T cells. However, there is growing evidence of its most beneficial role in patients with hepatitis B virus (HBV) viral loads below 10^6 cp/mL, patients with high alanine transferase levels and hepatitis B e-antigen (HBeAg)-negative patients.

A systematic review and meta-analysis were conducted of trials of therapeutic vaccination for chronic hepatitis B. The study concluded that therapeutic vaccines did not appear to be efficacious except for reduction in hepatitis B DNA detection at the end of the follow-up of patients with therapeutic vaccines and standard of care compared to those who did received only standard of care treatment. But this study was limited by the small number of randomized controlled trials and suboptimal vaccines.

Q11. Is there any therapeutic vaccine for Hepatitis C?

Ans. It has been noticed that in hepatitis C patients with insufficient immunity, the disease progresses towards chronicity. These patients are seen to lack specific T cell responses and interferon-α (IFN-α) are generally absent in patients who progress to chronic inflammation and fibrosis. Thus, redirection of immune response could halt or reverse liver fibrosis progression. It has been observed that immune responses against the E1 envelope protein are especially weak or absent. Therefore, vaccines directed against the E1 envelope are prime candidates. A development of polyepitope vaccine will have the potential advantages of targeting all patient segments and lower costs. There are five different vaccines in different phases of trials.

Q12. What is the status of therapeutic vaccines for use in autoimmune diseases?

Ans. Autoimmune diseases are conditions wherein the body mounts an immunological response against self-antigens because of loss of immunotolerance.

The response to self-antigens resembles normal protective immune responses to viruses and pathogens, involving T helper 1 (Th1) cells and IFN. The goal of therapeutic vaccines in autoimmune diseases is to shift the immune response to a Th2 type, IL-4, and IL-10 mediated or T regulatory cell, which induce an anti-inflammatory response. Various platforms are being investigated like DNA vaccines, whole autoreactive T cells, DC vaccines, and B cell-based immunogenic vaccines.

For rheumatoid arthritis (RA) an autologous modified DC vaccine (Rheumavax) pulsed with a mixture of four citrullinated peptide antigens (cit-vimentin), in a phase I trial, resulted in reduction in anti-cyclic citrullinated peptide (CCP) antibody titers. In another vaccine trial DEN-181, a nanoparticulate liposome formulation that encapsulates autoantigenic peptide and nuclear factor kappa B (NF-κB) inhibitor, 1,25 dihydroxycholciferol was used to target DCs. The vaccine was found to be safe and modulated antigen-specific T cells in RA patients of appropriate human leukocyte antigen (HLA) type.

Vaccines are being tried for diabetes type-1. DiaPep277, a 24 amino-acid peptide derived from human heat-shock protein 6, has been demonstrated to modulate immunological attack on β-cells in the nonobese diabetic (NOD) mouse model of type 1 diabetes and also activates regulatory T cells by interacting with their Toll-like receptor. The results have been encouraging and further phase trials are being planned.

Q13. What is the scope of therapeutic vaccines for neurological disorders like multiple sclerosis and Alzheimer's?

Ans. Therapeutic vaccines are being tried for multiple sclerosis also. Glatiramer acetate (Copaxone), a peptide that resembles myelin basic protein (MBP), has been licensed by USFDA for the management of multiple sclerosis.

A lot of research has undergone to find a vaccine for Alzheimer's as this disease kills more people than breast cancer and prostate cancer combined. Initial vaccines caused encephalitis in quite a few patients. Now they are working on a more specific vaccine that will produce antibodies to attack amyloid plaques but will not have inflammation as a side effect. UB-311 is a peptide composed of amino acids 1-14 in the beta amyloid protein. The vaccine works by targeting two proteins commonly found in the brain associated with Alzheimer's disease, beta-amyloid, and tau. In a phase 2a trial of 43 mild to moderate patents, it showed 96% response of patient's immune system to treatment.

Q14. Is there any role of Bacillus Calmette–Guérin (BCG) vaccine as a therapeutic vaccine?

Ans. Bacillus Calmette–Guérin vaccines such as RUTI- and *M. vaccae*-based vaccines are promising therapeutic vaccines for use in patients infected with TB to prevent recurrence of the disease after successful treatment and also to reduce the duration of treatment with antitubercular drugs. DAR-901 is being developed as both a prophylactic and a therapeutic vaccine.

A systemic analysis and meta-analysis for the role of BCG in treatment of type I diabetes mellitus (DM) concluded that though glycosylated hemoglobin tended to improve, the benefit was not significant to suggest its therapeutic role.

The BCG vaccine has also found to benefit patients with malignancy such as stage II colon cancer. BCG vaccine suppressed Th2-type immune response has found to improve lung function in adults with moderate-to-severe asthma.

Intravesical BCG is approved for treatment and prophylaxis of urothelial carcinoma in situ of the urinary bladder and for prophylaxis of primary or recurrent stage Ta and/or T1 urothelial carcinoma. In a meta-analysis, intravesical BCG showed a 27% reduction in the risk of disease progression. The role of BCG vaccination in Covid-19, is being actively investigated.

Q15. Are therapeutic vaccines the future of cancer treatment?

Ans. Going by the current levels of vaccines, probably not. The current vaccines at best can keep the diseases under control. The viruses hide in the cells of the body where the antibodies cannot penetrate. The primary benefit might be in better controlling the disease progressions and preventing relapses. By doing so we can reduce the exposure to chemotherapeutic drugs and thus reducing their side effects. So, as of date vaccines are best used for prevention than cure.

■ SUGGESTED READING

1. Balfour HH. Epstein–Barr Virus Vaccines. In: Plotkin SA, Orenstein WA, Offit PA (Eds). Vaccines, 7th edition. Philadelphia, PA: WB Saunders; 2018. pp. 295-300.
2. Chang YC, Lin CJ, Hsiao YH, Chang YH, Liu SJ, Hsu HY. Therapeutic Effects of BCG Vaccination on Type 1 Diabetes Mellitus: A Systematic Review and Meta-Analysis of Randomized Controlled Trials. J Diabetes Res. 2020;2020:8954125.
3. Choi IS, Koh YI. Therapeutic effects of BCG vaccination in adult asthmatic patients: a randomized, controlled trial. Ann Allergy Asthma Immunol. 2002;88(6):584-91.
4. Fatima S, Kumari A, Das G, Dwivedi VP. Tuberculosis vaccine: A journey from BCG to present. Life Sci. 2020;252:117594.
5. Gutowska-Owsiak D, Ogg GS. Therapeutic vaccines for allergic disease. NPJ Vaccines. 2017;2:12.
6. Hatherill M, White RG, Hawn TR. Clinical Development of New TB Vaccines: Recent Advances and Next Steps. Front. Microbiol. 2020;10:3154. doi: 10.3389/fmicb.2019.03154.
7. Kantoff PW, Higano CS, Shore ND, et al. Sipuleucel-T immunotherapy for castration-resistant prostate cancer. N Engl J Med. 2010;363:411-22.
8. Lim SG, Agcaoili J, De Souza NNA, Chan E. Therapeutic vaccination for chronic hepatitis B: A systematic review and meta-analysis. J Viral Hepat. 2019;26(7):803-17.
9. Melero I, Gaudernack G, Gerritsen W, Huber C, Parmiani G, Scholl S, et al. Therapeutic vaccines for cancer: an overview of clinical trials. Nat Rev Clin Oncol. 2014;11(9):509-24.
10. Michel ML, Deng Q, Mancini-Bourgine M. Therapeutic vaccines and immune-based therapies for the treatment of chronic hepatitis B: perspectives and challenges. J Hepatol. 2011;54(6):1286-96.
11. Mosolits S, Nilsson B, Mellstedt H. Towards therapeutic vaccines for colorectal carcinoma: a review of clinical trials. Expert Rev Vaccines. 2005;4(3):329-50.
12. Mylvaganam GH, Silvestri G, Amara RR. HIV therapeutic vaccines: moving towards a functional cure. Curr Opin Immunol. 2015;35:1-8.

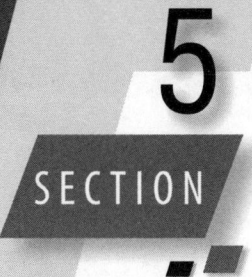

SECTION 5
Miscellaneous Topics

○ **Ethical Issues and Vaccine Refusal**
   Jagdish Chinnappa

○ **National Immunization Program**
   Harish K Pemde, Kamlesh Harish

CHAPTER 40: Ethical Issues and Vaccine Refusal

Jagdish Chinnappa

PART 1: ETHICAL ISSUES IN VACCINOLOGY

Q1. What are general principles of ethics that are applicable in the practice of vaccinology?

Ans. Ethical principles are universal in all areas of clinical practice but have a unique and important role while considering the choice and administration of vaccines. The main ethical principles to consider are:

- *Beneficence*: Will administering the vaccine produce either individual or collective good to the patient or community? Here again one has to determine what would be of maximal benefit?
- *Nonmaleficence*: Minimizing harm is paramount in interventions when dealing with children. Any vaccine that is likely to produce significant harm should be avoided.
- *Autonomy*: The choice of vaccine is always determined by parental choice. Discussion with parents about the pros and cons and the vital role of vaccines in preventing disease is important. The principle of autonomy is exemplified by informed consent. In most clinical situations, implied consent is assumed.
- *Justice*: Maximum good for the maximum children in a community even though there may be some adverse reactions is the basis for this principle.

In addition to these basic principles, there are other ethical issues that should be considered such as veracity (truth telling), confidentiality, and conflict of interest.

Q2. What are the common ethical conflicts that can occur in the practice of vaccinology?

Ans. Ethical conflicts rarely occur between what is right and wrong; they occur when there is clash between two of the above principles.

Let's take the example of diphtheria, pertussis, and tetanus (DPT) versus diphtheria, tetanus, and pertussis (DTaP) as the first dose that a baby gets. Beneficence clearly is in favor of DPT while nonmaleficence is in favor of DTaP. This is where autonomy or shared decision-making between parent and clinician will resolve the issue.

Or, for example, an adolescent who does not want to take the second dose of human papillomavirus (HPV) because the first dose was too painful. Here is a conflict between autonomy and beneficence. Here again, communication is the key where assent from the adolescent is mandatory prior to vaccine administration.

Q3. Can there be a situation where ethical principles clash with the law?

Ans. The overriding principles when dealing with children are beneficence and nonmaleficence. Sometimes what is ethically correct may not have legal sanction.

For example, the parents of a 14-year-old boy request HPV vaccine as there is a strong history of malignancies in the family. Though this is ethically acceptable, it is not legal and cannot be administered.

Q4. Is there a difference in ethical principles as it applies to clinical practice versus public health vaccination?

Ans. In office practice beneficence, nonmaleficence and autonomy are important considerations, while in public health programs such as oral polio vaccine (+OPV), measles and rubella (MR), and DPT, the overriding principle is Justice.

Here the government can compel vaccination as it is for the public good.

The ethical principle here is often referred to as the "harm principle" first enunciated by John Stuart Mill which states that "the only purpose for which power can be rightfully exercised over any member of a civilized community, against his will, *is to prevent harm to others*, his own good either physical or moral is not sufficient warrant".

Unvaccinated persons can be viewed as harming society. For serious and highly communicable diseases, "there is a role for compulsory vaccination".

Q5. If a parent refuses to administer either an individual vaccine or vaccines as a whole or wants to alter schedules, what should the doctor do?

Ans. Parents and pediatricians are considered as cofiduciaries who act in the best interest of the child.

If the parent does not seem to be acting in the best interest of the child, the doctor should establish rapport and seek reasons for the same. If after repeated counseling, the parent still refuses vaccination, this should be clearly documented. The doctor should continue to care for the child and monitor health carefully with the knowledge that the child is incompletely immunized.

Parents often change their decisions and it is important to be nonjudgemental.

Q6. What is vaccine friendly environment to convince parents that they are acting in the best interest of the child?

Ans. The key ethical concerns parents have should be dispelled in all office practices.

Complete transparency in the vaccine administration process right from providing adequate information prior to administration, providing choices, making shared decisions, administration of the vaccine in a nonthreatening way to provide it with least pain, and support after the vaccination go a long way in building vaccine confidence.

Communication by all staff about the importance of vaccines strengthens confidence.

Industry-related promotional material should never be seen in areas where vaccines are administered. They open the door to potential conflict of interest suspicions.

Q7. Are there other ethical concerns that one may encounter in practice?

Ans. The principles outlined above are relevant to clinical practice. There may be situations where clinicians may act as researchers of vaccines or help decide policy issues. Ethical principles in these situations are complex and may need expert ethical consultations.

■ SUGGESTED READING

1. El Amin AN, Parra MT, Kim-Farley R, Fielding JE. Ethical Issues Concerning Vaccination Requirements. Public Health Rev. 2012;34:207-26.
2. Giubilini A. The Ethics of Vaccination. Berlin, Germany: Springer; 2019.
3. Hendrix KS, Sturm LA, Zimet GD, Meslin EM. Ethics and Childhood Vaccination Policy in the United States. Am J Public Health. 2016;106(2):273-8.
4. Javitt G, Berkowitz D, Gostin LO. Accessing mandatory HPV vaccination: Who should call the shots? J Law Med Ethics. 2008;36:384-95.
5. Malone KM, Hinman AR. Vaccination mandates: The public health imperative and individual rights. New York: Oxford University Press; 2003. pp. 262-84.
6. Ulmer JB, Liu MA. Ethical issues for vaccines and immunization. Nat Rev Immunol. 2002;2(4):291-6.

PART 2: VACCINE HESITANCY

Q1. What is the classification of families that bring their children for vaccine administration?

Ans. Families that bring their children for vaccine administration fall under one of three categories:
1. Vaccine supporters and nonobjectors
2. Vaccine hesitant parents
3. Antivaccine lobby

Most families belong to the first variety and administer vaccines according to the advice of their doctor or health care system.

Families that belong to the last category are strongly antivaccers and will not administer vaccines. They are small in number and extend tremendous influence through the media.

The groups in the middle are hesitant, they are ambivalent and unsure and mostly confused. They can be swayed either way depending on the information that is given to them.

Q2. Why is there confusion?

Ans. Confusion rests on three main belief systems:
1. *Beneficence*: This disease is so rare, and we have not seen it; so, will the vaccine be of any benefit?
   This is the usual argument of hesitant parents. One needs to emphasize that the disease is rare because of vaccination and can resurface at any time (give examples of measles, pertussis, and diphtheria)
   Another argument is let the child go through natural illness; it will protect him.
   Such belief systems need to be handled gently with authentic data in visual form.
2. *Nonmaleficence*: Vaccines can harm my child. There are so many chemicals in the vaccine that it can cause long-term problems such as autism and developmental issues. These myths need to be dispelled with correct information.
3. *Autonomy*: Who is the government to decide which vaccine I should give my child? I should be able to choose. These arguments are common (especially during pulse polio campaigns). The value of vaccines in the public health system should be emphasized.

Q3. What are the key elements to dispel this confusion?

Ans. The key elements to dispel this confusion are confidence, trust, and information **(Flowchart 1)**.

"Confidence" is "the mental attitude of trusting in or relying on a person or thing.

The definition of trust is the "optimistic acceptance of a vulnerable situation in which the trustor believes the trustee will care for the trustor's interest.

In the context of vaccination, confidence implies trust in the vaccine (the product), trust in the vaccinator or other health professional (the provider), and trust in those who make the decisions about vaccine provision (the policymaker).

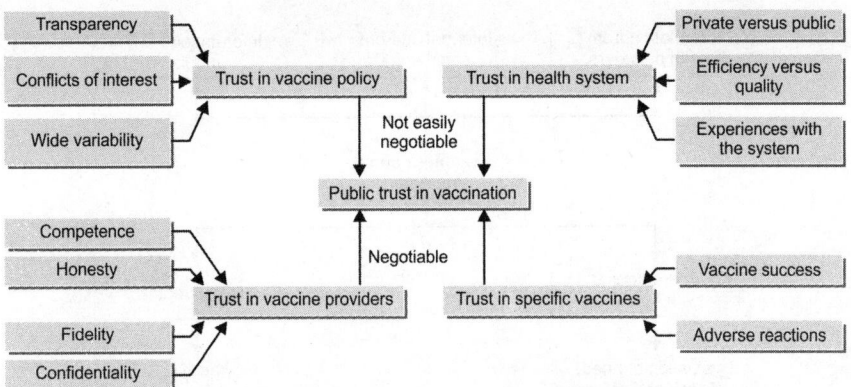

Flowchart 1: Public trust in vaccination.

Source: Adapted with permission from Gopichandran V. Public trust in vaccination: an analytical framework. Indian J Med Ethics. 2017;2(2)NS:98-104.

Q4. What about information?

Ans. Information from trusted sources makes a great impact in the trustworthiness of the system.

Vaccine information is available from many sources (media, community, healthcare workers, and others). Information thus obtained may increase or decrease the trust in vaccines.

Most antivaccine groups spread their messages by three strategies:
1. The messages are visual and spread by social media supporting pictures.
2. They have emotional content. The messages usually show a distraught mother with a tag line "if only I knew….".
3. They are repetitive. This helps in reinforcing the message.

Contrast this to a vaccine advocate who spreads messages with boring text and statistics and may be infrequent and ambivalent.

Q5. What are some of the other factors?

Ans. Other social factors play a significant role and should be considered.

Convenience: If the vaccine is administered at inconvenient times or at distant places, there may be a hesitancy. Costs of travel and wage loss also need to be considered.

Religious and cultural factors may also play a significant role **(Flowchart 2)**.

Q6. How should we counter hesitancy in practice?

Ans. Hesitancy in practice should be countered by building rapport. Key to this is listening and understanding the incorrect belief systems that the parent

Flowchart 2: Vaccine hesitancy.

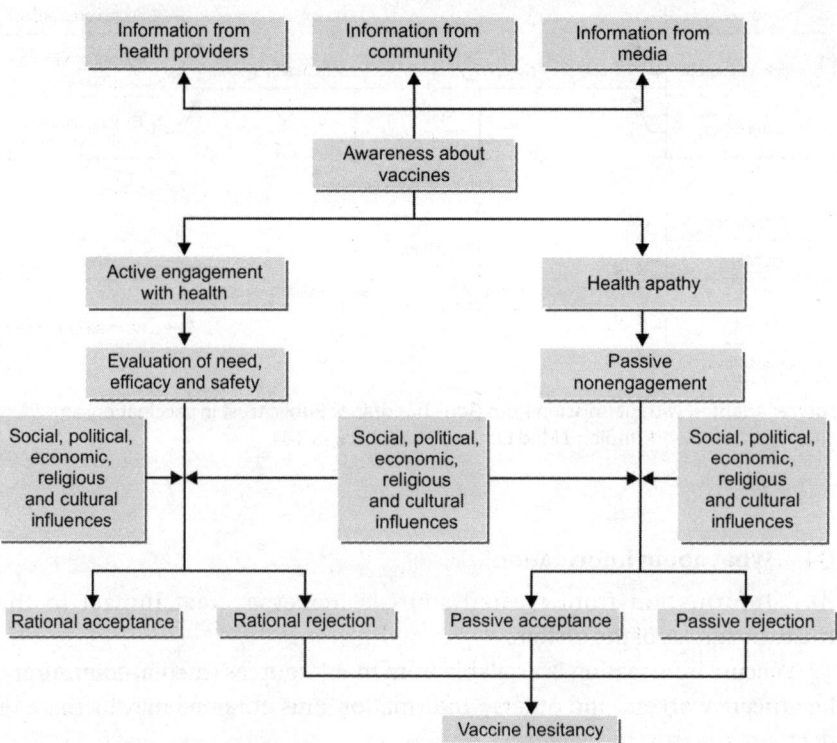

Source: Adapted with permission from Gopichandran V. Public trust in vaccination: an analytical framework. Indian J Med Ethics. 2017;2(2)NS:98-104.

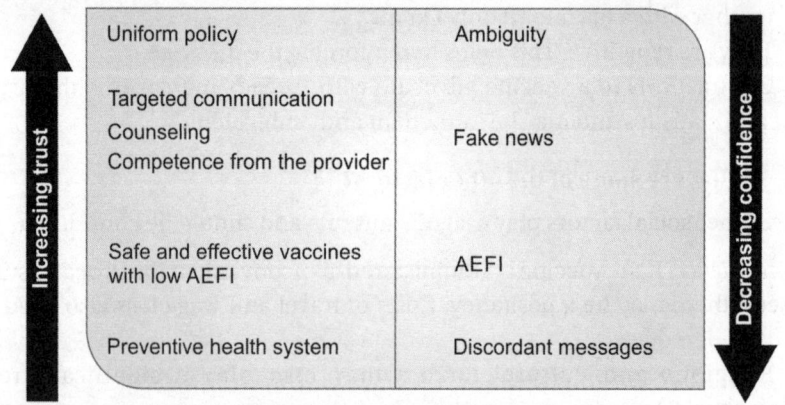

Fig. 1: Building trust in vaccines.
(AEFI: adverse event following immunization)

may have. Targeted (visual, emotional, and repetitive) communication and counseling with competence, clarity, and patience will help make shared decision-making easier **(Fig. 1)**.

SUGGESTED READING

1. Gopichandran V. Public trust in vaccination: an analytical framework. Indian J Med Ethics. 2017:2(2)NS:98-104.
2. Griffiths S. (2019). The rise of vaccine hesitancy. [online] Available from https://www.nuffieldbioethics.org/blog/the-rise-of-vaccine-hesitancy. [Last accessed October, 2020].
3. Gupta M, Kaushal K, Sharma N, Gupta A, Bashar AM, Dalpath S, et al. Newer vaccines (measles-rubella, human papillomavirus, rotavirus, and pneumococcal conjugate vaccine) Experience from Northern India. Int J Non-Commun Dis. 2018;3:S25-30.
4. Kumar D, Noor N, Kashyap V. Vaccine hesitancy—Issues and possible solutions. J Med Allied Sci. 2018;8(2):55-8.
5. Larson HJ, Clarke RM, Jarrett C, Eckersberger E, Levine Z, Schulz WS, et al. Measuring trust in vaccination: A systematic review. Hum Vaccin Immunother. 2018;14(7):1599-609.
6. Laxminarayan R, Ganguly NK. India's Vaccine Deficit: Why More Than Half Of Indian Children Are Not Fully Immunized, And What Can—And Should—Be Done. Health Aff (Millwood). 2011;30(6):1096-103.
7. Suri S. Reducing Infectious Diseases in Children: Tracking India's Progress and Outlining the Challenges. ORF Special Report No. 86. New Delhi: Observer Research Foundation; 2019.

CHAPTER 41

National Immunization Program

Harish K Pemde, Kamlesh Harish

Q1. What are the achievements of India's national immunization program?

Ans. Immunization currently prevents 2–3 million deaths worldwide. The annual number of deaths in under five children fell from 3.4 million to 1.2 million in India between 1990 and 2015. Immunization is one of the several factors behind this reduction in these deaths. Global measles mortality has reduced by nearly 75% in past 20 years.

India achieved eradication of poliomyelitis and elimination of neonatal tetanus recently.

Universal Immunization Program (UIP) of India has been found to increase height-for-age (0.50 z-score, p = 0.001) and weight-for-age z-scores (0.29 z-scores, p = 0.002) in children under 4 years of age. A recent study found that UIP of India was associated with 0.2–0.3 additional schooling grades.

Q2. What are the salient features of National Immunization Program of India?

Ans.
- Expanded Program on Immunization was launched in 1978. It was renamed as Universal Immunization Program in 1985 when its reach was expanded beyond urban areas. In 1992, it became part of Child Survival and Safe Motherhood Program and in 1997 it was included in the ambit of National Reproductive and Child Health Program. Since the launch of National Rural Health Mission in 2005, UIP has always been an integral part of it.
- Universal Immunization Program is one of the largest public health programs targeting close of 2.67 crore newborns and 2.9 crore pregnant women annually.
- It is one of the most cost-effective public health interventions and largely responsible for reduction of vaccine preventable under-5 mortality rate.
- Under UIP, immunization is provided free of cost against 12 vaccine preventable diseases:
  - *Nationally against nine diseases*: Diphtheria, pertussis, tetanus, polio, measles, rubella, severe form of childhood tuberculosis, hepatitis B

and meningitis, and pneumonia caused by *Haemophilus influenzae* type B
- *Subnationally against three diseases*: Rotavirus diarrhea, pneumococcal pneumonia, and Japanese encephalitis (JE); of which rotavirus vaccine and pneumococcal conjugate vaccine (PCV) are in process of expansion while JE vaccine is provided only in endemic districts.

- The two major milestones of UIP have been the elimination of polio in 2014 and maternal and neonatal tetanus elimination in 2015.
- *Mission Indradhanush (MI)* was launched in December 2014 and aimed at increasing the full immunization coverage to children to 90%.
- Under this drive, focus is given on pockets of low immunization coverage and hard to reach areas where the proportion of unvaccinated and partially vaccinated children is highest.
- A total of six phases of MI have been completed covering 554 districts across the country.
- While the first two phases of MI resulted in 6.7% increase in full immunization coverage in a year, a recent survey carried out in 190 districts covered in *Intensified MI (IMI)* (fifth phase of MI) shows 18.5% points increase in full immunization coverage as compared to National Family Health Survey-4 (NFHS-4) survey carried out in 2015–2016.
- National Cold Chain Training Centre (NCCTE), Pune and National Cold Chain & Vaccine Management Resource Centre (NCCVMRC)-National Institute of Health and Family Welfare (NIHFW), New Delhi have been established to provide technical training to cold chain technicians in repair and maintenance of cold chain equipment.
- The Government of India has rolled out an electronic Vaccine Intelligence Network (eVIN) system that digitizes the entire vaccine stock management, their logistics and temperature tracking at all levels of vaccine storage—from national to the subdistrict.
- This enables program managers to have real time view of the vaccine stock position and their storage temperature across all the cold chain points providing a detailed overview of the vaccine cold chain logistics system across the entire country.
- eVIN is to be scaled up to entire country.
- National Cold Chain Management Information System (NCCMIS) to track the cold chain equipment inventory, availability, and functionality.
- Adverse Events Following Immunization (AEFI) reporting and causality assessment happens in almost all districts. Serious AEFI are reported through District Immunization Officer to state and national authorities. Causality assessment is done at state and national levels and the results are reviewed by National AEFI Committee for feeding the national policy making.

Q3. What is the current goal of national immunization program?

Ans. The current goal of the national immunization program is "steering the country's vision into action to achieve *90% full immunization coverage* in all districts of the country and sustain the coverage through immunization system strengthening". The IMI 2.0 program (from December 2019 to March 2020) was entrusted to provide the main stimulus for achieving this. Now, with Covid-19 pandemic, achieving and maintaining full immunization coverage of 90% or more will be quite challenging.

Q4. What is the hierarchy of governance in national immunization program?

Ans. National Immunization Program of India is governed by National Health Mission (NHM). Additional Secretary and Managing Director (ASMD of NHM) heads the NHM and he/she reports to the Secretary, Department of Health and Family Welfare, Govt. of India. A team of Joint Secretaries manages various health programs, and one joint secretary looks after Child Health and Immunization program. Joint Secretary reports to ASMD.

Secretary Health at state leads the health programs including immunization program. State immunization program is managed by State NHM Chief [different designations are given in different states and generally, it is MD-NHM (Managing director–NHM)]. State Immunization Officer is the technical person who manages the immunization program in the state under the guidance of MD-NHM and Health Secretary. In many states, a post of Commissioner Health/Health Commissioner is also there who acts as a bridge between Secretary Health and MD-NHM.

District Immunization Officer manages the immunization program at district level under the Chief Medical and Health Officer or Civil Surgeon (states may have different designations for the chief of health department at state level.

Further, it is the Block Medical Officer (BMO) or MO at primary healthcare center (PHC) and Accredited Social Health Activist (ASHA) and Anganwadi workers (AWWs) at field level support the delivery of services under immunization program.

Q5. What is the National Immunization Schedule under Universal Immunization Program?

Ans. National Immunization Schedule is a vaccination plan that all children and pregnant women should follow and complete to ensure protection against vaccine-preventable diseases. This schedule includes name of vaccine, recommended age/s of administration, total doses required, route and site of administration, and volumes of doses **(Table 1)**.

Table 1: National Immunization Schedule (according to age).

Age	Vaccines given
Birth	Bacillus Calmette-Guérin (BCG), oral polio vaccine (OPV)-0 dose, hepatitis B birth dose
6 Weeks	OPV-1, pentavalent-1, rotavirus vaccine (RVV)-1***, fractional dose of inactivated polio vaccine (fIPV)-1, pneumococcal conjugate vaccine (PCV)-1***
10 weeks	OPV-2, pentavalent-2, RVV-2***
14 weeks	OPV-3, pentavalent-3, fIPV-2, RVV-3***, PCV-2***
9–12 months	Measles and rubella (MR)-1, JE-1*, PCV-Booster***
16–24 months	MR-2, Japanese encephalitis (JE)-2*, diphtheria, pertussis and tetanus (DPT)-booster-1, OPV–booster
5–6 years	DPT-Booster-2
10 years	Tetanus and adult diphtheria (Td)
16 years	Td
Pregnant mother	Td1, 2 or Td booster**

* JE in 231 endemic districts
** One dose if previously vaccinated within 3 years
*** Rotavirus vaccine and PCV in selected states/districts as per details below:
- *Rotavirus*: Andhra Pradesh, Assam, Haryana, Himachal Pradesh, Jharkhand, Madhya Pradesh, Odisha, Rajasthan, Tamil Nadu, Tripura, and Uttar Pradesh.
- PCV: Bihar, Himachal Pradesh, Madhya Pradesh, Uttar Pradesh (12 districts) and Rajasthan (9 districts). *These may vary as more states are likely to add these vaccines.*

Q6. How new vaccines are introduced in UIP and how is immunization schedule decided?

Ans. The decision on inclusion of vaccines is taken by the Ministry of Health and Family Welfare, Government of India, on recommendation of National Technical Advisory Group on Immunization (NTAGI). Schedule for administration of different vaccines is decided based on the operational aspects of national immunization program; and the recommendations provided by WHO-recommended schedules, vaccine position papers, as well as the Strategic Advisory Group of Experts (SAGE).

This is a complex process. The below given criteria are considered for an informed decision-making about the introduction of new vaccine in UIP.
- Disease burden (incidence/prevalence, absolute number of morbidity/mortality, and epidemic/pandemic potential)
- Safety and efficacy of the vaccine under consideration
- Affordability and financial sustainability of the vaccination program, even if the initial introduction is supported by the external funding agency
- Program capacity to introduce a new antigen, including cold chain capacity
- Availability of a domestic or external vaccine production capacity

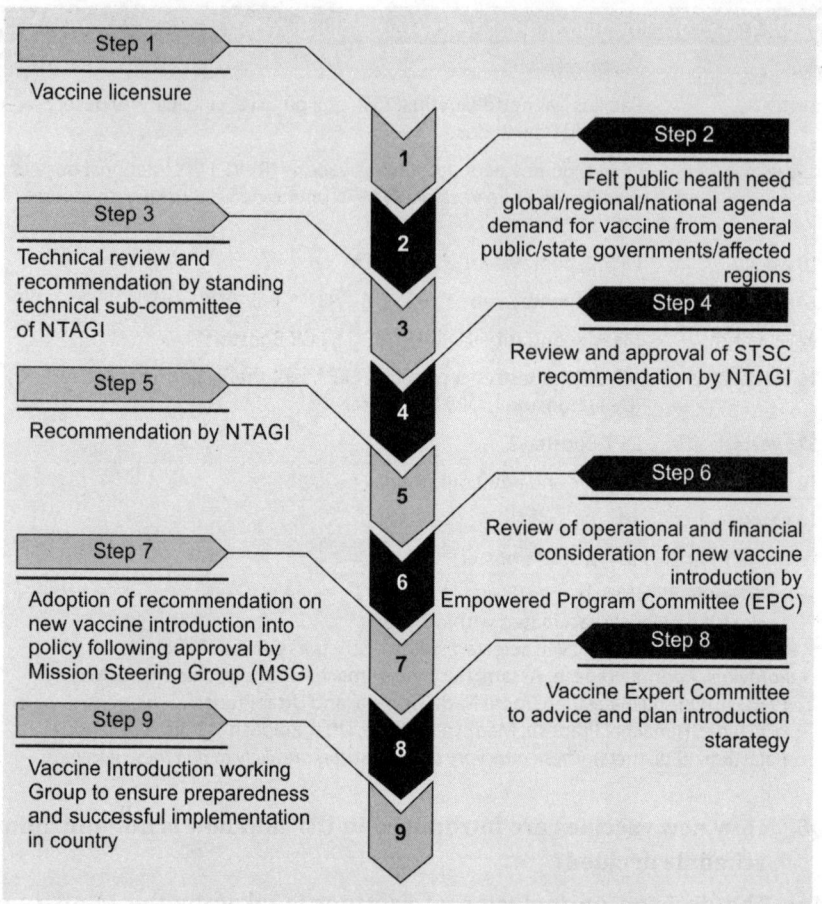

Fig. 1: Steps for introduction of new vaccine in India.
(NTAGI: National Technical Advisory Group on Immunization; STSC: Safety Trained Supervisor Construction)

- The cost effectiveness of the vaccination program and also of the alternatives other than vaccination.

This process is given in **Figure 1**.

Q7. What are the upper age limits for various vaccines in UIP?

Ans. According to National Immunization Schedule, some vaccines have an upper age limit for administration and these vaccines should not be administered once that age limit is crossed.

The vaccines should be given till the following ages as per UIP guidelines:
- *Bacillus Calmette-Guérin (BCG)*: Up to 1 year of age
- *Oral polio vaccine*: Up to 5 years (OPV zero dose till 15 days of birth)
- *Measles/MR*: Up to 5 years (in MR campaigns, vaccine is given to 9 months to 15 years age group)

- *Diphtheria, pertussis and tetanus*: Up to 7 years
- *Japanese encephalitis*: Up to 15 years

Only the above-mentioned vaccines have upper age limits. Efforts should be made to ensure that all vaccines are given at the recommended ages, or closer to it.

For pentavalent, inactivated polio vaccine (IPV), PCV, and rotavirus vaccines, if at least one dose is given before 1 year of age, then remaining doses can be administered and schedule must be completed irrespective of the age of child. If the first dose is not administered before one year of age, then these vaccines cannot be administered to the child under UIP.

Q8. Why are the vaccines in national immunization program given at a specific site?

Ans. Each vaccine is normally administered at the same and specific site on the body to maintain uniformity and to help determine vaccination history by asking from beneficiary or caretaker (in case immunization card is not available or lost). Specific sites of administration also help parents and caretakers recall previous vaccinations during the follow-up visits and household surveys **(Fig. 2)**.

Q9. When several vaccines are to be given in the same visit then what should be the sequence of administration of various vaccines?

Ans. During 6th, 10th, 14th weeks and 9 months, when multiple vaccines are to be administered, it is preferable for health workers/vaccinators to follow the sequence as given below **(Fig. 3)**, for the sake of programmatic consistency and uniformity.

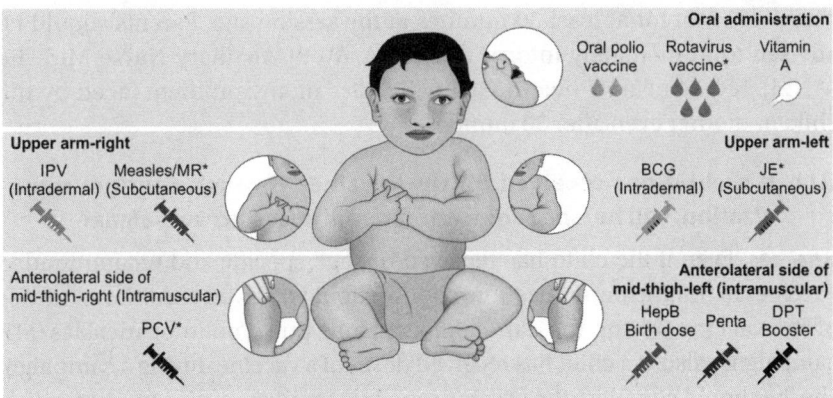

Fig. 2: Site of vaccine administration.
(BCG: Bacillus Calmette-Guérin; DPT: diphtheria, pertussis and tetanus; IPV: inactivated polio vaccine; JE: Japanese encephalitis; PCV: pneumococcal conjugate vaccine; MR: measles and rubella)

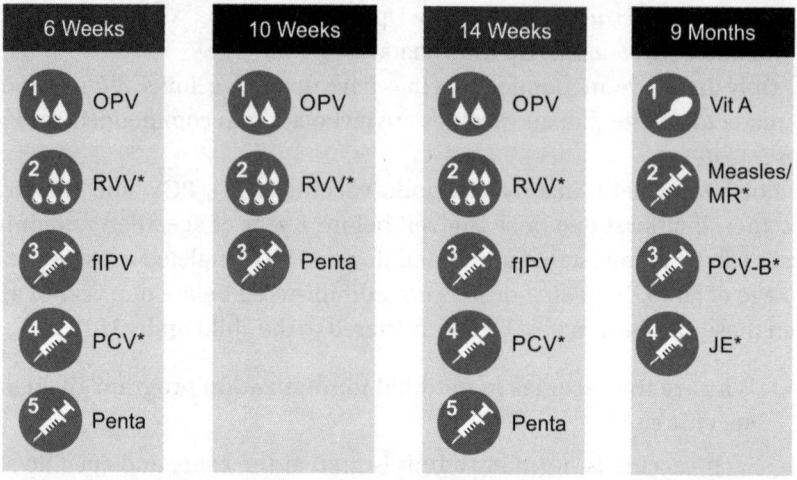

Fig. 3: Sequence of vaccine administration.
*Wherever applicable
(fIPV: fractional dose of inactivated polio vaccine; JE: Japanese encephalitis; MR: measles and rubella; OPV: oral polio vaccine; PCV: pneumococcal conjugate vaccine; RVV: rotavirus vaccine)

Q10. What are the four key messages which should be given to parents at the time of vaccination?

Ans. As per the national guidelines, the four key messages that need to be delivered by health worker to parents and caregivers are:
1. What vaccine was given, and what disease it prevents
2. What minor adverse event could occur, and how to deal with them
3. When and where to come for the next visit
4. To keep the immunization card safe and to bring along for the next visit

After vaccination, the health workers should ensure that the parents/caregivers wait for at least 30 minutes at the session site. Parents should be advised to immediately inform the ASHA/AWW/Auxiliary Nurse Midwife (ANM)/MO of nearest health facility, in case of any problem faced by the child or mother even after 30 minutes.

Q11. If a child has received all the vaccines through routine immunization, will he/she require additional doses in campaigns?

Ans. Yes. Even if the child has received the age-specific and recommended vaccines in routine immunization, she/he should be given "additional" doses of the vaccine during the campaigns such as pulse polio or measles/MR campaigns. Also, if a child has received doses of a vaccine during a campaign, she/he should complete the vaccine schedule through routine immunization as well.

These additional doses during campaigns can be given/administered irrespective of days since last dose was received. For example, if a child has received second dose of OPV 3 weeks before, she/he can still receive an additional dose during the pulse polio campaign.

■ SUGGESTED READING

1. Anekwe TD, Kumar S. The effect of a vaccination program on child anthropometry: evidence from India's Universal Immunization Program. J Public Health. 2012;34(4):489-97.
2. Liu L, Oza S, Hogan D, Perin J, Rudan I, Lawn JE, et al. Global, regional, and national causes of child mortality in 2000-13, with projections to inform post-2015 priorities: an updated systematic analysis. Lancet. 2015;385(9966):430-40.
3. Ministry of Health & Family Welfare. (2011). National Vaccine Policy. [online] Available from: https://nhm.gov.in/images/pdf/programmes/immunization/Guidelines/National_Vaccine_Policy.pdf. [Last accessed October, 2020].
4. Ministry of Health & Family Welfare. (2017). FAQs on Immunization for Program Managers. [online] Available from: https://nhm.gov.in/New_Updates_2018/NHM_Components/Immunization/Guildelines_for_immunization/FAQ_on_Immunization_for_Program_Manager-English.pdf. [Last accessed October, 2020].
5. Ministry of Health & Family Welfare. Immunization Handbook for Medical Officers 2016. New Delhi: Ministry of Health & Family Welfare; 2016.
6. Nandi A, Kumar S, Shet A, Bloom DE, Laxminarayan R. Childhood vaccinations and adult schooling attainment: Long-term evidence from India's Universal Immunization Programme. Soc Sci Med. 2020;250:112885.
7. NHM. (2018). National Immunization Schedule. [online] Available from https://nhm.gov.in/New_Updates_2018/NHM_Components/Immunization/report/National_Immunization_Schedule.pdf. [Last accessed October, 2020].
8. NHM. Immunization. [online] Available from: https://nhm.gov.in/index1.php?lang=1&level=2&sublinkid=824&lid=220. [Last accessed October, 2020].

Annexure
Vaccines marketed in India

Vaccine	Brand name	Company
BCG VACCINE	TUBERVAC BCG	SERUM
	ONCO BCG	CIPLA
CHICKENPOX	VARILIX	GSK
	VARIPED	MSD
	NEXIPOX	NOVO
	ZUVICELLA	ZUVENTUS
CHOLERA VACCINES	SHANCHOL	SANOFI
DTaP + IPV+HIB VACCINE	PENTAXIM	SANOFI
DTaP + IPV+HIB+HEP-B VACCINE	HEXAXIM	SANOFI
	INFANRIX HEXA	GSK
DTP + IPV+HIB+HEP-B VACCINE	EASY SIX PFS	PANACEA
DPT+HIB+HEP-B VACCINE	PENTAVAC SD	SERUM
	PENTAVAC PFS	SERUM
	EASY FIVE PFS	PANACEA
	COMBIFIVE VIAL	BIOLOGICAL E.
	COMVAC-5 PFS	BHARAT BIOTEC
DPT+HIB VACCINE	QUADROVAX SD	SERUM
	QUADROVAX PFS	SERUM
	EASY FOUR	PANACEA
HEP-A VACCINE	HAVRIX 720 PFS	GSK
	HAVRIX 720 VIAL	GSK
	BIOVAC A	WOCKHARD
	AVAXIM-80	SANOFI
HEP-B VACCINE	REVAC-B 1mL	BHARAT BIOTECH
	REVAC-B 0.5 mL	BHARAT BIOTECH
	REVAC-B MCF PFS	BHARAT BIOTECH
HEP-B VACCINE	GENEVAC-B 0.5 mL	SERUM
	GENEVAC-B 1 mL	SERUM
	GENEVAC-B 10 mL	SERUM
HEP-B VACCINE	BEVAC 1 mL	BIOLOGICAL E.
	BEVAC 0.5 mL	BIOLOGICAL E.
HPV VACCINE	GARDASIL VIAL	MSD
	CERVARIX PFS	GSK

ANNEXURE: Vaccines marketed in India

Vaccine	Brand name	Company
INFLUENZA VACCINE	INFLUVAC 0.5 mL	ABBOTT
	INFLUVAC TETRA 0.5 mL	ABBOTT
	FLUARIX TETRA 0.5 mL	GSK
	FLUQUADRI 0.5 mL	SANOFI
	VAXIFLU-4 0.5 mL	ZYDUS CADILA
JE VACCINE	JEEV 3 mcg PFS	BIOLOGICAL
	JEEV 6 mcg VIAL	BIOLOGICAL
	JE-SHIELD	ABBOTT
	JENVAC PFS	BHARAT BIOTECH
MENINGOCOCCAL VACCINE	MENACTRA	SANOFI
	MENVEO	GSK
MMR VACCINE	TRESIVAC	SERUM
	TRESIVAC PFS	SERUM
	PRIORIX MONODOSE	GSK
PNEUMOCOCCAL POLYSACCHRIDE VACCINE	PNEUMOVAX-23 PFS	MSD
PNEUMOCOCCAL CONJUGATE VACCINE	PREVENAR-13	PFIZER
	SYNFLORIX PFS	GSK
	PNEUMOSIL	SERUM
POLIO VACCINE	BI-POLIO—20 DOSES	BHARAT BIOTECH
	BI-POLIO—10 DOSES	PANACEA
IPV VACCINE	POLIOVAC	SERUM
ANTIRABIES VACCINE	RABIVAX-S	SERUM
	CHIRORAB	CHIRON
	VAXIRAB-N	ZYDUS CADILA
ANTIRABIES IMMUNOGLOBULIN	RABISHIELD 100 IU	SERUM
	RABISHIELD 50 IU	SERUM
	BERIRAB-P 300 IU	BHARAT SERUM
	TWINRAB 1500 IU	ZYDUS CADILA
	TWINRAB 600 IU	ZYDUS CADILA
ROTAVIRUS VACCINE	ROTARIX	GSK
	ROTASIL	SERUM
	ROTATEQ ORAL	MSD
	ROTAVAC	BHARAT BIOTEC
	ROTASURE	ABBOTT

ANNEXURE: Vaccines marketed in India

Vaccine	Brand name	Company
RUBELLA VACCINE	R VAC	SERUM
TETANUS DIPHTHERIA VACCINE	TD VAC	SERUM
	BE-Td	BE VACCINES
Tdap VACCINE	BOOSTRIX	GSK
	ADACEL	SANOFI
TYPHOID POLYSACCHARIDE VACCINE	TYPBAR PFS	BHARAT BIOTECH
	TYPBAR VIAL	BHARAT BIOTECH
	TYPBAR 2.5 mL VIAL	BHARAT BIOTECH
TYPHOID CONJUGATE VACCINE	TYPBAR TCV	BHARAT BIOTECH
	ZYVAC TCV	ZYDUS CADILA
	ENTEROSHIELD	ABBOTT
	TYPHIBEV	BIOLOGICAL E.
YELLOW FEVER VACCINE	STAMARIL	SANOFI

Index

Page numbers followed by *f* refer to figure and *t* refer to table.

A

Accidental needle stick injury 159
Acellular pertussis 140
  vaccine 138, 139, 140*t*
Acquired immunodeficiency syndrome 26, 351
Acute lower respiratory infections 197
Acute lung injury, transfusion related 114
Acute respiratory
  distress syndrome 190
  syndrome coronavirus 345
  tract infection 191
Adenovirus
  advantages of 364
  vaccines 337
Adolescent Vaccination Program 304
Adrenaline 100
Adventitious viruses 364
Adverse Event Following Immunization 50, 72, 75*f*, 77*f*, 79, 94, 100, 206, 266, 382
  types of 72
Advisory Committee on Immunization Practices 38, 146, 183, 197, 235, 251, 267, 295
Aedes aegypti mosquito 347
Alanine aminotransferase 311
Alcoholism 309
Allergens 3
Allergic disorders 368
Allogenic vaccines 369
Aluminum 328
  hydroxide 136
  oxide-based nanocarriers 330
  phosphate 136
Alzheimer's disease 368, 373
Anaphylactic allergic reaction 200, 287
Anemia, severe 109
Antibody 3
  affinity 16
  dependent enhancement 357
  functions of 8*f*
  mediated organ transplant rejection 109
  titers 364
Anti-cyclic citrullinated peptide 372
Anti-D immune globulins 107
Antigen 3
  combination 20
  dose of 19, 46
  polysaccharide vaccine 215
  presenting cells 8
Anti-hepatitis vaccine 226
Anti-pertussis toxin 302
Antirabies
  immunoglobulin 394
  vaccine 394
Antiretroviral therapy 371
Antiviral therapy 291
Anxiety 78
Asplenia 87
Asthma 309
Ataxia-telangiectasia 82
Atherosclerosis 368
Attack rate, secondary 27
Autism, association of 208
Autoimmune
  diseases 372
  disorders 110
  lymphoproliferative disorder 109
Auxiliary nurse midwives 74

B

Bacillus-Calmette-Guérin 42, 119, 124, 339, 388, 389
  reaction, classical 121
  scar 124
  severe complications of 121
  vaccination
    complications of 121
    contraindications of 122
  vaccine 119, 123, 373, 393
    administration of 120
    dosage of 120
    role of 373
Bacteria 3
Bacterial infection, prevention of 113
B-cell activation 12
Bell's palsy 252
Bethesda system 240
Bioencapsulation 331
Blepharitis 290
Blindness 290

Index

Blood
  dyscrasias 170
  transfusion 47
Bloody diarrhea 78
B-lymphocyte 5
  deficiency disorders 82
Body mass index 191
Bordetella pertussis 302, 336
Botulism immunoglobulin 110
Bovine rotavirus pentavalent vaccine 164, 165
Breast cancers 369
Breastfeeding 169
Burkitt lymphoma 370

C

Canadian Adverse Events Following Immunization Surveillance System 95
Cancer
  cells 369
  clinical applications in 369
  colorectal 369
Catch-up vaccination 167, 209
Cell-mediated immune response 122
Centers for Disease Control and Prevention 248, 277
Central Drugs Standard Control Organisation 359
Central nervous system 270
Cerebrospinal fluid 183
Cervical cancer 301
  problem 241
Cervical intraepithelial neoplasia 240
Chickenpox 2, 228, 304, 312
  vaccine 393
Chikungunya virus 350
Chlamydia 324
Chlorpheniramine 100
Cholera 26, 279, 317
  vaccines 279, 281, 342, 393
Circumsporozoite protein 335
Cirrhosis 152, 311
Citrobacter freundii 217, 220
Clostridioides 113
Cochlear implants 183
Cold chain 54
  elements of 55
  equipment, specifications of 63t
  management 54
  representation of 54f
Colitis 113
Communicable diseases 378
Complement-mediated serum bactericidal activity 264

Complete blood count 114
Complex regional pain syndrome 252
Conjugate vaccine 179, 217, 264
  advantage of 177
Convulsions 78
Corneal ulceration 290
Coronavirus disease 2019 5, 124
Cough 266
COVID-19 5, 124, 125
  pandemic 365
  risk of 355
  vaccines 355, 357, 358, 360, 363, 365, 366
    accelerated development 356f
    efficacy of 366
    technology 358t
CoWIN 367
Culex tritaeniorhynchus 270
Cytokines 326
Cytomegalovirus immune globulins 110
Cytotoxic cells 6

D

Dendritic cell 9
  role of 10f
  vaccines 369
Dengue
  vaccine, status of 349
  viruses 347-349, 357
Deoxyribonucleic acid 151, 153, 239, 291, 324, 326, 345, 347, 369
  vaccine 12, 326
  basics of 325
Diabetes mellitus 155, 309
Diarrhea 266
  severe 78
Diarrheal diseases 162
DiGeorge syndrome 82
Digital data loggers 65, 66f
Digital maximum-minimum thermometers 65, 66f
Diphtheria 30, 112, 302, 306
  and tetanus 136
    toxoids 102
  clinical presentation 113
  immunoglobulins 110
  pertussis, and tetanus 135, 136, 377, 384, 389
    vaccine for 135
  pertussis, and vaccine
    efficacy of 137
    role of adjuvants in 136
  tetanus and
    acellular pertussis 42
    whole-cell pertussis 42

tetanus toxoids 137
and whole-cell pertussis 136, 138, 139*t*
tetanus, and acellular pertussis 136, 138, 139*t*
toxoid 140, 146, 265
and acellular pertussis 42
nontoxic variety of 146
Disability-adjusted life years 25
Disodium phosphate anhydrous 294
Dog bite cases 257
Drug Controller General of India 248, 275
Dysgammaglobulinemia 170

E

Ebola virus 346, 346*t*, 356
disease 345
prevention of 345
infection 346
vaccine 346
Efficacy data
long-term 293*t*
short-term 293*t*
Egg allergy 201
Electronic vaccine intelligence network 68
Encephalitis 190, 208, 290
syndrome, acute 270
Endemic disease 26
Endocarditis 174
Enteroviral infections 109
Enzyme-linked immunosorbent assay 180, 280
Epinephrine 100
Epitope 3, 4*f*
Epizootic disease 26
Epstein-Barr virus infection 109, 370
Equine rabies immunoglobulin 257
Escherichia coli 341

F

Fabricius bursa 5, 45
Fainting 78
Fatty liver disease 311
Filamentous hemagglutinin 136, 140
Fimbrial hemagglutinin 136
Flavivirus 282
Fluorescent antibody 230
Follicular dendritic cells 16, 19
Follicular lymphoma 370
Food and Drug Administration 160, 334, 345
Freeze sensitive vaccines 56
Fungal ligand 5

G

Gastroenteritis 163, 164
Gastrointestinal loss 109
Gastrointestinal tract 171
Geometric mean
antibody titer 246
concentrations 178
titers 231, 274
Germinal center response 15*f*
Gliomas 369
Global Advisory Committee on Vaccine Safety 95, 252
Glycoconjugate 335
Glycoprotein enzyme-linked immunosorbent assay 230, 231
Graft-versus-host disease 85
Granulomatous disease, chronic 83
Guillain-Barré syndrome 74, 109, 195, 200, 208, 252, 266

H

H1N1
influenza 26, 356
strain 190, 191
H3N2 strain 191
Haemophilus influenzae 7, 31, 144, 178, 180, 213, 385
B
disease 148
infection 144
vaccine 146-148, 248
Hand, foot and mouth disease 334
Hansenula polymorpha 153
Healthcare professionals, vaccinations of 311
Hearing loss 290
Heart
and light sensitive vaccines 56
disease
chronic 309
congenital 212
Helicobacter pylori 368
Hemagglutinin 189
Hematopoietic stem cell transplantation 81, 85*t*, 113, 158, 234
Hemoglobinopathies 183
Hemolytic anemia, autoimmune 109
Hemophagocytic lymphohistiocytosis 109
Hepatic transaminases 114
Hepatitis 150
A 15, 52, 86, 111, 222, 304
infection 222
vaccine 40, 41, 223-226, 303
virus 35, 150, 304
autoimmune 311

B 15, 42, 52, 78, 84, 104, 150, 151, 304, 311
  candidate vaccine 333
  carriers 226
  immunoglobulin 109, 158-160
  infections, chronic 371
  problem 150
  vaccine 88, 153, 154, 157, 159, 161, 328, 393
  virus 150, 151, 151*f*, 152, 160, 333, 349, 372
C 311, 372
  virus 150
D virus 150
E virus 150
infection 223
syndromes, acute 150
vaccine 46
Hepatocellular carcinoma 152
Herpes viruses 323
Herpes zoster 232, 290
  history of 312
  risk of 229
  vaccination 310
Highly active antiretroviral therapy 157
Holoendemic disease 26
Human cytomegalovirus disease 340
Human diploid cell vaccine 256
Human immunodeficiency virus 87, 155, 170, 207, 234, 323, 333
  immunization in 88*t*
  infection 113, 121, 287, 315
  vaccines, clinical trials for 352, 353
Human leukocyte antigen 373
Human papillomavirus 42, 239, 240, 302, 307, 323, 378
  bivalent 243
  infection 240, , 242, 250
    risk factors for 240
    symptoms of 239
  vaccine 239, 242, 244, 245, 249, 318, 393
    contraindications for 252
    effects of 250
    use of 303
Human rabies immunoglobulin 257
Hyperendemic disease 26
Hyperhemolytic crisis 109
Hyperimmune globulins 107-109
Hyperpyrexia 138
Hypertension 309, 318, 368
Hyperventilation 78
Hypogammaglobulinemia 113, 170
Hypotensive-hyporesponsive episodes 138
Hypothyroidism 318
Hypotonic-hyporesponsive episodes 49

I

Immune
  deficiencies 110
  dysfunction 323
  globulins 108
  response 17
    conjugated vaccines 15
  system, function of 3
  thrombocytopenia 109
Immunity 3, 10*f*
  active 11
  adaptive 4*f*
  cell-mediated 8, 121, 290, 325
  cellular 8
  herd 30, 30*t*
  humoral 7
  innate 4*f*
Immunization 3
  anxiety-related reaction 72
  documentation of 52
  error-related reaction 72
  schedule 146
  technical support unit 68
Immunodeficiency
  primary 107, 108
  severe combined 121, 49, 170
Immunogenicity 208, 217
Immunoglobulin 3, 7, 107, 256
  A 234
  administration of 115*t*
  G 151, 231, 234, 304
  types of 7
  use of 108
Immunosuppression 49
In vitro dendritic cell 325
Inactivated influenza vaccine 42, 195
  contraindications for 196
  efficacy of 196
  side effects of 195
Inactivated polio vaccine 42389
  fractional dose of 390*f*
Indian Academy of Pediatrics 38, 76, 146, 169, 195, 200, 235, 258
Indian Council of Medical Research 272
Indian Medical Association 76
Indian Neonatal Rotavirus Live Vaccine 165
Indian Rotavirus Strain Surveillance Network 163
Indirect fluorescent antibody 231
Infections 109

Inflammatory bowel disease 208
Inflammatory disorders 110
Influenza 189, 191, 192, 304, 312, 318, 323
    complications of 190
    disease burden of 190
    management of 192
    prevention of 192
    severe 191
    treatment of 192
    type B 194
    vaccine 192-195, 200, 328, 394
        composition of 193
        types of 192
    viruses 351
Integrated digital thermometers 65, 65*f*
International Certificate of Vaccination 285
International Health Regulations 285
Intradermal rabies vaccination 259
Intravenous immunoglobulin 230
    G 107
    doses of 110
    use of 108
Invasive bacterial infection surveillance 175
Invasive pneumococcal disease 89, 174, 180
    surveillance of 175

J

Japanese encephalitis 39, 270, 270, 304, 317, 389, 390*f*
    control 271
    disease burden of 271
    prevention of 273
    vaccine 270, 274, 276, 317, 394
        Program 272
    virus 270, 347
Joint pain 266

K

Kawasaki disease 109, 124
Killed oral whole-cell-bivalent vaccine 280, 281
Kolar strain vaccine, salient features of 275

L

Lactobacillus acidophilus 224
Lassa fever virus 345
Leukemia 170
    acute lymphatic 236
    chronic lymphocytic 109

Leukocyte adhesion deficiency 83
Live-attenuated hepatitis A vaccine 224
Live-attenuated influenza vaccine 198, 199
    contraindications of 200
    side effects of 199
Live-attenuated vaccines 11, 12
Live-attenuated yellow fever vaccine 276
Liver
    cancer, primary 150
    disease
        alcoholic 311
        chronic 226, 309
Low birth weight 159
Lung cancers 369
Lymphocyte antigen 370
Lymphoid tissue
    gut-associated 331
    nasal-associated 329
Lymphomas 170
Lyssavirus 254

M

Macrophage activation syndrome 109
Major histocompatibility complex 6
Malaria 26, 323, 368
    vaccines 334, 335
Malignant cells 3
Mannide monooleate 328
Maternal antibodies 21
Measles 30, 384, 389
    containing vaccine 211
    postexposure prophylaxis 109
    prevention 205
Measles and rubella 390*f*
    vaccination campaigns 211
Measles, mumps, and rubella 42, 52, 208, 230, 304
    and varicella 231
    and varicella 318
        vaccine 213
    vaccine 36, 204, 206, 288, 316
        contraindications for 207
        immunogenicity of 207
Measles, pertussis, and diphtheria 301, 380
Measles, varicella containing vaccine 115*t*
Medical equipment 100
Medical termination of pregnancy 234
Melanoma 369
Membrane antigen 230
Memory B cells 16
Meningitis 174
    belt 303
Meningococcal conjugate vaccine 264, 265, 315

Meningococcal polysaccharide vaccine 15, 265
Meningococcal serogroup B vaccine 268
Meningococcal vaccination 303
Meningococcal vaccine 263, 266, 304, 394
    protection for 264
Mental retardation 212
Messenger ribonucleic acid 347
Microarray patch 331
Microneedle technologies 331
Mission Indradhanush 385
Monoclonal antibodies 107, 256
Mucosal vaccination 329
Mucosal vaccine delivery system, concept of 330
Multidose vial policy 68
Multifocal motor neuropathy 109
Multi-organ failure 190
Multiple myloma 108
Multiple sclerosis 233
Multistage vaccine 335
Mumps 30
Muscle 266
Myasthenia gravis 109
Mycobacterial disease 121
Mycobacterium
    avium 122
    indicus pranii 371
    intracellulare 122
    marinum 122
    tuberculosis 119, 323, 339
    vaccae 371
Myocarditis 190
Myositis 190

N

Nasopharyngeal carriage 174, 175
Nasopharyngitis 266
National Immunization Program 38, 124, 149, 153, 161, 168, 184, 263, 301, 306, 384, 386
National Immunization Schedule 387*t*
National Institute of Allergy and Infectious Diseases 347
National Regulatory Authority 93, 94, 360
National TB Control Program, revised 119
National Vector Borne Disease Control Program 272
Natural infection 152
Natural killer T cells 6
Natural varicella 229
Neisseria meningitides 146, 263, 312, 323
Neonatal alloimmune thrombocytopenia 109

Neonatal rotavirus vaccine 338
Neuraminidase 189
Neuritis 233
Neurologic disease 287
Neurological diseases 368
Neurological disorders 373
Neutralizing antibodies 349
Neutropenia, autoimmune 109
New tuberculosis vaccine 339
New vaccine
    development 324
    technologies 323
Nipah
    glycoprotein 345
    viral disease 347
    virus 345, 347
        disease, prevention of 347
Nonavalent Human papillomavirus vaccine 246
Noncommunicable diseases 368
Non-human adenovirus vectors 364
Noninvasive diseases 174
Nonpneumococcal conjugate vaccine 175
Nonsterile injection 73
Nonsteroidal anti-inflammatory drugs 284, 291
Novel virus 345
    vaccine against 345

O

Obesity 368
Ocular palsy 290
Ocular zoster 290
Optimum immunization schedule 37
Oral cholera vaccine 279, 304, 336
Oral polio vaccine 127, 390*f*
    birth dose of 130
    characteristics of 126
    monovalent 127
    types of 126
Oral poliovirus vaccine 42, 126, 156, 169, 378
    bivalent 127
Oral rehydration solution 162
Oral typhoid vaccine 216
Oral vaccine 280
Oseltamivir 192
Osteomyelitis 174
Otitis media, acute 180

P

Packing cold box 69
Pain relief 48

Paralytic polio, vaccine-associated 127
Paralytic poliomyelitis, vaccine associated 77
Parasites 3
Paratope 3, 4f
Paratyphoid
   A vaccine 215
   B vaccine 215
   vaccine 215
      development of 221, 342
Parvovirus infection, chronic 109
Passive immunity 11
Peramivir 192
Pertussis 30, 302, 307
   toxin 136, 140
Phagocytic function disorders 83
Pichia pastoris 349
Plasmodium falciparum 335
Platelet alloimmunization 109
Pneumococcal bacteremia 174
Pneumococcal conjugate vaccine 42, 103, 174, 176, 177, 179, 181, 184, 389, 390, 394
   efficacy of 180
Pneumococcal disease 174, 176
Pneumococcal infections 183
Pneumococcal polysaccharide vaccine 15, 176, 184, 394
Pneumococcal serotype 174
Pneumococcal vaccine 182-184, 184t, 304
   status of newer 187
   types of 176
Pneumococcus 174
Pneumonia 174, 180, 290
Polio 30, 126, 384
   endgame 129
   eradication 127
   status of 126
   vaccine 40, 126, 316, 394
Polyepitope vaccine, development of 372
Polymerase chain reaction 135, 197, 232, 244
Polysaccharide 335
   antigens 18
   vaccine 14, 14f, 264, 315
      efficacy of 264
Population level effects of vaccination, types of 29
Postexposure prophylaxis 111, 209, 337
Posthematopoietic cell transplantation 108
Postherpetic neuralgia 290
Postlicensure surveillance 94
Post-marketing surveillance, types of 95
Post-transfusion purpura 109
Post-transplant lymphoproliferative disorder 370
Postural orthostatic tachycardia syndrome 251
Postvaccination observation area, requirements of 99
Pregnancy 49
Prehematopoietic cell transplantation 108
Premature newborns, severe sepsis in 109
Programmatic vaccine deliveries 331
Prophylaxis, pre-exposure 111, 258, 337
Protection, serologic correlate of 218
Protein
   antigens 18
   loss, severe 109
Pseudomonas aeruginosa 217, 218
Purified chick embryo cell vaccine 256
Purified duck embryo vaccine 256
Pyrexia 266

Q

Quadrivalent influenza vaccine 194, 201
   efficacy of 197
Quadrivalent meningococcal conjugate vaccine 103, 304
Quadrivalent vaccine 250
Quality-adjusted life years 25
Quillaja saponaria 294

R

Rabies 113, 254, 255, 312
   immunoglobulins 110, 256
   in dogs 255
   transmit 254
   vaccine 254, 259, 337
Randomized controlled trial 33, 217
Rapid schedule 154
Recombinant zoster vaccine 86
   contraindications for 295
Recurrent infections 109
Re-exposure prophylaxis 256
Renal disease, chronic 156
Renal failure, chronic 155
Renal loss 109
Replacement phenomenon 175
Respiratory infection, acute 196
Respiratory syncytial virus 335
Resuscitation, cardiopulmonary 79
Reverse vaccinology 324
Rhabdomyolysis 190
Rhabdovirus 254
Rheumatoid arthritis 109
Ribonucleic acid 270, 324
   vaccines 12, 324
Ringer's lactate 80
Rituximab therapy 84

Rotaviral diarrhea 167
Rotavirus 104, 162-164, 167, 338
   diarrhea 33
      cause of 163
   disease 162, 163
   gastroenteritis, severe 166
   infection 162, 163
   strains of 163
   vaccination 33
   vaccine 42, 78, 162, 164, 165, 167-171, 172t, 338, 390, 394
      dose of 166, 169
Routine vaccination 276
Rubella 30, 113, 384, 389
   control 204, 212
   syndrome, congenital 207, 212, 213
   vaccine 395

S

Saccharomyces cerevisiae 153
Salmonella
   minnesota 294
   paratyphi infection 342
   typhi 218
Septicemia 174
Seroconversion 28
   rate 218t
Serogroups 263
Seropositivity 28
Seroprotection 28
Serum
   creatinine 114
   glucose 114
Severe acute respiratory syndrome coronavirus 2 26, 124
Severe and serious adverse events following immunization 73
Sexual transmission 152
Sexually active 246
Shake test 67
   negative 67f
Shigella vaccine 341
Shingles 290
   prevention study 292
   vaccine 307
Sickle-cell disease 183
Simple febrile seizures 138
Smallpox 30, 261
   vaccine 90
Soft tissue infections 174
Solid organ transplant 81, 234
Spontaneous bacterial peritonitis 307
Squamous intraepithelial lesions 240
Standard immunoglobulins 107

Staphylococcus aureus 324, 342
Streptococcus pneumoniae 89, 177, 178, 323, 324
Strokes 290
Subcutaneous immunoglobulins 107
Subcutaneous immunotherapy 368
Subcutaneous vaccines 44
Sublingual immunotherapy 368
Supplemental immunization activity 128, 210
Swine flu 201
Synthetic peptide vaccines 324
Systemic inflammatory response 190
Systemic lupus erythematosus 109, 233
Systemic vascular inflammatory diseases 109

T

T cell
   activation 12
   dependent vaccines 15
   independent immune response 13
   types of 6
T helper cell 5, 122
T lymphocytes 5
Talimogene laherparepvec 369
Temperature monitoring devices 65
Termination of pregnancy 249
Tetanus 112, 302, 307
   immunoglobulin 110
      dose for 141t
   prophylaxis 141
   toxoid 140, 146, 301
      doses of 142
Tetanus, diphtheria 42, 136, 306
   and acellular pertussis 136
      vaccine 395
   vaccine 395
T-helper cells 6
Therapeutic tuberculosis vaccines 371
Therapeutic vaccines 368, 373
   applications of 371
   role of 368
   scope of 373
   status of 372
Thrombocytopenia 233
T-lymphocyte deficiency disorders 82
Toll-like receptors 9, 14
Toxic shock syndrome 109
Traditional vaccine development 356
Trained immunity 5
Transforming growth factor 6, 7
Travelers, vaccination for 272, 314
Treponema pallidum 108

Index

Triplex vaccine 340
Trivalent influenza vaccines 194
Tuberculosis 26, 40, 119, 368
   and pertussis 323
Tuberculous skin testing 123
Tumor cells 370
Typhoid
   conjugate vaccine 215, 217, 304, 395
   fever 215
   polysaccharide vaccine 395
   vaccine 41, 215, 221
      developments in 342
      types of 215
   VI polysaccharide vaccine 216

U

United States Food and Drug
      Administration 274
Univalent varicella vaccine 86
Universal Immunization Program 168,
      169, 210, 273, 384
   vaccines in 388
Upper respiratory tract infection 266
Urine analysis 114

V

Vaccination 3, 284, 299
   area, requirements of 99
   clinics 98
   documentation of 50, 51
   procedure 43, 50
   recommendations for 85t
   records, nonavailability of 52
   schedule 19, 37
Vaccine 17, 88
   adjuvant-delivery system 331
   administration 43, 379
      schedule for 235, 390f
      site of 389f
   adverse effects of 281
   adverse event reporting system 96, 251
   candidates 358
   carrier 70, 70f
   concept, vector-based 327
   delivery 331
   derived poliovirus 128
   development 351
   documentation of 51
   dose, part of 45
   doses of 20t
   effectiveness 29
   efficacy 29, 310t, 348
   failure 36
      primary 36
      secondary 36
   hesitancy 379
   immunogenicity of 28, 230
   impact 30
   in fridge, storage of 60, 61
   plant-based 331
   preventable diseases 306, 314
   product-related reaction 72
   quality defect-related reaction 72
   recipient, documentation of 50
   safety 92
      network 95
   sensitivity of 56t
   simultaneous administration of 47
   Sputnik V 359
   storage of 57
      temperature for 57t
   subunit 11, 350
   temporary storage of 69
   types of 11, 264
      combination 104
   vial monitor 64
      interpretation of 64f
Vaccine-preventable disease 301
   disease epidemiology of 22
   surveillance 33
Vaccinia immune globulins 110
Vaccinology
   practice of 377
   role in 327
Varicella 52, 228, 304, 312
   epidemiology of 228
   history of 312
   infection 109
Varicella vaccination 233, 236, 237
   adverse effects of 233
   impact of 232
Varicella vaccine 228-230
   effect of 232
   use of 235
Varicella zoster
   immunoglobulin 110
   virus 111, 231
Vasculitis 233
Vasovagal syncope 72
Vesicular stomatitis virus 327, 346
Vibrio cholerae 279
   infection 317
Viral vector vaccines 337, 350, 351
Virosomes 328
Virus 3
   infection 357
Viscerotropic disease 287

Vitamin E 328
Vomiting 78, 266

W

West Nile virus 347
    vaccine 348*t*
Whole-cell inactivated typhoid 215
Whole-cell pertussis vaccine 102, 138
Wiskott-Aldrich syndrome 82
World Health Organization 39, 55, 126, 135, 144, 163, 193, 194, 204, 222, 225, 256, 263, 270, 271, 281
WRSS1 vaccine 341

X

X-linked agammaglobulinemia 82

Y

Yellow fever 90, 282-284, 286, 287, 304
    clinical features of 283
    vaccination 286, 288
    vaccine 82, 86, 282, 284, 286, 288, 315, 316, 347, 395
        adverse effects of 287
    virus, transmission cycles of 282*f*

Z

Zanamivir 192
Zika virus 347, 357
    vaccine 347*t*
Zostavax 292
Zoster 290
    vaccine 290, 292, 297, 307, 311